Recent Results in Cancer Research 65

Fortschritte der Krebsforschung
Progrès dans les recherches sur le cancer

Lymphoid Neoplasias II

Clinical and Therapeutic Aspects

Edited by
G. Mathé M. Seligmann M. Tubiana

With 71 Figures and 102 Tables

Springer-Verlag
Berlin Heidelberg New York 1978

CNRS International Colloquium.
Held in Paris on June 22–24, 1977

Professor GEORGES MATHÉ
Institut de Cancérologie et d'Immunogénétique
Hôpital Paul-Brousse, 14–16, Avenue Paul-Vaillant-Couturier
F-94800 Villejuif

Professor MAXIME SELIGMANN
Laboratory of Immunochemistry and Immunopathology
INSERM (U 108), and Laboratory of Cytology
Research Institute on Blood Diseases, Hôpital Saint-Louis
2, Place du Docteur-A. Fournier, F-75010 Paris

Dr. MAURICE TUBIANA
Department of Radiation, Institut Gustave-Roussy
16bis, Avenue Paul-Vaillant-Couturier, F-94800 Villejuif

Sponsored by the Swiss League against Cancer

ISBN-13 : 978-3-642-81251-4 e-ISBN-13 : 978-3-642-81249-1
DOI : 10.1007 / 978-3-642-81249-1

Library of Congress Cataloging in Publication Data. Main entry under title: Lymphoid neoplasias. (Recent results in cancer research; 64–65) Papers presented at a CNRS international colloquium, held in Paris, June 22–24, 1977, sponsored by the Swiss League against Cancer. Bibliography: p. Includes index. CONTENTS: 1. Classification, categorization, natural history.—2. Clinical and therapeutic aspects. 1. Lymphoma—Congresses. I. Mathé, Georges, 1922– . II. Seligmann, Maxime, 1927– . III. Tubiana, Maurice, 1920– . IV. France. Centre national de la recherche scientifique. V. Schweizerische Nationalliga für Krebsbekämpfung und Krebsforschung. VI. Series. RC261.R35 vol. 64–65, etc. [RC280.L9] 616.9'94'008s [616.9'94'46] 78–19077.

Typeset by CCC at William Clowes & Sons Limited, London and Beccles

2125/3140-5 43210

Contents

List of Contributors

B. AMOR, Service de Thérapeutique Fonctionnelle de l'Hôpital Cochin, 7, Rue du Faubourg Saint-Jacques, F-75014 Paris

P. BATAINI, Fondation Curie, Section Médicale, 26, Rue d'Ulm, F-75005 Paris

A. BELPOMME, Service de Rhumatologie de l'Hôpital Cochin, 27, Rue du Faubourg Saint-Jacques, F-75014 Paris

D. BELPOMME, Institut de Cancérologie et d'Immunogénétique, Hôpital Paul-Brousse, and Institut Gustave-Roussy, 14–16, Avenue Paul-Vaillant-Couturier, F-94800 Villejuif

G. BONADONNA, Istituto Nazionale dei Tumori, Via G. Venezian 1, I-20133 Milan

K. BREMER, Hämatologische Abteilung, Medizinische Klinik und Poliklinik, Universitätsklinikum Essen (Gesamthochschule), Hufelandstraße 55, D-4300 Essen 1

G. BRITTINGER, Hämatologische Abteilung, Medizinische Klinik und Poliklinik, Universitätsklinikum Essen (Gesamthochschule), Hufelandstraße 55, D-4300 Essen 1

J. BRUGERE, Section Médicale, Fondation Curie, 26, Rue d'Ulm, F-75005 Paris

B. CAILLOU, Institut Gustave-Roussy, 16bis, Avenue Paul-Vaillant-Couturier, F-94800 Villejuif

B. CARLMARK, Division of Hematology, Medical Department, Karolinska Hospital, Stockholm 60, Sweden

S. K. CARTER, Northern California Cancer Program, 1801 Page Mill Road, Bldg. b, Suite 200, Palo Alto, CA 94304/USA

R. CASTELLANI, Istituto Nazionale dei Tumori, Via G. Venezian 1, I-20133 Milan

B. A. CHABNEV, Branches of Medicine and Clinical Pharmacology, Division of Cancer Treatment, National Cancer Institute, Bethesda, MD 20014/USA

P. CHARBORD, Institut de Recherches de Radiobiologie Clinique, Institut Gustave-Roussy, 16 bis, Avenue Paul-Vaillant-Couturier, F-94800 Villejuif

J. CHAUVERGNE, Fondation Bergonié, Cancer Center, 180, Rue Saint-Genès, F-33076 Bordeaux Cédex

H. L. DAVIS, Wisconsin Clinical Cancer Center, 701-G University Hospital, 1300 University Ave., Madison, WI 53706/USA

F. DELBARRE, Service de Rhumatologie de l'Hôpital Cochin, 27, Rue du Faubourg Saint-Jacques, F-75014 Paris

M. DELGADO, Institut de Cancérologie et d'Immunogénétique, Hôpital Paul-Brousse, and Département d'Hématologie de l'Institut Gustave-Roussy, 14–16, Avenue Paul-Vaillant-Couturier, F-94800 Villejuif

A. DELRIEU, Service de Rhumatologie de l'Hôpital Cochin, 27, Rue du Faubourg Saint-Jacques, F-75014 Paris

A. DE MASCAREL, Fondation Bergonié, Cancer Center, 180, Rue Saint-Genès, F-33076 Bordeaux Cédex

R. DEPIERRE, Service de Néphrologie, Hôpital Paul-Brousse, 14, Avenue Paul-Vaillant-Couturier, F-94800 Villejuif

F. DE VASSAL, Institut de Cancérologie et d'Immunogénétique, Hôpital Paul-Brousse, and Département d'Hématologie de l'Institut Gustave-Roussy, 14–16, Avenue Paul-Vaillant-Couturier, F-94800 Villejuif

J. P. DROZ, Institut de Recherches de Radiobiologie Clinique, Institut Gustave-Roussy, 16bis, Avenue Paul-Vaillant-Couturier, F-94800 Villejuif

J. DUMONT, Section Médicale, Fondation Curie, 26, Rue d'Ulm, F-75005 Paris

M. DURAND, Fondation Bergonié, Cancer Center, 180, Rue Saint-Genès, F-33076 Bordeaux Cédex

B. G. M. DURIE, Section of Hematology and Oncology, and The University of Arizona Cancer Center, The University of Arizona, Tucson, AZ 85724/USA

A. ENNUYER, Fondation Curie, Section Médicale, 26, Rue d'Ulm, F-75005 Paris

F. FEUILHADE DE CHAUVIN, Institut de Cancérologie et d'Immunogénétique, 14–16, Avenue Paul-Vaillant-Couturier, F-94800 Villejuif

R. I. FISHER, National Cancer Institute, Division of Cancer Treatment, Bethesda, MD 20014/USA

D. FRIES, Service de Néphrologie, Hôpital Paul-Brousse, 14, Avenue Paul-Vaillant-Couturier, F-94800 Villejuif

M. GIL, Institut de Cancérologie et d'Immunogénétique, Hôpital Paul-Brousse, 14–16 Avenue Paul-Vaillant-Couturier, F-94800 Villejuif

D. R. GOFFINET, Division of Radiotherapie, Department of Radiology, Stanford University School of Medicine, Stanford, CA 94305/USA

M. Hayat, Institut de Cancérologie et d'Immunogénétique, Hôpital Paul-Brousse, and Département d'Hématologie de l'Institut Gustave-Roussy, 16, Avenue Paul-Vaillant-Couturier, F-94800 Villejuif

T. S. Herman, Section of Hematology and Oncology, The University of Arizona, Health Sciences Center, Tucson, AZ 85724/USA

B. Hœrni, Fondation Bergonié, Cancer Center, 180, Rue Saint-Genès, F-33076 Bordeaux Cédex

G. Hœrni-Simon, Fondation Bergonié, Cancer Center, 180, Rue Saint-Genès, F-33076 Bordeaux Cédex

D. Hollard, Service d'Hématologie clinique, Centre Hospitalier Régional et universitaire de Grenoble, F-38700 La Tronche

N. Jaffe, Sidney Farber Cancer Institute, Children's Hospital Medical Center, 44 Binney Street, and Harvard Medical School, Boston, MA 02115/USA

C. Jasmin, Institut de Cancérologie et d'Immunogénétique, Hôpital Paul-Brousse, and Département d'Hématologie de l'Institut Gustave-Roussey, 14–16, Avenue Paul-Vaillant-Couturier, F-94800 Villejuif

C. Jaulerry, Head and Neck Unit, Section Médicale, Fondation Curie, 26, Rue d'Ulm, F-75231 Paris Cédex 05

S. E. Jones, Section of Hematology and Oncology, Department of Internal Medicine, University of Arizona College of Medicine, Tucson, AZ 85724/USA

H. S. Kaplan, Cancer Biology Research Laboratory, Department of Radiology, Stanford University School of Medicine, Stanford, CA 94305/USA

B. Lachet, Cea-Ceng, Département de Recherche Fondamentale, Laboratoire de Biologie Végétale, 85 X, F-38041 Grenoble Cédex

C. Lagarde, Fondation Bergonié, Cancer Center, 180, Rue Saint-Genès, F-33076 Bordeaux Cédex

P. Lasser, Département de Chirurgie, Institut Gustave-Roussy, 16bis, Avenue Paul-Vaillant-Couturier, F-94800 Villejuif

J. Lamarche, Centre Hospitalier de Sherbrooke, Sherbrooke, Quebec, Canada

J. P. Le Bourgeois, Département des Radiations, Institut Gustave-Roussy, 16bis, Avenue Paul-Vaillant-Couturier, F-94800 Villejuif

B. Le Mevel, Centre Réné-Gauducheau, Quai Moncousu, F-44000 Nantes

H. Leopold, Abteilung für Strahlentherapie der Universität Freiburg im Breisgau, Hugstetter Straße 55, F-7800 Freiburg i. Br.

M. Lepine-Martin, Centre Hospitalier Universitaire de Sherbrooke, Sherbrooke, Quebec, Canada

B. Longpre, Centre Hospitalier Universitaire de Sherbrooke, Sherbrooke, Quebec, Canada

D. Machover, Institut de Cancérologie et d'Immunogénétique, Hôpital Paul-Brousse, 14–16, Avenue Paul-Vaillant-Couturier, F-94800 Villejuif

D. Maraninchi, Institut Gustave-Roussy, and Institut de Recherche de Radiobiologie Clinique, and 16bis, Avenue Paul-Vaillant-Couturier, F-94800 Villejuif

H. Martin, Laboratoire d'Anatomie Pathologique, Centre Hospitalier Regional et Universitaire de Grenoble, F-38700 La Tronche

G. Mathé, Institut de Cancérologie et d'Immunogénétique, Hôpital Paul-Brousse, and Département d'Hématologie de l'Institut Gustave-Roussy, 14–16, Avenue Paul-Vaillant-Couturier, F-94800 Villejuif

A. Mazabraud, Fondation Curie, Section Médicale, 26, Rue d'Ulm, F-75005 Paris

M. Meignan, Département des Radiations, Institut Gustave-Roussy, 16bis, Avenue Paul-Vaillant-Couturier, F-94800 Villejuif

C. Menkes, Service du Rhumatologie de l'Hôpital Cochin, 27, Rue due Faubourg Saint-Jacques, F-75014 Paris

M. Michallet, Service d'Hématologie clinique, Centre Hospitalier Régional et Universitaire de Grenoble, F-38700 La Tronche

J. L. Misset, Institut de Cancérologie et d'Immunogénétique, Hôpital Paul-Brousse, and Département d'Hématologie de l'Institut Gustave-Roussy, 14–16, Avenue Paul-Vaillant-Couturier, F-94800 Villejuif

N. Morardet, Institut Gustave-Roussy, and Institut de Recherche de Radiobiologie Clinique, 16bis, Avenue Paul-Vaillant-Couturier, F-94800 Villejuif

S. B. Murphy, Division of Hematology-Oncology, St-Jude Children's Research Hospital, 332 North Lauderdale, P.O. Box 318, Mamphis, TN 38101/USA

M. Musset, Institut de Cancérologie et d'Immunogénétique, Hôpital Paul-Brousse, and Département d'Hématologie de l'Institut Gustave-Roussy, 16bis, Avenue Paul-Vaillant-Couturier, F-94800 Villejuif

K. Musshoff, Abteilung für Strahlentherapie der Universität Freiburg im Breisgau, Hugstetter Straße 55, D-7800 Freiburg i. Br.

C. E. Myers, Branches of Medicine and Clinical Pharmacology, Division of Cancer Treatment, National Cancer Institute, Bethesda, MD 20014/USA

G. Narduzzi, Istituto Nazionale dei Tumori, Via G. Venezian 1, I-20133 Milan

E. Ösby, Division of Hematology, Medical Department, Karolinska Hospital, Stockholm 60, Sweden

C. Parmentier, Institut de Recherches de Radiobiologie Clinique and Institut Gustave-Roussy, 16bis, Avenue Paul-Vaillant-Couturier, F-94800 Villejuif

F. PENE, Département des Radiations, Institut Gustave-Roussy, 16bis, Avenue Paul-Vaillant-Couturier, F-94800 Villejuif

P. POUILLART, Institut de Cancérologie et d'Immunogénétique, 14–16, Avenue Paul-Vaillant-Couturier, F-94800 Villejuif

P. REIZENSTEIN, Division of Hematology, Medical Department, Karolinska Hospital, Stockholm 60, Sweden

M. RIBAS-MUNDO, Departmento de Medicina Interna, Cátedra de Patología y Clínica Médicas, Universidad Autónoma de Barcelona, Barcelona/Spain

P. RIBAUD, Unité Fred-Siguier, Institut de Cancérologie et d'Immunogénétique, Hôpital Paul-Brousse, and Départements d'Hématologie, de Radiothérapie et de Pathologie de l'Institut Gustave-Roussy, F-94800 Villejuif

P. RICHAUD, Fondation Bergonié, Cancer Center, 180, Rue de Saint-Genès, F-33076 Bordeaux Cédex

F. RILKE, Istituto Nazionale dei Tumori, Via G. Venezian 1, I-20133 Milan

M. ROCHON, Centre Hospitalier Universitaire de Sherbrooke, Sherbrooke, Quebec, Canada

S. A. ROSENBERG, Division of Oncology, Department of Medicine, Stanford University School of Medicine, Stanford, CA 94305/USA

S. E. SALMON, Section of Hematology and Oncology, and The University of Arizona Cancer Center, Health Sciences Center, Tucson, AZ 85724/USA

R. SCHAERER, Service d'Hématologie clinique, Centre Hospitalier Régional et Universitaire de Grenoble, F-38700 La Tronche

G. SCHWAAB, Head and Neck Department, Institut Gustave-Roussy, 16bis, Avenue Paul-Vaillant-Couturier, F-94800 Villejuif

L. SCHWARZENBERG, Institut de Cancérologie et d'Immunogénétique, Hôpital Paul-Brousse, 14–16, Avenue Paul-Vaillant-Couturier, F-94800 Villejuif

B. SERROU, Centre Paul-Lamarque, Clinique Saint-Eloi, F-34000 Montpellier

F. SIMON, Service de Rhumatologie de l'Hôpital Cochin, 27, Rue du Faubourg Saint-Jacques, F-75014 Paris

J. J. SOTTO, Service d'Hématologie clinique, Centre Hospitalier Regional et Universitaire de Grenoble, F-38700 La Tronche

M. F. SOTTO, Laboratoire d'Hématologie, Centre Hospitalier Régional et Universitaire de Grenoble, F-38700 La Tronche

P. SPINELLI, Istituto Nazionale dei Tumori, Via G. Venezian 1, I-20133 Milan

C. TENTAS, Institut de Cancérologie et d'Immunogénétique, Hôpital Paul-Brousse, and Départements d'Hématologie, de l'Institut Gustave-Roussy, 16bis, Avenue Paul-Vaillant-Couturier, F-94800 Villejuif

M. TUBIANA, Département des Radiations, Institut Gustave-Roussy, 16bis, Avenue Paul-Vaillant-Couturier, F-94800 Villejuif

B. VAN DER WERF-MESSING, Rotterdam Radiotherapy Institute, and Erasmus University Rotterdam, Groene Hilledijk 301, Rotterdam 24, The Netherlands

D. D. VON HOFF, Medicine Branch, Clinical Oncology, Division of Cancer Treatment, National Cancer Institute, Bethesda, MD 20014/USA

C. VROUSOS, Service de Radiothérapie, Centre Hospitalier Régional et Universitaire de Grenoble, F-38700 La Tronche

R. C. YOUNG, National Cancer Institute, Division of Cancer Treatment, Bethesda, MD 20014/USA

Part I

Clinical Aspects: Staging and Therapeutic Implications

Introductory Remarks

M. Tubiana

The aim of these last two sessions is to assess to what extent recent pathologic and biologic considerations can be used for diagnosis and treatment. This morning's session is devoted to staging. Staging constitutes one of the major advances of the last decade for malignant lymphoma. As a result of speculations about the propagation of this disease, laparotomy was introduced by the Stanford group. In turn, laparotomy and modern staging have provided important information on the natural history of malignant lymphoma. In particular, the incidence of occult involvement of spleen in Hodgkin's disease or of bone marrow in non-Hodgkin's lymphoma is much higher than previously suspected.

Much information has now been collected, and in light of 10 years' experience, we must now ask ourselves two questions: 1) what do we expect from staging laparotomy and 2) in which patients is staging laparotomy legitimate, i.e., when do the benefits outweigh the cost? The complications of laparotomy are not negligible, in particular for aged patients. Furthermore, laparotomy increases the therapeutic burden; for instance, the incidence of side-effects after abdominal irradiation is higher for those patients who have had laparotomy, a point that shall be discussed this afternoon.

Staging has three purposes: to provide prognostic indicators, to provide guidance for treatment, and to treat the spleen. Since a few papers will be devoted to staging in non-Hodgkin's lymphomas, I shall illustrate those points with Hodgkin's disease data. A controlled clinical trial was carried out by the radiotherapy-chemotherapy group of EORTC from 1971–1976. The protocol was the following. All patients with Hodgkin's disease, clinical stages I and II located above the diaphragm, were randomized between staging laparotomy and splenectomy or no laparotomy. After laparotomy, irrespective of the results of the pathologic study of the spleen and the biopsy of the para-aortic lymph nodes, an irradiation of the para-aortic lymph nodes was carried out. For those patients without laparotomy, an irradiation of the spleen was also performed. Subsequently, for those patients with mixed cellularity or lymphoid depletion histologic types, chemotherapy was performed regardless of the results of the staging laparotomy. This trial had two aims: 1) to compare splenectomy and splenic irradiation and 2) to assess the prognostic significance of the information provided by laparotomy. This is why, in order to reach these goals, all patients received the same treatment without taking into account the results of the splenectomy or the para-aortic lymph node biopsy. Two hundred and ninety-five patients were included in this cooperative trial, and only one patient had another treatment protocol because the liver biopsy was positive.

The preliminary results of the trial will be published by the EORTC Radiotherapy-Chemotherapy group, and I shall only briefly summarize them. There is no difference in the survival or the incidence of recurrence between the two groups: 1 death and 21 recurrences out of 114 patients with laparotomy and 2 deaths and 21 recurrences out of 108 patients without laparotomy. Splenectomy and spleen irradiation appear to be equivalent. In the group with laparotomy, it is interesting to compare patients with or without spleen involvement. In those patients without spleen involvement (68 patients), six recurrences were located in an irradiated area, none in a nonirradiated lymphatic area, and six were extranodal recurrences. In the group with spleen involvement (26 patients), the incidence of recurrence in an irradiated area was comparable (two patients), but the recurrence in nonirradiated lymphatic area was much higher (five patients); on the other hand, the incidence of extranodal recurrence was not increased (two patients). These data show that spleen involvement has a significant prognostic value. But contrary to what was expected, they suggest that it is more an indicator of lymphatic spread than of extranodal dissemination.

On the basis of these data and the statistical analysis of a previous controlled clinical trial, a new trial was designed with the aim of distinguishing two groups of clinical stages in Hodgkin's disease: one with a favorable prognosis, for which a minimal treatment might be sufficient to obtain a high proportion of cure, and another group, for which a more aggressive treatment including multiple courses of polychemotherapy is performed, despite its side-effects on gonads and bone marrow. In the first group are included clinical stages I and II with all the following requirements: age below 40 years, a good histologic subgrouping (lymphoid predominance or nodular sclerosis), ESR below 70 mm/h, and pattern of presentation with mediastinal involvement (for clinical stage II). All these patients are submitted to diagnostic laparotomy and splenectomy. They are included in the good group only if they remain at pathologic stage I or II after laparotomy.

Laparotomy is not performed for the other patients for whom polychemotherapy seems to be required anyway. Hence, in this new trial, laparotomy is used for selecting a group of patients with a good prognosis and for whom a minimal treatment might be sufficient. It is hoped that it will make it possible to avoid polychemotherapy or irradiation of the pelvis in some young patients and consequently reduce damage to the gonads and decrease the genetic burden.

Unfortunately, many years will be necessary to evaluate the validity of this approach, Nevertheless, it stresses the present tendency toward reducing, at least for some patients, the cost of treatment.

Cellular Renewal Kinetics of Malignant Non-Hodgkin's Lymphomas

K. BREMER

To maintain the cellularity of the human lymphatic system at its normal level, the rates of lymphocyte production and death apparently must be equal. This steady-state equilibrium is the result of complex regulatory mechanisms of the micro- and macroenvironment including direct cellular interactions, antigenic stimulation, and biochemical and humoral influences [39]. To give rise to the development of malignant lymphomas, the production rate of the neoplastic lymphocytes must exceed their death rate. In contrast, if malignant transformation of lymphocytes is associated with higher death rates than production rates, these neoplastic cells eliminate themselves due to this suicidal proliferative constellation. These considerations may elucidate the decisive importance of lymphocyte proliferation kinetics for the development of malignant non-Hodgkin's lymphomas (NHL).

Proliferating Lymphoma Cells

Using labeled DNA precursors such as ^{3}H-thymidine (^{3}H-T), recent studies of lymphocyte proliferation kinetics in man confirmed previous animal-derived data showing that usually only large basophilic lymphoid cells (immunoblasts, large germinal center cells = centroblasts, plasmoblasts, large and medium-sized lymphocytes = lymphoblasts) actively synthesize DNA and divide, also giving rise to smaller cell variants of limited or no proliferation capacity [39, 40].

Cell Cycle Parameters of Lymphoma Cells

For normal human large basophilic lymphoid cells, an average generation time of about 24 h and DNA synthesis time of usually 10–12 h have been determined (Table 1). These two cell cycle parameters, which are of great importance for characterization of cellular proliferation kinetics, exhibited considerable time variation in normal cells and even more in the different lymphoma cells. With the exception of Burkitt's lymphoma cells, however, the generation time of NHL cells generally revealed a tendency to be prolonged, whereas the majority of the DNA synthesis times of the neoplastic cells were found to be within the normal range. This indicates that the prolonged generation time is mainly caused by an extended postmitotic G_1-phase. Furthermore, to initiate growth of malignant lymphomas, it must be postulated that this prolonged cellular generation time is overcompensated by an even longer than normal life span of these neoplastic lymphocytes; thus, the production rate of lymphoma cells exceeds their death rate.

Table 1. DNA synthesis time (T_S) and generation time (T_G) of large lymphoid proliferating human lymphoma cells

Diseases	T_S[a] (h)	T_G[a] (h)	References
Normal	10 (7–12)	24 (8–40)	[14, 26–28, 31, 41]
Burkitt's Lymphoma	10 (7–12)	24 (22–26)	[5, 13, 31]
Chronic lymphocytic leukemia	12 (11–14)	28 (22–96)	[8, 14, 37]
Reticulum cell sarcoma	10 (8–24)	48 (15–480)	[18, 21, 26]
Lymphosarcoma	12 (10–14)	48 (38–160)	[18, 26, 30]
Acute lymphoid leukemia	26 (10–47)	48 (17–215)	[20, 23, 42]
Multiple myeloma	18 (1–20)	57 (33–156)	[11, 17]

[a] Estimated average times, ranges given in parentheses.

Growth Fraction

In addition to the duration of the generation time, the number of newly produced cells also depends upon the absolute size of the proliferating cell compartment within each cell population, i.e., the growth fraction. Usually it is relatively small, e.g., comprising 1%–5% of the lymph node cells of resting or activated normal human lymph nodes as well as of lymph nodes from patients with chronic lymphocytic leukemia (CLL) [39, 40]. However, in other lymphomas, the growth fraction may increase considerably up to values of about 40% [40] or even represent the majority of all lymphoma cells [13]. Since these proliferating cells are almost exclusively large and medium-sized lymphocytes, a considerable correlation may exist between the size of the growth fraction and the percentage of large lymphoid cells within each lymphoma cell population.

Cellular Composition of Lymph Nodes

Up to 10% of normal lymph node cells represent large basophilic cells, all of which usually proliferate [37, 39, 40]. Similar percentages of "lymphoblasts" have been noticed in CLL lymph nodes, but not all of them synthesized DNA [36, 37]. In contrast, in patients with germinal

Table 2. Estimated composition of non-Hodgkin's lymphoma cell populations according to cell size[a]

Disease	Cellular distribution		
	Small[b]	Medium-sized[c]	Large[d]
Normal	+++	++	+
Chronic lymphocytic leukemia	++++	++	+
Lymphoplasmacytoid lymphoma	+++	++	+
Germinal center cell tumors			
Small type, diffuse	−−	++++	−−
Follicular = nodular form	++	+++	++
Large type, diffuse	−−	++	++++
Burkitt's	−−	++++	−−
Lymphoblastic lymphoma, acute lymphoid leukemia	++	+++	+ (+)
Immunoblastic lymphoma	−−	−−	++++

[a] Data according to H. Stein, personal communication.
[b] Similar to blood lymphocytes.
[c] Similar to small germinal center cells.
[d] Similar to large germinal center cells and immunoblasts = transformed lymphocytes.

center cell-derived lymphomas, including Burkitt's tumors [19, 33], and with lymphoblastic or immunoblastic lymphomas, up to 100% of the lymph node cells have to be classified as medium-sized or large lymphoid cells (Table 2); however, the proliferating fraction of these large cells (=growth fraction) varies considerably, indicating some limitations of this correlation hypothesis in these lymphomas [40].

Lymphocyte Production

Since the total number of neoplastic cells of each lymphoma patient considerably exceeds normal cellularity of the human lymphatic system of 10^{11}–10^{12} lymphocytes [38], the absolute number of newly synthesized large cells is again significantly higher in lymphoma patients than in normal ones, although the generation times of the neoplastic cells seem to be longer than in normal patients. Thus, despite prolonged generation times, the production of lymphoma cells is increased because of increased absolute numbers of dividing lymphoma cells (Table 3). This kinetic constellation seems to be valid not only in the smaller sized lymphomas such as CLL and lymphoplasmacytoid lymphomas (LPL), in which an increased cell production has been observed [8, 24, 36, 37, 40], but also in the lymphomas composed of larger cells. In CLL patients, it has been shown that not only the production of short-lived and long-lived lymphocytes is markedly increased by a factor of 5–50 [24, 40] but also that their average life span is prolonged [6, 24, 25, 36]. At present, unfortunately, analogous studies of lymphocyte production in other NHL lymphomas are not available.

Table 3. Increased lymphocyte (ly) production in patients with non-Hodgkin's lymphomas

Parameter	Normal	Non-Hodgkin's lymphomas (e.g., CLL[a], LPL[b])
Cellularity of lymphatic system	10^{11}–10^{12} ly	10^{12}–10^{15} ly
% of large lymph node cells	~10%	~10%
Total number of large "blasts"	~10^{10}	~10^{13}
Generation time of dividing ly	Normal	Prolonged
Total number of proliferating ly	Normal	Increased
Ly production: daily input of newly produced ly into blood	30–50 ly/μl	300–1500 ly/μl

[a] CLL: chronic lymphocytic leukemia.
[b] LPL: lymphoplasmacytoid lymphoma.

Proliferation Kinetics of Lymphoma Cells

As pointed out above, in most patients of externally unaffected lymphoma growth, cell production exceeds cell death. This net cell gain can be the result of four kinetically different situations:

1. Cell production normal and cell death reduced;
2. Cell production increased and cell death reduced;
3. Cell production increased and cell death normal;
4. Cell production greatly increased and cell death increased.

Because in CLL the numbers of newly produced lymphocytes are increased and the cell death rates are reduced due to a prolonged life span of the CLL lymphocytes [6, 24, 25, 36, 40], the proliferative constellation 2 must be attributed to CLL. Similarly, in other NHL of low-grade malignancy such as multiple myeloma, LPL, and centrocytic lymphoma according to the Kiel classification [10, 19, 33], the total number of newly produced neoplastic cells within each lymphoma patient is apparently also increased. Therefore, the proliferative constellation 2, or perhaps constellation 3, is applicable to these NHL of low-grade malignancy. Further kinetic studies are necessary to clarify this point.

Proliferative constellation 4 was found to be valid in Burkitt's lymphoma [13] because the greatly enhanced production of Burkitt's lymphoma cells is subjected to an increased death rate of about 70%. Analogously, kinetic constellation 4 may also be postulated for other high-grade NHL such as immunoblastic, lymphoblastic, and centroblastic lymphomas [10, 19, 33], all of which are mainly composed of large-sized, proliferating cell types suggestive of greatly increased production rates by large growth fractions associated with high death rates of the lymphoma cells.

The high cell death rates in the high-grade NHL are possibly due to unspecific factors such as a decreased supply of oxygen, energy, and substrates inhibiting further lymphoma cell proliferation within this disadvantageous microenvironment and finally resulting in cell death. In contrast, in the NHL of low-grade malignancy, the majority of the newly produced lymphoma cells may be capable of some "maturation" by entering into the G_0-phase [6, 8, 36]. This cytokinetically resting stage may be associated with a prolonged life-span of the respective neoplastic cells as shown in CLL. Because the lymphoma cells are considered as immunologically incompetent [6], most of these neoplastic G_0 cells may not reenter the proliferative cell cycle in contrast to the normal lymphocytes [6, 39] and thus apparently die as G_0 cells.

Furthermore, the prognostic superiority of the nodular NHL compared with all other diffuse lymphoma entities [4, 15, 34] seems to be related to the uniquely favorable proliferation kinetics of these NHL cells, possibly to the proliferative constellation 1. Although in these NHL, 20%–50% of the lymphoma cells represent large germinal center cells (centroblasts) (see Table 2), their proliferation is apparently slowed down and/or inhibited by unknown mechanisms (factors) possibly associated with the organ-like structures (nodularity, sclerosis) of these lymphomas imitating germinal center formation. On the other hand, since terminal "transformation" of low-grade NHL into high-grade NHL has been observed [19, 29], the kinetic constellations 1, 2, or 3 may change into constellation 4.

Prognostic Significance of Lymphoma Cell Proliferation Kinetics

Several recent analyses of NHL patient survival data [4, 15, 32, 34] have shown that the survival expectancies of these high-grade malignant lymphomas with the apparent constellation 4 are in fact the shortest or poorest compared with the statistically significantly higher survival probability of other NHL subtypes, e.g., the low-grade malignant lymphomas, as has been revealed by a retrospective analysis by the Kiel Lymphoma Group (Fig. 1). This different survival prognosis, particularly between low-grade and high-grade NHL, is considered to correlate with and depend upon the proliferative constellation of the cellular renewal kinetics of the respective lymphoma cells. Furthermore, although these NHL entities of high-grade malignancy with the kinetic constellation 4 have a similarly poor prognosis [4, 15, 34], they carry different surface markers; thus, the majority of cases with Burkitt's lymphoma and immunoblastic lymphoma must be regarded as monoclonal B-cell proliferations, whereas most cases with lymphoblastic lymphomas or acute lymphoid leukemia represent null or T-cell

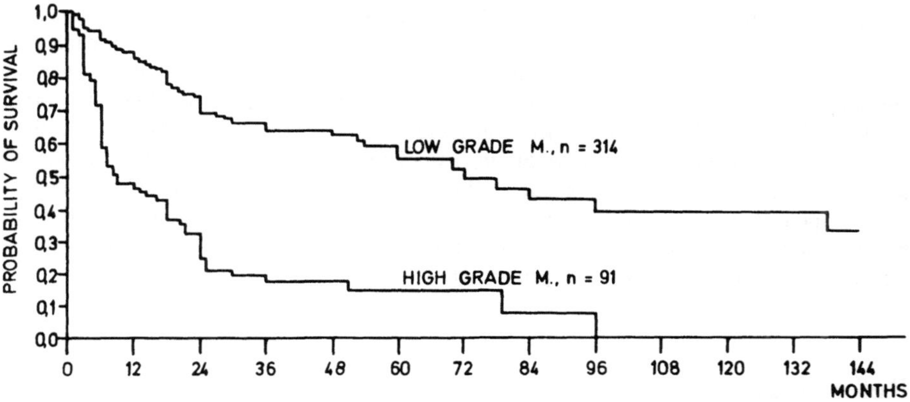

Fig. 1. Retrospective survival data analysis of 405 patients with non-Hodgkin's lymphomas diagnosed according to the Kiel classification; $p<0.001$

neoplasias [19, 29, 33, 34]. In addition, the nodular forms of the NHL exhibit significantly better prognosis than the corresponding diffuse variants [4, 15, 34], although most of these lymphomas are of B-cell origin [19, 29, 33]. The data in the recent literature are controversial about the prognostic superiority of B-, T-, or null cell variants of certain histologic subtypes [1, 2]. Because there is no apparent correlation between the prognosis and the B- or T-cell properties of the lymphoma cells, it is supposed that the main factors in determining survival probability of NHL patients are not their B- or T-cell surface marker characteristics but the proliferation kinetics of the respective lymphoma cells.

Therapeutic Implications of Lymphoma Cell Proliferation Kinetics

The lymphocyte proliferation kinetics are considered to be of decisive influence on the results of the various therapeutic regimens applied to NHL. Thus, the adequate therapeutic attack for the disseminated NHL of low-grade malignancy presumably with the proliferative constellation 2 or perhaps 1 or 3 may consist of procedures depleting the accumulated masses of neoplastic cells (e.g., leukapheresis) combined with the various methods of radiotherapy (splenic or extracorporeal irradiation of the blood, regional, extended field or total nodal irradiation, and total body irradiation) and/or moderate aggressive cytostatic treatment [12, 16, 22, 34, 35]. In the disseminated NHL of high-grade malignancy with the proliferative constellation 4, the best therapeutic results will be achieved by highly aggressive combination chemotherapy regimens [3, 7, 9, 15]. The validity of these suggestions is again supported by recent survival data analyses [3, 7, 9, 34].

Summary

Although the DNA synthesis times of the dividing NHL cell types were found to be within the normal range (7–12 h), the generation times of these neoplastic lymphocytes seem to be prolonged. However, even with a normal percentage of proliferating lymphoma cells (=growth fraction), the total number of mitotically active neoplastic lymphocytes is considerably increased in each NHL due to extensive enlargement of the total cellularity of each patient's lymphatic system. Therefore, in each NHL patient, the total number of newly produced lymphoma cells is significantly increased. According to the Kiel classification of the NHL, the NHL of low-grade malignancy are considered to be characterized by the proliferative constellation of an enhanced cell production associated with reduced or normal cell death rates, whereas in the NHL of high-grade malignancy, increased cell death rates seem to be overcompensated by even higher cell renewal rates. These differences in the cellular proliferation kinetics of the NHL are supposed to be of higher prognostic and clinical significance than their B- or T-cell properties.

References

1. Belpomme, D., Mathé, G., Davies, A. J. S.: Clinical significance and prognostic value of the T-B immunological classification of human primary acute lymphoid leukaemias. Lancet *1977 I*, 555–558
2. Bloomfield, C. D., Kersey, J. H., Brunning, R. D., Gajl-Peczalska, K. J.: Prognostic significance of lymphocyte surface markers in adult non-Hodgkin's malignant lymphoma. Lancet *1976 II*, 1330–1333
3. Bonadonna, G., Lattuada, A., Banfi, A.: Recent trends in the treatment of non-Hodgkin's lymphomas. Eur. J. Cancer *12*, 661–673 (1976)
4. Brittinger, G., Bartels, H., Bremer, K., Dühmke, E., Gunzer, U., König, E., Stein, H. (Kieler Lymphomgruppe): Klinik der malignen Non-Hodgkin-Lymphome entsprechend der Kiel Klassifikation: Centrocytisches Lymphom, centroblastisch-centrocytisches Lymphom, lymphoblastisches Lymphom, immunoblastisches Lymphom. In: Maligne Lymphome und monoklonale Gammopathien. Löffler, H. (ed.) München: Lehmann 1976, Haematol. Bluttransfus., Vol. XVIII, pp. 211–223
5. Cooper, E. H., Frank, G. L., Wright, D. H.: Cell proliferation in Burkitt tumours. Eur. J. Cancer *2*, 377–384 (1966)
6. Dameshek, W.: Chronic lymphocytic leukemia—an accumulative disease of immunologically incompetent lymphocytes. Blood *29*, 566–584 (1967)
7. De Vita, V. T., Canellos, G. P., Chabner, B., Schein, P., Hubbard, S. P., Young, R. C.: Advanced diffuse histiocytic lymphoma, a potentially curable disease. Lancet *1975 I*, 248–250
8. Dörmer, P., Trepel, F., Schick, P.: DNS-Synthese und Wachstumsfraktion von Lymphoblasten bei chronischer lymphatischer Leukämie. Blut *31*, 180 (1975)
9. Durant, J. R., Loeb, V., Jr., Dorfman, R., Chan, Y.-K.: 1,3- bis (2-chloroethyl)-1-nitrosourea (BCNU)-, cyclophosphamide-, vincristine-and prednisone- (BCOP). A new therapeutic regimen for diffuse histiocytic lymphoma. Cancer *36*, 1936–1944 (1975)
10. Gerard-Marchant, R., Hamlin, I., Lennert, K., Rilke, F., Stansfeld, A. G., Van Unnik, J. A. M.: Classification of non-Hodgkin's lymphomas. Lancet *1974 II*, 406–408
11. Harris, E. B., Hoelzer, D.: DNA synthesis time in leukaemic cells as measured by the double labelling and the percentage labelled mitoses methods. Cell Tissue Kinet. *4*, 433–441 (1971)
12. Huguley, C. M.: Chronic myelocytic and chronic lymphocytic leukemia. Cancer *30*, 1583–1587 (1972)
13. Iversen, O. H., Iversen, U., Ziegler, J. L., Bluming, A. Z.: Cell kinetics in Burkitt lymphoma. Eur. J. Cancer *10*, 155–163 (1974)
14. Jaksic, B., Pagliardi, G. L., Pegoraro, L.: Kinetics of phytohemagglutinin stimulated lymphocytes in chronic lymphocytic leukemia. Cell Tissue Kinet. *9*, 419–428 (1976)
15. Jones, S. E.: Clinical features and course of the non-Hodgkin's lymphomas. Clin. Haematol. *3*, 131–160 (1974)
16. Kaufman, J. H., Ezdinli, E., Aungst, C. W., Stutzman, L.: Lymphosarcoma. A comparison of extended to conservative chemotherapy. Cancer *37*, 1283–1292 (1976)
17. Killmann, S. A., Cronkite, E. P., Fliedner, T. M., Bond, V. P.: Cell proliferation in multiple myeloma studied with tritiated thymidine in vivo. Lab. Invest. *11*, 845–852 (1962)
18. Klein, H. O., Lennartz, K. J., Gross, R., Eder, M., Fischer, M.: In-vivo- und in-vitro-Untersuchungen zur Zellkinetik und Synchronisation menschlicher Tumorzellen. Dtsch. Med. Wochenschr. *97*, 1273–1282 (1972)
19. Lennert, K., Mohri, N., Stein, H., Kaiserling, E.: The histopathology of malignant lymphoma. Brit. J. Haematol. *31* (suppl. II), 193–203 (1975)

20. MAUER, A. M., FISHER, V.: Characteristics of cell proliferation in four patients with untreated acute leukemia. Blood *28*, 428–445 (1966)
21. OHARA, K., FRIED, J., DOWLING, J. R., BITTAR, E. S., CLARKSON, B. D.: Studies of cellular proliferation in human leukemia: VII. Cytokinetic behavior of neoplastic cells in a patient with reticulum cell sarcoma in a leukemic phase. Cancer *28*, 862–885 (1971)
22. PORTLOCK, C. S., ROSENBERG, S. A., GLATSTEIN, E., KAPLAN, H. S.: Treatment of advanced non-Hodgkin's lymphomas with favorable histologies: Preliminary results of a prospective trial. Blood *47*, 747–756 (1976)
23. SAUNDERS, E. F., LAMPKIN, B. C., MAUER, A. M.: Variation of proliferative activity in leukemic cell populations of patients with acute leukemia. J. Clin. Invest. *46*, 1356–1363 (1967)
24. SCHICK, P.: Lymphozytenkinetik bei lymphatischen Systemerkrankungen (chronische lymphatische Leukämie, Lymphogranulomatose). Verh. Dtsch. Ges. Inn. Med. *79*, 154–158 (1973)
25. SCHIFFER, L. M.: Kinetics of chronic lymphocytic leukaemia. Ser. Haematol. I. *3*, 3–23 (1968)
26. SCHIFFER, L. M.: Human lymphocyte proliferation. DNA synthesis time. Cell Tissue Kinet. *4*, 585–595 (1971)
27. SCHIFFER, L. M.: Observations on the in-vitro measurement of human lymphocyte DNA synthesis time. Cell Tissue Kinet. *4*, 597–599 (1971)
28. SCHIFFER, L., MIGLIORATO, D. A.: Characterization of One Human Lymphocyte Population. In: 7th Leukocyte Culture Conference. Quebec, June 6–11, 1972
29. SELIGMANN, M., BROUET, J.-C., PREUD'HOMME, J. L.: The immunological diagnosis of human leukemias and lymphomas: an overview. In: Immunological Diagnosis of Leukemias and Lymphomas. THIERFELDER, S., RODT, H., THIEL, E. (eds.) Berlin-Heidelberg-New York: Springer 1977, Haematol. Blood Transfus., Vol. XX, pp. 1–16
30. SHEEHY, P. F., FRIED, J., DOWLING, J. R., CLARKSON, B. D.: Studies of cellular proliferation in human leukemia. VIII. The generation time and growth fraction in lymphosarcoma in a leukemic phase during advanced and early relapsing disease. Cancer *36*, 203–210 (1975)
31. SMITH, H., MURRAY, D., GÖKCEN, M.: Life cycle of lymphoid cells in vitro. Eur. J. Cancer *6*, 269–271 (1970)
32. STACHER, A., WALDNER, R., THEML, H.: Klinik der malignen Non-Hodgkin-Lymphome entsprechend der Kieler Klassifikation: Lymphoplasmozytoides Lymphom (LPL) und chronisch lymphatische Leukämie (CLL). In: Maligne Lymphome und monoklonale Gammopathien. LÖFFLER, H. (ed.) München: Lehmann 1976, Haematol. Bluttransfus., Vol. XVIII, pp. 199–209
33. STEIN, H.: Klassifikation der malignen Non-Hodgkin-Lymphome aufgrund gemeinsamer morphologischer und immunologischer Merkmale zwischen normalen und neoplastischen lymphatischen Zellen. Immun. Infekt. *4*, 52–69, 95–109 (1976)
34. Symposium on Non-Hodgkin's lymphomata. PECKHAM, M. J. (ed.), Br. J. Cancer *31* (suppl. II), 60–72, 168–173, 174–186, 187–200, 208–216, 386–401, 402–412, 441–449, 450–455, 456–464, 465–473, 474–480, 497–504 (1975)
35. THEML, H., BEGEMANN, H.: Die Bedeutung kinetischer und immunologischer Daten fürlin pathomechanisches Verständnis und eine kritische Therapie von Lymphomen. In: Lymphozyt und klinische Immunologie. THEML, H., BEGEMANN, H. (eds.) Berling-Heidelberg-New York: Springer 1975, pp. 140–147
36. THEML, H., TREPEL, F., SCHICK, P., KABOTH, W., BEGEMANN, H.: Kinetics of lymphocytes in chronic lymphocytic leukemia: Studies using continuous ^{3}H-thymidine infusion in two patients. Blood *42*, 623–636 (1973)
37. TREPEL, F.: Zellproliferation in malignen Lymphomen. In: Leukämien und maligne Lymphome. STACHER, A. (ed.) München: Urban und Schwarzenberg 1973, pp. 212–218
38. TREPEL, F.: Number and distribution of lymphocytes in man. A critical analysis. Klin. Wochenschr. *52*, 511–515. (1974)
39. TREPEL, F.: Das lymphatische Zellsystem: Struktur, allgemeine Physiologie und allgemeine Pathophysiologie. In: Handbuch der Inneren Medizin, 2. Band: Blut und Blutkrankheiten. BEGEMANN, H. (ed.) Berlin-Heidelberg-New York: Springer 1976, Vol. III: Leukocytäres und retikuläres System I, pp. 1–191
40. TREPEL, F., SCHICK, P.: Proliferation und Wachstum von lymphatischen Zellpopultionen bei malignen Lymphomen. In: Maligne Lymphome und monoklonale Gammopathien. LÖFFLER, H. (ed.). München: Lehmann 1976, Haematol. Bluttransfus. Vol. XVIII, pp. 33–47
41. WAGNER, H. P., ECKMANN, L.: Proliferative characteristics of thoracic duct lympoid cells in man. Abstract volume, XIII Congr. Intern. Soc. Hematol. München, 1970, p. 206
42. WAGNER, H. P., COTTIER, H., CRONKITE, E. P.: Variability of proliferative patterns in acute lymphoid leukemia of children. Blood *39*, 176–186 (1972)

Clinical Staging and New Therapeutic Approaches in Multiple Myeloma

S. E. SALMON and B. G. M. DURIE

Introduction

The application of quantitative measurements in clinical oncology has been a major objective in our clinical research program. We believe that use of such techniques, plus reasonably enlightened empiricism, extrapolation from data on drug action, and availability of effective new drugs could result in major improvement in end results of cancer treatment. Such comments are particularly germane to multiple myeloma because substantial improvements in end results beyond those which can be obtained with alkylating agent-prednisone combinations have yet to be uniformly achieved. Our kinetic approach has already increased our understanding of the clinical phases of myeloma. We believe that we are now beginning to see clear-cut evidence of ways in which clinical staging and kinetic data have not only led to new clinical trials but have also begun to improve results of treatment. Some of our observations on staging, kinetics of response, and drug sensitivity are being put to the test in a large-scale clinical trial initiated in the Southwest Oncology Group (SWOG) in 1977. Newer observations in our own institution suggest that an individualized approach to treatment based on measured drug sensitivity may also prove feasible.

Clinical Staging and Prognostic Factors

Clinical staging has been widely accepted as essential for optimal treatment of many types of cancer (e.g., Hodgkin's disease). Various groups of workers have investigated factors which influence prognosis in multiple myeloma. Important features which have been identified include the performance status, the presence or absence of renal insufficiency, the M-component type and subtype, the extent of bone lesions, the hemoglobin level, and the serum concentrations of albumin and calcium as well as a number of less critical features [3, 5, 8]. At the University of Arizona, we have recently analyzed the presenting clinical features, response to treatment, and survival in a group of patients with multiple myeloma who have had direct measurements of myeloma tumor mass with techniques detailed elsewhere in this volume [14, 18, 22]. Data on the clinical features were correlated with the immunologically measured tumor mass using stepwise, multivariate regression techniques. Based on this analysis, we have proposed a staging system for patients with multiple myeloma which is outlined in Table 1. It can be seen that patients are divided into three stages based on clinical parameters which correlate with measured cell mass, response to treatment (with alkylating agent-prednisone combinations), and survival. These groups are subclassified A or B based upon the presence or absence of relatively normal renal function. We observed a clear relationship between stage and survival as illustrated in Fig. 1. The validity of the staging system has been confirmed in retrospective analyses by ALEXANIAN et al. [3].

Table 1. Myeloma staging system[a]

Stage	Criteria	Measured myeloma cell mass (cells × $10^{12}/m^2$)[b]
I	*ALL* of the following: Hemoglobin value > 10 g/100 ml Serum calcium value normal (⩽12 mg/100 ml) On x-ray, normal bone structure (scale 0) or solitary bone plasmacytoma only Low M-component production rates IgG value <5 g/100 ml IgA value <3 g/100 ml Urine light chain M-component on electrophoresis <4 g/24 h	<0.6 (Low)
II	Fitting neither Stage I nor Stage III	0.6–1.20 (Intermediate)
III	*One or More* of the following: Hemoglobin value <8.5 g/100 ml Serum calcium value >12 mg/100 ml Advanced lytic bone lesions (scale 3) High M-component production rates IgG value >7 g/100 ml IgA value >5 g/100 ml Urine light chain M-component on electrophoresis >12 g/24 h	>1.20 (High)

Subclassification
A: relatively normal renal function (serum creatinine value <2.0 mg/100 ml)[c]
B: abnormal renal function (serum creatinine value ⩾2.0 mg/100 ml)

Examples
Stage IA: low cell mass with normal renal function
Stage IIIB: high cell mass with abnormal renal function

[a] See Durie and Salmon 1975 [8].
[b] 10^{12} cells: approximately 1 kg or 2.2 lbs; m^2: square meter of body surface area.
[c] If the serum creatinine is not available, the blood urea nitrogen (BUN) value may be used as an indicator of renal function. (A BUN value of 30 mg/100 ml is roughly equal to a serum creatinine value of 2 mg/100 ml).

Additionally, Bergsagel and co-workers [21] have shown the critical importance of clinical stage and renal function in cases of Bence Jones myeloma. Alternative techniques, using regression equations to predict tumor cell number, have been detailed elsewhere [8, 19]. A number of institutions and co-operative groups are now applying our staging system prospectively in relation to ongoing myeloma chemotherapy trials. In several instances, patient entry into protocol randomization is first stratified by tumor mass grade to assure that major prognostic factors are balanced in various treatment groups.

Application of Kinetic Principles to Clinical Trials

An important application of clinical staging and tumor kinetic concepts has been in the area of large-scale clinical trials in which detailed measurement of kinetic parameters is not always feasible. The approach that we have used is to quickly stage patients prior to treatment and follow tumor regression serially with the M-component marker as determined by electrophoresis. In IgG myeloma, it is important to correct for concentration-dependent changes in M-component metabolism [23]. This is most readily accomplished with a programmable pocket

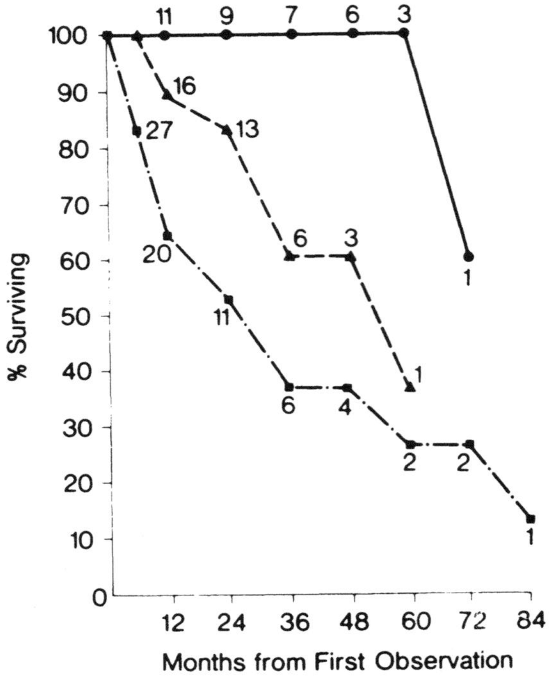

Fig. 1. Relationship of measured myeloma cell mass to survival (shown as actuarial survival by the method of KAPLAN and MEIER, J. Am. Stat. Assoc. *53*: 457–582, 1958.) Low cell mass: <0.6 × 10^{12} cells/m² BSA (●——●); intermediate cell mass: 0.6–1.2 × 10^{12} cells/m² BSA (▲- - -▲); high cell mass: >1.2 × 10^{12} cells/m² (■—·—■). [Reproduced with permission from DURIE and SALMON, Cancer, *36*, 842 (1975)] [8]

calculator [19] or slightly less well with a nomogram [14]. The major clinical phases of myeloma are summarized in Fig. 3. In responsive patients, induction chemotherapy (e.g., with melphalan-prednisone) results in a fall in the tumor mass in the range of 75%–90% (for most patients) over the first 6–8 months of treatment. A remission "plateau phase" is reached shortly thereafter wherein additional therapy does not result in a further tumor mass reduction. Entry into this plateau phase appears to follow a "reverse Gompertzian" curve as long as the treatment is given in a constant dose on a constant schedule [23]. Finally, a relapse phase eventuates in which a subclone is expressed which is either kinetically or biochemically resistant to the treatment program.

Clinical tumor mass staging yields certain additional insights with respect to results of treatment. When a patient with multiple myeloma starts off with a very high cell mass, even after a one or two log (very excellent) cell kill, the remaining tumor cell mass may be higher than in a patient starting off with a low tumor mass at the time of initial diagnosis. Based on the studies of SKIPPER (22), which indicated that biochemically resistant cells occur with a frequency of only 1 out of 10^6 or 10^7 cells in a tumor population, one would predict that patients presenting with a high cell mass would have a higher chance of harboring a resistant mutant clone (even after an excellent response to treatment) than patients presenting with a low cell mass. This indeed corresponds with findings of ALEXANIAN et al. [3] and ourselves [8] that patients with initial high cell mass have a shorter duration of remission than other patients.

The major clinical phases of disease are induction therapy, the plateau phase, and relapse. These are depicted schematically in Fig. 2. We have recently analyzed the tritiated thymidine labeling index (LI) in the induction, remission, and relapse phases of disease in a series of patient studies at the University of Arizona [9]. The overall findings are as follows: patients who show the best and most durable responses to treatment appear to fall into the group who initially present with a low LI (1–3%) and who do not have a significant (twofold) rise in the LI by the end of induction therapy. It must be mentioned, however, that many responsive patients

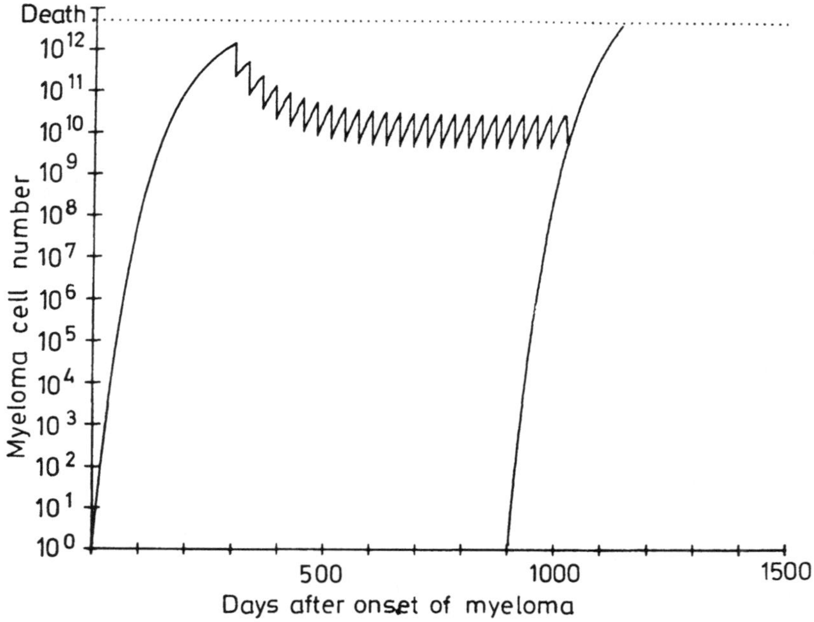

Fig. 2. Theoretic illustration of the natural history of multiple myeloma, based on Gompertzian kinetics. In this instance, the tumor cell generation time is fixed at 2.35 days (growth rate at time 0 $A_0 = 0.295$) throughout the entire course from initation of the monoclone (one malignant cell) to the time of death in relapse. If pulse chemotherapy had not been initiated (day 300) when the cell mass was 1.5×10^{12} cells, the tumor theoretically would have plateaued at 6.5×10^{12} cells (a supralethal level for this patient). The value for the retardation constant α is fixed at 0.01 for the original monoclone throughout the period prior to diagnosis and through the period of partial remission. The pharmacologically and kinetically resistant subclone responsible for relapse is finally selected (presumably from a series of less effective mutants) 630 days after the initiation of chemotherapy. Although the mutant cell also has an initial doubling time of 2.35 days, the value for α is reduced to 0.009. The lethal tumor burden in this example, 5×10^{12} cells, is reached by the subclone in 250 days with a final doubling time of 15 days at the time of death. The theoretic plateau for the subclone is 10^{14} cells, as it is almost completely unaffected by feedback mechanisms

have transitory rises in LI within 7–10 days of individual courses of pulse chemotherapy, but these generally do not remain elevated. In contrast, patients who present with a higher LI, or who have a twofold or greater rise in LI during induction therapy, generally either fail to achieve 75% tumor regression or relapse quickly after achieving an initial remission status. The minority of patients who present with stage III myeloma with a high LI have a particularly poor prognosis and generally survive less than 6 months with standard treatment. New approaches will be required to treat such cases. Patients who achieve durable remissions continue to manifest a low LI during the plateau phase of disease and a rising LI may be an early predictor of relapse; however, not all patients who relapse have significant rises in the LI. Over the past 5 years, we and others have tried to add cycle-active agents to standard alkylating agent-prednisone regimens in an effort to eradicate the cycling myeloma cells. Drugs tested have been methotrexate, cytosine arabinoside, azathioprine, hydroxyurea, and vincristine. While many of these agents may not have been tested at optimal doses or schedules, only vincristine has shown some evidence of specificity for cycling myeloma cells. The effects of vincristine have been a modest 25%–50% further reduction in tumor cell mass [15]. Analyses of survival in recent SWOG studies that have employed vincristine show an approximate 10% increase in survival of those patients who received vincristine in their treatment regimens versus those who did not [4]. It thus appears that we currently lack cycle-active agents which have a high degree of specificity for cycling myeloma cells. Our recent in vitro studies of human myeloma stem cells (performed with DR. HAMBURGER) do suggest that in most cases the colony-forming myeloma cells are in cycle [10]. This was established with tritiated thymidine (^{3}H-T) suicide experiments. In these studies, a 1-h exposure to high specific activity ^{3}H-T resulted in a 50%–75% reduction in survival of myeloma colony-forming units. The only exceptions were two stage III myeloma cases with 75%–90% marrow replacement with tumor. In those cases, the myeloma stem cells appeared to be in G_0, and would therefore not be susceptible to cycle-active drugs.

Treatment of the Relapse Phase of Myeloma

A major problem in myeloma therapy with use of conventional alkylating agents has been that even though treatment is continued for 1–4 years, most patients eventually become refractory to treatment and renewed myeloma growth occurs. We reasoned that since myeloma was a "low growth fraction tumor", cycle-nonspecific agents, which are not cross-resistant with melphalan or cyclophosphamide, should be tried in combination in the relapse phase of disease. We selected adriamycin (A) and BCNU (B) because both met these criteria and had some evidence of activity in myeloma for either induction [BCNU (16)] or relapse [adriamycin (2)]. A low dose schedule, utilizing 30 mg/M^2 of each of these two agents was used every 3 weeks in our Arizona pilot study [1]. In this study, 7 of 13 patients (53%) responded to "BA". An example of an excellent response to "BA" treatment is shown in Fig. 3. BCNU as a single

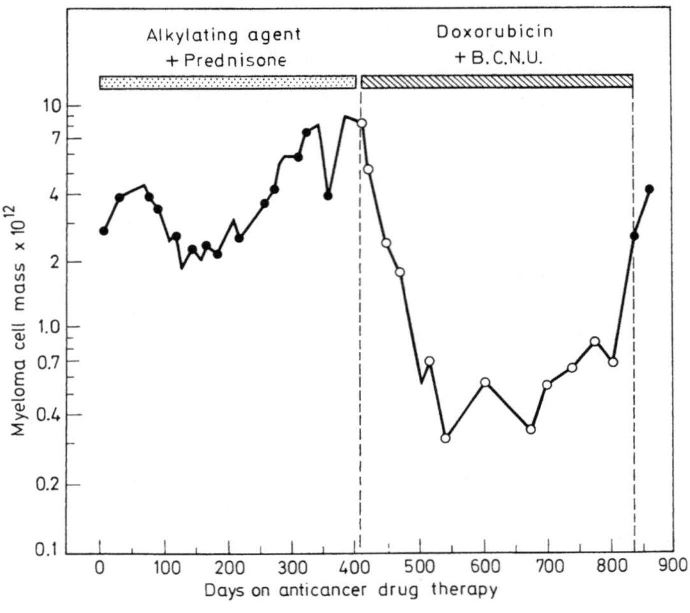

Fig. 3. Myeloma cell mass determinations on a patient while on alkylating agent and prednisone therapy or adriamycin/BCNU treatment (Reproduced with modification from ALBERTS et al., Lancet *1976* i, 926 [1], with permission from the authors)

agent has a very low response rate in the relapse phase and adriamycin has no more than a 20% transitory response rate [2, 16]. Thus the response to the combination of these agents appears to represent an example of true drug synergism. The Southwest Oncology Group has recently conducted a large-scale clinical trial of the same combination with the addition of vincristine (V) and prednisone (P) in protocol 7432 (VBAP) coordinated by Dr. Bonnet.
In the SWOG experience, 29 of 62 evaluable patients (46%) who had previously responded to melphalan/cyclophosphamide-prednisone and later relapsed were successfully reinduced into remission with VBAP [7].
We have recently analyzed the ^{3}H-T LI data on patients in our own institution who were treated with VBAP. Of extreme interest, 11 of 14 relapse patients (79%) who responded to VBAP manifested significant rises in LI prior to VBAP. In contrast, of ten relapse patients who failed to respond to VBAP, only one had a significant rise in LI prior to initiation of VBAP ($p < .05$). Thus the BA and the VBAP treatments appear to be about equivalent in activity and appear to be particularly effective in patients with cytokinetically active myeloma with a higher growth fraction. To our knowledge, this may be the first example where cell kinetic information may be predictive of response to treatment with a specific regimen of anticancer drugs. SWOG is also studying VBAP for previously untreated patients in protocol 7418. While that study is still going on, it is clear that VBAP has activity in remission induction as well.

Development of a New Clinical Trial

Based on many of the above clinical, pharmacologic, and cytokinetic observations, a new SWOG clinical trial (protocol 7704) was designed to test many of these concepts prospectively. The Southwest Oncology Group has implemented quantitative criteria for staging and follow-up of tumor mass in patients with multiple myeloma. These criteria have been applied prospectively in SWOG studies since 1973, and retrospectively for the period from 1965–1973. Combinations of melphalan (M) and prednisone (P), with or without cyclophosphamide (C), adriamycin (a), vincristine (v), and BCNU (B) have induced a significant therapeutic effect in 45%–50% of evaluable patients, using criteria based on a reduction of myeloma protein production (and tumor mass) by more than 75% within 6 months. An additional 25% of the patients treated achieved at least at 50% reduction in tumor mass so that, overall, approximately 70% of patients now achieve significant palliation of multiple myeloma with our treatment regimens. Using the more stringent criteria (75% regression) at those four institutions where the largest number of SWOG patients were treated (57% of all patients), investigators found that 69% of evaluable patients responded to VMCP and 61% to VCAP. This experience suggested that we may be achieving better results with multiple-drug combinations than with melphalan-prednisone alone. However, the group had not made a direct prospective comparison of a simple regimen (e.g., melphalan-prednisone) with the newer multidrug regimens to firmly conclude this. We have established that survival time for groups of patients correlated directly with the degree of myeloma protein mass reduction, regardless of the induction regimen. With protocol 7418, SWOG introduced shorter cycles of treatment (i.e., every 3 weeks) with either CAP, VCAP, VMCP, or VBAP. Our 1-year survival experience has clearly improved with this strategy, with 80% of patients surviving at 1 year (statistical report, SWOG minutes, October 1976). Additionally, we have shown VBAP to be a useful regimen for patients in relapse from alkylating agents in protocol 7432. VBAP contains several drugs (BCNU and adriamycin) which are not cross-resistant with conventional alkylating agents. In our new protocol (7704), we attempt to further extend and compare our experience with multidrug combinations with a simple melphalan-prednisone regimen for induction and follow the induction phase with maintenance with either VMCP alone or in combination with the immunotherapeutic agent, levamisole. In view of the fact that VMCP and VCAP were both excellent treatment arms, and VBAP proved useful in VMCP relapse patients, it appeared logical to attempt to alternate two of these regimens (VMCP and VCAP) and try two of them in a three-cycle series (VMCP-VBAP) in an effort to retard the acquisition of drug resistance by myeloma cells. The identical rationale has been used in the development of new treatments for Hodgkin's disease by BONADONNA, who is alternating the noncross-resistant ABVD regimen with MOPP [6]. A notable feature of recent SWOG studies has been the development of progressively shorter intervals between intermittent pulse courses of treatment. While initial melphalan-prednisone regimens were repeated every 4–6 weeks, the interval between pulse treatments was shortened to 4 weeks in protocol 7305 and to 3 weeks in protocol 7418. This shortening has been achieved with the same drug doses as in the 4-week schedule without increased toxicity. This scheduling was developed after Gompertzian kinetic modeling studies suggested that a q 3-week schedule would result in an approximate one log greater cell kill if drug doses were held constant [17].

The schema for this protocol is summarized in Table 2. It is obviously too early to have results available from this study, however, the study design should clearly permit us to tell whether application of these concepts can improve end results in a large population of previously untreated myeloma patients. A significant cohort of these patients will have serial kinetic data obtained (M-component marker and LI), which should allow us to evaluate the effects of these different treatment regimens on myeloma kinetics.

Table 2. Chemoimmunotherapy of Multiple Myeloma (SWOG 7704) (all treatment cycles started every 21 days)

Induction	Induction for a minimum of 6 months to a maximum of 1 year to achieve CR[a]		Maintenance (1 year)
Limb 1: regular alternating combinations	VMCP (one cycle)—VCAP (one cycle) Continued alternation every 3 weeks	CR→ PR→Continued Rx NR or prog.→new agents	
Limb 2: sequential alternating combinations	VMCP (3 cycles)—VBAP (3 cycles) Alternation from VMCP to VBAP (etc.) after every 3 cycles of each combination	CR→ PR→continued Rx NR or prog.→new agents	VMCP VMCP + levamisole
Limb 3: single combination	MP—cycles every 3 weeks	CR→ PR→continued Rx NR or prog.→new agents	

CR = greater than 75% tumor regression
PR = greater than 50% but less than 75% tumor regression
NR = less than 50% tumor regression

[a] Upon achieving CR, and after a minimum of 6 months, patients are randomized to maintenance therapy.

VMCP		*VCAP*		*VBAP*	
Vincristine	1 mg iv, day 1	Vincristine	1 mg iv, day 1	Vincristine	1 mg iv, day 1
Melphalan	6 mg/m²/d, po days 1–4	Cytoxan	125 mg/m²/d, po days 1–4	BCNU	30 mg/m², iv, day 1
Cytoxan	125 mg/m²/d, po days 1–4	Adriamycin	30 mg/m², iv, day 1	Adriamycin	30 mg/m² iv, day 1
Prednisone	60 mg/m²/d, po days 1–4	Prednisone	60 mg/m²/d, po days 1–4	Prednisone	60 mg/m²/d, po days 1–4

In Vitro Prediction of Drug Sensitivity

Perhaps the most promising new approach to myeloma therapy which has arisen in our clinical research program has been based on the development of a soft agar colony-forming assay for human myeloma stem cells [10, 11]. PARK et al. had previously developed a similar assay for mouse myeloma stem cells [13], and OGAWA et al. [12] showed that differential drug sensitivity was present between different mouse myeloma lines. Furthermore, the in vitro colony-forming assay results were predictive of in vivo results in the same myeloma line.

Using our in vitro human myeloma stem cell assay, we have tested anticancer drug sensitivity of patient marrows with a 1-h exposure to pharmacologically achievable concentrations of various agents. Thus far, we have conducted studies with BCNU, adriamycin, and melphalan in five patients who were previously untreated or were drug responsive and in two patients in relapse who had received these agents previously. We observed an eightfold range in sensitivity to BCNU, with the relapse patients being least sensitive. Our studies of adriamycin sensitivity showed that tumor stem cell killing occurs with as little as .01 µg/ml of the agent. Patients in relapse from adriamycin were the least sensitive and a 20-fold overall range in sensitivity was manifest. Even in previously untreated patients, increasing doses of adriamycin beyond the .05 µg/ml dosage did not routinely increase lethality to myeloma stem cells. This suggests that a fraction of the tumor stem cells may be biochemically resistant to this agent even prior to exposure. Our studies of melphalan showed more than a 25-fold range in differential sensitivity. Several untreated patients had complete inhibition of colony formation at the lowest dose tested (.05 µg/ml) [20].

These preliminary studies suggest to us that in vitro drug sensitivity of myeloma stem cells may be predictive of in vivo results in humans. Our plan is to continue surveying drug sensitivity in various treatment groups but also to initiate predictive trials for patients in relapse whom standard agents no longer benefit. Such trials will clearly be arduous as they will involve high risk cases with very poor prognoses. Indeed, the assay currently requires a 2–3-week incubation period for results so that many of these patients will require substantial supportive care before results are available. However, if we can successfully identify differences in sensitivity and select new agents which can reinduce remission in this setting, it will be reasonable to also consider subsequently applying this approach in previously untreated myeloma patients. In our view, this approach could provide the same type of selectivity of agents as is currently employed in the analogous clinical problem of selection of appropriate antibiotics for treatment of difficult or resistant bacterial infections.

Acknowledgements

This work was supported in part by grants from the United States Public Health Service (CA 14102, CA 13612, CA 17094, and CA 21839). B. G. M. DURIE is a Scholar of The Leukemia Society of America.

References

1. ALBERTS, D. S., SALMON, S. E.: Adriamycin (NSC-123127) in the treatment of alkylator-resistant multiple myeloma: a pilot study. Cancer Chemother. Rep. *59*, 345–350 (1975)
2. ALBERTS, D. S., DURIE, B. G. M., SALMON, S. E.: Doxorubicin/B. C. N. U. chemotherapy for multiple myeloma in relapse. Lancet *I*, 926–928 (1976)
3. ALEXANIAN, R., BALCERZAK, S., BONNETT, J. D., GEHAN, E. A., HAUT, A., HEWLETT, J. S., MONTO, R. W.: Prognostic factors in multiple myeloma. Cancer *36*, 1192–1201 (1975)
4. ALEXANIAN, R., SALMON, S., BONNETT, J., GEHAN, E. A., et al.: Combination therapy for multiple myeloma. Cancer *40*, 2765–2771 (1977)

5. Bergsagel, D. E.: Plasma Cell Myeloma: Prognostic Factors and Criteria of Response to Therapy. In: Cancer Therapy: Prognostic Factors and Criteria of Response. Staquet, M. J. (ed.) New York: Raven Press, 1975, pp. 73–87, 1975
6. Bonadonna, G., Zucali, R., Delena, M.: Combined chemotherapy (MOPP VS ABVD) plus radiation therapy in advanced Hodgkin's disease. ASCO Proceedings (abstract) p. 260, (Toronto) 1976
7. Bonnett, J. D.: Minutes of Myeloma Committee, Southwest Oncology Group Minutes, June 1977. Personal commun.
8. Durie, B. G. M., Salmon, S. E.: A clinical staging system for multiple myeloma. Correlation of measured myeloma cell mass with presenting clinical features, response to treatment, and survival. Cancer *36*, 842–854 (1975)
9. Durie, B. G. M., Vaught, L., Salmon, S. E.: Prognostic significance of tritiated thymidine labeling Index (LI) in multiple myeloma and acute myeloid leukemia. AACR Proceedings (abstract) p. 80, (Denver) (1977)
10. Hamburger, A. W., Salmon, S. E.: Primary bioassay of human myeloma stem cells. J. Clin. Invest. *60*, 846–854 (1977)
11. Hamburger, A. W., Salmon, S. E.: Primary bioassay of human tumor stem cells. Science *197*, 461–463 (1977)
12. Ogawa, M., Bergsagel, D. E., McCulloch, E. A.: Chemotherapy of mouse myeloma: quantitative cell culture predictive of response *in vivo*. Blood *41*, 7–15 (1973)
13. Park, C. H., Bergsagel, D. E., McCulloch, E. A.: Mouse myeloma tumor stem cells: a primary cell culture assay. J. Natl. Cancer Inst. *46*, 411–416 (1971)
14. Salmon, S. E.: Immunoglobulin synthesis and tumor kinetics of multiple myeloma. Semin Hematol. *10*, 135–147 (1973)
15. Salmon, S. E.: Expansion of the growth fraction in multiple myeloma with alkylating agents. Blood *45*, 119–129 (1975)
16. Salmon, S. E.: Nitrosoureas in multiple myeloma. Cancer Treat. Rep. *60*, 789–794 (1976)
17. Salmon, S. E., Durie, B. G. M.: Application of Cell Kinetics to Chemotherapy for Multiple Myeloma. In: Growth Kinetics and Biochemical Regulation of Normal and Malignant Cells (The University of Texas System Cancer Center M. D. Anderson Hospital and Tumor Institute 29th Annual Symposium on Fundamental Cancer Research, 1976), Drewinko, B., Humphrey, R. M. (eds.) Baltimore: Williams and Wilkins Co., pp. 865–878, (1977)
18. Salmon, S. E., Smith, B.: Immunoglobulin synthesis and total body tumor cell number in IgG multiple myeloma. J. Clin. Invest. *49*, 1114–1121 (1970)
19. Salmon, S. E., Wampler, S. B.: Multiple myeloma: quantitative staging and assessment of response with a programmable pocket calculator. Blood *49*, 379 (1977)
20. Salmon, S. E., Hamburger, A. W., Soehnlen, B., Durie, B. G. M., Alberts, D. S., Moon, T. E.: Quantitation of differential sensitivity of human tumor cells to anticancer drugs. N. Engl. J. Med. *298*, 1321–1327 (1978)
21. Shustik, C., Bergsagel, D. E., Pruzanski, W.: Kappa and lambda light chain disease: Survival rates and clinical manifestations. Blood *48*, 41–51 (1976)
22. Skipper, H. E.: Thoughts on cancer chemotherapy and combination modality therapy (1974). J. Am. Med. Assoc. *230*, 1033–1035 (1974)
23. Sullivan, P. W., Salmon, S. E.: Kinetics of tumor growth and regression in IgG multiple myeloma. J. Clin. Invest. *51*, 1697–1706 (1972)

Staging of Myeloma. A Preliminary Study of Staging Factors and Treatment in Different Stages

E. ÖSBY, B. CARLMARK, and P. REIZENSTEIN

Introduction

Almost all tumors originating in the lymphatic cell system, except myelomas, are staged. The intensity and type of treatment is usually adapted to the stage of the disease. In more malignant or advanced stages, fairly intense combination chemotherapy is often used. In myelomas, treatment has often been less intense. Often a single cytostatic is used. Since myelomas are not usually staged, this is true even for advanced stages and malignant forms. However, staging procedures for myeloma have been proposed [4, 5]. For such a procedure to be clinically relevant, prognostic differences between the different stages have to be established. The present purpose was to study whether initial clinical parameters can be found which are correlated to the prognosis in myeloma. In addition, a differentiated program for treatment of the different stages is proposed, and some preliminary treatment results are reported.

Patients and Methods

Patients

All myeloma patients seen at the hematology division between January, 1972 and May, 1977 were studied. There were 21 men aged 45–78 years (median 60 years) and 29 women aged 49–80 years (median 66 years). The age distribution is seen in Fig. 1.

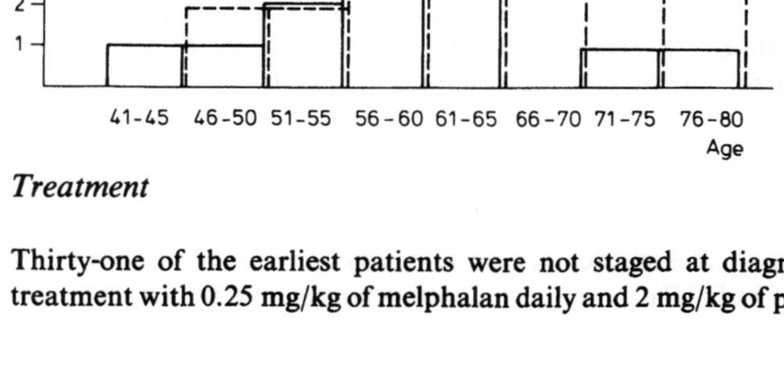

Fig. 1. Age distribution. The dominance of women (broken lines) in the older age groups and that of men (unbroken lines) in the younger ones is seen

Treatment

Thirty-one of the earliest patients were not staged at diagnosis but given "standardized" treatment with 0.25 mg/kg of melphalan daily and 2 mg/kg of prednisone daily for 4 days about every 6th week according to ALEXANIAN [1]. These patients were staged retrospectively. In five additional nonstaged patients, melphalan was inadvertently replaced by small oral doses of cytoxan. These patients are excluded. Eleven of the latest patients were staged and given "individualized" treatment. In stage I this was as described above. In stage II, 300–500 mg of cytoxan were given i.v. daily for 3 days every 3–6 weeks. In stage III, 2 mg vincristine were given on day 1, 300–500 mg cytoxan daily for 3 days, and 2 mg/kg prednisone daily for 3 days every 3–6 weeks. Three additional patients in stage II and III died before proper treatment could be given.

Staging

An attempt was made, using a partial regression method, to identify clinical parameters influencing the prognosis and thus the staging. The correlation was studied between survival and 13 different clinical and laboratory values (Table 1) in 16 deceased patients. It is possible to do this type of study only in deceased patients, but it is recognized that the result is biased since surviving patients are excluded. A modification of the method described by SALMON [4, 5] was thus obtained (Table 3).

Clinical Laboratory Studies

Customary methods were used for estimations of hemoglobin (normal values: men 140–170 g/liter; women 120–150 g/liter), serum creatinine (normal values: 60–120 μmol/liter), erythrocyte sedimentation rates (ESR, normal: 2–15 mm/h), serum electrophoresis (normal: IgM 0.4–2.0 g/liter, IgG 7–14 g/liter, IgA 0.8–3.8 g/liter), and qualitative estimations of light chains in the urine (courtesy Assist. Prof. A. NORMAN, Central Chemistry Laboratory). Skeletal x-rays were used to establish localized myeloma infiltrates. Generalized osteopenia without localized lesions was graded equally to a single myeloma infiltrate.

Plasma Cells in Bone Marrow

The degree of differentiation of the plasma cells in the bone marrow was judged subjectively by one investigator and graded I (mature) and II (immature). The number of plasma cells in the bone marrow smears was not counted; only a simple estimate of limited or extensive infiltration was made.

Minimum Intestinal Calcium Absorption

This was measured according to the whole body counting technique previously described by SJÖBERG et al. [13]. After an overnight fast and a background measurement in the whole body counter, 3–4 μCi of ^{47}Ca in a carrier dose of 135 mg $CaCl_2$ was administered orally. A measurement 14 days later estimated the retained activity, which is added to the excreted activity in the urine during the first 3 days to give the minimum absorption.

Skeletal Calcium Uptake

A method to measure the skeletal uptake of calcium has previously been described by ARMAN and REIZENSTEIN [3]. About 4 μCi of $^{47}CaCl_2$ is injected intravenously, and the radioactivity is recorded over one hand with a 3 in. × 2 in. NaI crystal, 10 min and 240 min after the injection. The hand and the crystal are fixed in a plastic holder to standardize the counting geometry. The counted activity is referred to the injected activity and the results expressed as counts per second (cps) per given μCi.

Results

Identification of Staging Parameters

Of the 13 clinical and laboratory parameters studied in 16 deceased patients (Table 1), the best correlation was found with the presence or absence of light chains in the urine. Statistically significant reductions in the residual variance could be obtained by introducing into the partial regression equation the quantity of the monoclonal fraction in the serum, apparently

Table 1. Clinical and laboratory parameters: correlation to prognosis studied by multiple regression analysis for possible staging use in 16 deceased patients (dependent variable: survival time)

Independent variable	Residual variance	F value
Variables found to reduce the residual variance		
Light chains in urine	17.1	*
Skeletal lesions (x-ray)	16.1	*
M-component in serum (quantitative)	14.6	*
Treatment[a]	12.8	**
ESR	11.8	**
Variables not reducing residual variance		
Serum creatinine		
Sex		
Frequency and maturity of plasma cells in marrow		
Serum calcium		
Age		
M-component (qualitative)		
Hemoglobin		

[a] = melphalan + prednisone; 2. 2 = cytoxan (+ vincristine + prednisone).

Table 2. Partial regression equation predicting survival in myeloma, all stages[a] (n = 16)

Expected survival (months) = 53.8 + 0.41(M-component, quantity, g/liter) − 18.8 (light chains, 0 = neg, 1 = pos) − 22.1 (skeletal lesions, 0 = neg, 1 = pos) − 0.13 (ESR, mm/h) + 14.5 (Treatment, 0 = melphalan + prednisone, 1 = cytoxan (+ vincristine + prednisone))
(Residual variance 11.8)

[a] Based only on dead patients.

independently of its nature, of skeletal lesions, the ESR, and the form of treatment given. No statistically significant further reduction could be achieved by including any of the other factors listed in Table 1. Thus, a partial regression equation predicting the expected survival could be obtained (Table 2).

Staging Procedure

Since the "staging factors" identified were almost identical to those previously described by Salmon [4, 5], the modification of Salmon's staging procedure given in Table 3 was used.

Table 3. Clinical staging of myeloma

Stage I
All of:
Hemoglobin > 100 g/liter
Serum calcium normal
Normal x-ray
Low M-component
Ig-G < 50 g/liter
Ig-A < 30 g/liter
Stage II
One or more of:
Solitary lytic bone lesions
Urinary light chains
Fitting neither I nor III
Stage III
One or more of:
Hemoglobin < 85 g/liter
Serum calcium > 3 mmol/liter
Multiple lytic bone lesions
High M-component
Ig-G > 70 g/liter
Ig-A > 50 g/liter

Staging and Calcium Metabolism

No difference was found between the intestinal minimum calcium absorption in stage I (29.8 ± 4.74 SE, in percentage of the given dose) and that in stage III (29.0 ± 3.71 SE, percentage). The skeletal calcium uptake was numerically but not statistically significantly higher in stage I (0.162 ± 0.0076 SE, cps/μCi) than in stage II + III (0.148 ± 0.0059 SE, cps/μCi).

Staging and Prognosis

The survival was statistically significantly ($p < 0.01$) better in stage I and numerically better in stage II than in stage III in the group of patients all given a standard treatment, independent of the stage (Fig. 2).

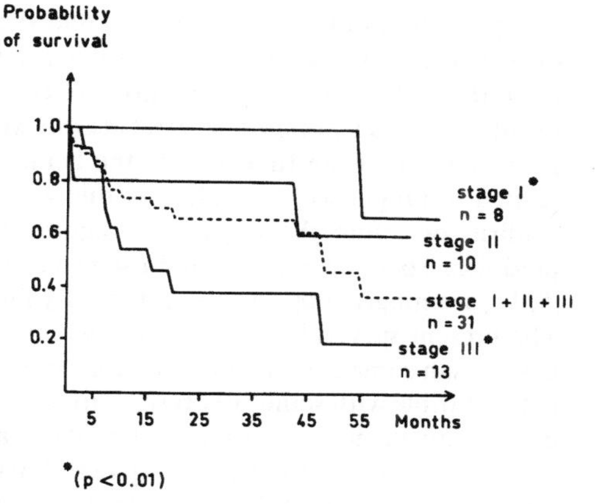

Fig. 2. Actuarial survival in a uniformly treated group of myeloma patients. Survival in stage I is statistically significantly ($p < 0.01$) longer than in stage III

Staging and Treatment

When the standard melphalan-prednisone treatment earlier given to stages II and III was replaced by the more intensive treatment assigned to these stages, the apparent probability to survive 2 years increased from 55% to 80% (Fig. 3). The median survival with standard treatment was 43 months but had not been reached by 53 months with the more intense treatment. However, none of these differences is statistically significant.

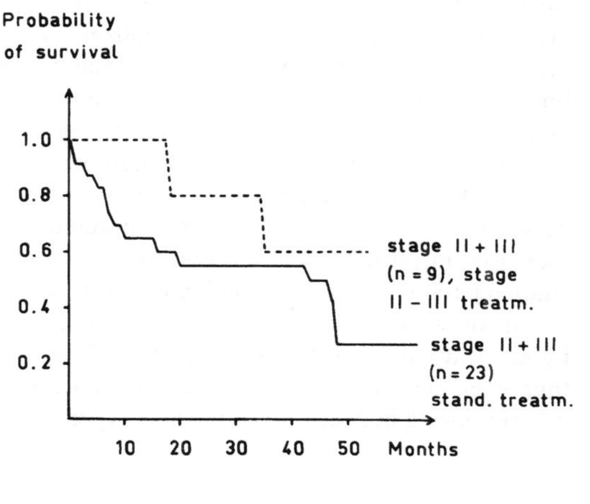

Fig. 3. Actuarial survival in stage II–III myeloma treated with melphalan-prednisone (unbroken line) and with more intensive chemotherapy (cytoxan-vincristine-prednisone, broken line)

Discussion

To study the correlation between survival and hopefully prognostic factors in a small patient group from which survivors are excluded may give deceptive results. Another study is planned when all 50 patients in the present group are dead. To study an earlier group of patients now deceased is not possible because of inadequacies in the laboratory studies before 1972.

The present finding that light chains and skeletal lesions are valuable as prognostic factors is expected [1, 4, 5] and reasonable. Previous results regarding the prognostic implications of the quantity of the monoclonal fraction are controversial [2, 4, 5, 14]. Some of the other present results are not only preliminary but also unexpected, and they must be interpreted with caution. It is thus surprising that neither the hemoglobin nor the serum creatinine are significantly related to prognosis [2, 9, 14], and this will be further studied. Similarly, we will attempt to confirm or refute the apparently significant (Table 2) superiority of cytoxan-vincristine-prednisone over melphalan-prednisone treatment. However, the cytokinetic studies by SALMON [5, 11] seemingly support this preliminary finding.

The present survival in nonstaged, melphalan-prednisone-treated patients, 66% at 2 years, is better than some early figures [10], for example 15% at 2 years [6]. However, the present figure is compatible with some later results, for example a 2-year survival at 51% [7, 8]. In stage II–III, patients given more intensive treatment had a preliminary 2-year survival of 80% in the present study. Compared to the figures given above for groups containing all stages, this must be regarded as promising. However, three patients in stage II and III were excluded because they died before proper treatment was given.

An attempt was made to study calcium metabolism in myeloma for two reasons. One was its possible use in prognosis. The present method of estimating skeletal calcium uptake had previously been found to be relevant and to distinguish the young from the ageing skeleton [3]. However, measurements are performed over the skeleton of the hand, and further studies are required to demonstrate whether local myeloma lesions in the hand explain the decreased skeletal radiocalcium uptake. All four hand x-rays performed were negative, but four patients were not examined. It is also possible that skeletal lesions in general reduce the skeletal radiocalcium uptake as it is measured in the hand. Previous studies showed that patients with femoral fractures had a lower radiocalcium uptake over the hand skeleton than patients of similar age without fractures. It is not yet possible to state whether this effect is caused by calcium trapping in the skeletal lesions, fracture, or myeloma, or if it is caused by general metabolic effects on calcium metabolism, or if a preexisting low skeletal calcium uptake increases the liability of developing traumatic or myelomatous skeletal lesions. Another reason for studying calcium metabolism in myeloma was that the differentiation between myeloma and hyperparathyroidism can be aided by calcium absorption studies. In hyperparathyroidism, intestinal calcium absorption has been shown to be increased [12], and parathormone is known to stimulate calcium absorption. In myeloma with skeletal lesions, on the other hand, hypercalcemia is frequent, but no stimulation of parathormone secretion occurs, and no increased intestinal calcium absorption is found. During the past years, several insufficiently studied patients, or patients with nonsecretory myeloma, or some where no myeloma cells were found in a marrow smear, have been seen in this division, where the diagnosis of hyperparathyroidism had been mistakenly made. One of the present myeloma patients had thus been parathyroidectomized. Calcium absorption studies may, therefore, be useful in differentiating between myeloma and hyperparathyroidism, but not in staging myeloma.

Summary

Attempts were made to find prognostic factors in myeloma. In 16 deceased patients, urinary light chains, skeletal lesions, and the quantity of the monoclonal protein fraction in the serum were correlated to prognosis, in contrast to the electrophoretic mobility of the monoclonal fraction, the hemoglobin, the serum creatinine value, the serum calcium, or the intestinal calcium absorption. Skeletal calcium uptake was only numerically higher in mild myeloma than in advanced myeloma. Since these findings partially agreed with the staging procedure previously proposed by SALMON, a modification of this procedure was used to stage 50 myeloma patients. Survival was statistically significantly shorter in stage III than in stage I. A differentiated treatment with melphalan-prednisone in stage I, cytoxan infusions in stage II, and vincristine-cytoxan-prednisone in stage III is proposed. A preliminary comparison of nine patients in stage II–III given intensive treatment with 23 given melphalan-prednisone suggests a numerically, but not as yet a statistically significant increase in survival in the intensively treated group, which seems to have an 80% 2-year survival.

References

1. ALEXANIAN, R., HAUT, A., KHAN, A. U., LANE, M., MCKELVEY, E. M., MIGLIORE, P. J., STICKEY, W. J., and WILSON, H. E.: Treatment for multiple myeloma. Combination chemotherapy with different melphalan dose regiments. JAMA *208*, 1680–1685 (1969)
2. ALEXANIAN, R., BALCERZAH, S., BONNET, J. D., GEHAN, E. A., HAUT, A., HEWLETT, J. S., and MONTO, R. W.: Prognostic factors in multiple myeloma. Cancer *36*, 1192–1201 (1975)
3. ARMAN, E., and REIZENSTEIN, P.: Hand radioactivity after intravenous injection of ^{47}Ca. Effect of age and femoral neck fracture. Geriatrics *26*, 155–165 (1971)
4. DURIE, B. G. M., and SALMON, S. E.: A clinical staging system for multiple myeloma. Cancer *36*, 842–854 (1975)
5. DURIE, B. G. M., and SALMON, S. E.: Cellular kinetics, staging, and immunoglobulin synthesis in multiple myeloma. Annu. Rev. Med. *26*, 283–288 (1975)
6. FEINLEIB, M., and MAC MATRON, B.: Duration of survival in multiple myeloma. J. Natl. Cancer Inst. *24*, 1259–1269 (1960)
7. GALTON, D. A. G., and PETO, R.: A progress report on the Medical Research Council's therapeutic trial in myelomatosis. Br. J. Haematol. *15*, 319–320 (1968)
8. HOBBS, J. R.: Growth rates and responses to treatment in human myelomatosis. Br. J. Haematol. *16*, 607–617 (1969)
9. HOBBS, J. R.: Monitoring myelomatosis. Arch. Intern. Med. *135*, 125–130 (1975)
10. INNES, J., and NEWALL, J.: Myelomatosis. Lancet *I*, 239–245 (1961)
11. SALMON, S. E.: Expansion of the growth fraction in multiple myeloma with alkylating agents. Blood *45*, 119–129 (1975)
12. SJÖBERG, H. E.: Retention of ^{47}calcium administered orally in patients with primary hyperparathyroidism. Horm. Metab. Res. *2*, 32–34 (1970)
13. SJÖBERG, H. E., REIZENSTEIN, P., and ARMAN, E.: Retention of orally administered ^{47}Ca in man measured in a whole-body counter. Scand. J. Clin. Lab. Invest. *26*, 67–71 (1970)
14. WALDENSTRÖM, J.: Diagnosis and treatment of multiple myeloma. New York, London, Grune and Stratton (1970)

Prognostic Factors and Treatment of Multiple Myeloma: Interest of a Cyclic Sequential Chemohormonotherapy Combining Cyclophosphamide, Melphalan, and Prednisone

D. BELPOMME, F. SIMON, P. POUILLART, B. AMOR, F. FEUILHADE DE CHAUVIN, A. BELPOMME, C. MENKES, A. DELRIEU, R. DEPIERRE, B. LE MEVEL, B. SERROU, D. FRIES, F. DELBARRE, and G. MATHÉ

Introduction

In 1889, KALHER succeeded in establishing the relationship between Bence Jones proteinuria [27], discovered in 1845, and the bone "tumor," called "multiple myeloma" by RUSTISKY in 1873 [51]. Later, in 1900, WRIGHT identified the plasmocytic nature of the tumoral proliferation. More recently, after GRABAR's discovery of immunoelectrophoresis procedures in 1953, several authors documented the immunologic significance of the disease [12, 22, 32, 39, 48]. It is now well-established that Kahler's disease is restricted to monoclonal primary plasmocyte tumor proliferations, usually associated with early dissemination of tumor cells in bone marrow and excretion, by these cells, of monoclonal immunologic products in the serum and urine.

In most cases, the immunologic component deals with monoclonal immunoglobulins of the IgG type, less frequently with the IgA type, and, rarely, with IgD or IgE type. In some cases, however, the excretion of immunologic products is restricted to κ or λ light chains, and this is known as BENCE JONES myeloma [26]. In other cases, there are, in fact, no detectable immunologic serum or urine abnormalities associated with the monoclonal plasmocyte tumor proliferation: those cases have been termed "nonexcreting myeloma" [17]. By definition, Kahler's disease is, therefore, quite distinct from: 1) plasmocytoma, which is only local plasmocyte tumor proliferation, 2) plasmocytic sarcoma, which is a primary plasmocyte tumor not necessarily located in bones, and 3) Waldenström's primary macroglobulinemia, which is associated with dysglobulinemia of the IgM type.

Although multiple myeloma is now a well-established clinical and immunogic entity, little progress has been made in the treatment of the disease. This tumor proliferation, in fact, raises several therapeutic difficulties: 1) myeloma usually occurs in patients of advanced age, 2) tumor volume is often considerable at the time of diagnosis [21, 45] with many cells in Go [19, 44, 47], since the kinetic of tumor proliferation follows the Gompertz equation [50], 3) the disease is often associated with severe bone marrow insufficiency, renal failure, and metabolic problems which tend to limit the use of chemotherapy, 4) the disease is an immunopathy, with humoral [12, 22, 37] and cellular [33, 37] immune deficiency which accounts for the particular sensibility of patients to infection [37, 54], and 5) clinically and biologically, the disease is relatively heterogenous, which accounts for the difficult standardization of treatment since a patient may be initially examined for rheumatologic, hematologic, or nephrologic symptoms by different specialists.

Although no decisive therapeutic progress has been made in recent years, several interesting procedures dealing with methodology and therapy have been developed:

1. The introduction in 1958 of melphalan [3, 7, 8, 9, 15, 20, 36, 49, 52] and, later on, of cyclophosphamide [10, 28, 29, 41, 42] has resulted in a significant therapeutic effect: cyclophosphamide has been shown to be associated with an improved survival comparable to that obtained with melphalan [10, 35, 40, 43]. Using either alkylating drug, the median survival of patients was raised 16–28 months, while the spontaneous median only ranged from 7–12 months (Table 1).

Table 1. Active drugs and combinations in multiple myeloma

Trials	Response rate (%)	Medial of survival (months)	Authors
Historical control	—	7–11	
PDN	—	7–11 (NS)	MASS (1962)
Urethane	—	7 (NS)	HOLLAND (1966)
MPH (C or I)	30–50%	18–26	ALEXANIAN (1969)
CPM	30–50%	18–26 (NS)	KORST et al. (1964)
BCNU	30–50%	18–26 (NS)	LEONE (1972)
PDN + MPH (C)	50–70%	22 (NS)	COSTA (1966) CUTTNER (1969)
PDN + MPH (I)	50–70% (NS)	22 (NS)	ALEXANIAN
PDN + MPH + PCZ (I)	69% (NS)	22 (NS)	ALEXANIAN (1972)

I: intermittent—PDN 2 mg/kg/day × 4–6 weeks, MPH 0.25 mg/kg/day × 4–6 weeks;
C: continuous—PDN 0.3–1.25 mg/kg/day: MPH 0.05 mg/kg/day.

2. Progress in intensive care has also led to some benefits, due to the use of chemotherapy in patients for whom such a therapeutic program could not be initially performed for metabolic or hematologic reasons.
3. Finally, more recently, the development of a clinical staging system, related to the total tumor mass [45, 46], has been reported to be of prognostic value [21]. This has led to a better definition of therapeutic indications.

The present study based on the retrospective survey of 120 multiple myeloma cases includes 1) an analysis of the main prognostic factors of the disease, with special attention to testing the prognostic value of the recently proposed staging classification [21] and 2) a type II therapeutic trial, using a sequential chemohormonotherapy. This regimen, which combines prednisone, melphalan, and cyclophosphamide, has been administered in 20 patients having a stage II or III myeloma, according to the previous prognosis classification. In this study, special attention has been paid to the comparison of this phase II trial with three comparable series of control patients. The results of the work bring out the following points: 1) as regards methodology, the need for an accurate classification method in order to obtain a comparable series of patients and 2) in therapeutic management, the advantage of using two alkylating agents instead of one at the beginning of the disease.

Materials and Methods

Patients

This study deals with 120 cases of multiple myeloma. From 1970–1976, patients were examined regularly in different departments[1]. Kahler's disease has been diagnosed on the basis of the usual immunohematologic criteria applying to the disease. In addition, a complete bone and kidney investigation has been systematically performed in patients before treatment. Distribution according to the different immunologic types of myeloma is as follows: IgG = 71 patients (59%), IgA = 26 patients (21%), Bence Jones κ or λ = 12 patients (11%), nonexcreting

1 Institut de Cancáerologie et d'Immunogénétique (Villejuif) (Pr. G. MATHÉ), Hôpital Cochin (Paris) (Pr. F. DELBARRE, Pr. B. AMOR), Hôpital Paul Brousse (Villejuif) (Pr. D. FRIES, Dr. R. DEPIERRE), Centre Réné Gauducheau (Nantes) (Dr. B. LEMEVEL), Centre Paul Lamarque (Montpellier) (Dr. B. SERROU).

Table 2. Immunologic heterogeneity of multiple myeloma (120 patients)

IgG	IgA	B.J.	Nonsecreting myeloma	Double IgG–IgA	IgD	Total
71[a]	26[b]	12[c]	8	2	1	120
59%	21%	10%	7%	1.5%	1%	100%

[a] $k/\lambda = 1$; [b] $k/\lambda = 3$; [c] $k/\lambda = 1.5$.

myeloma = 8 patients (6.5%), double peak myeloma (IgG + IgA) = 2 patients, and IgD myeloma = 1 patient (Table 2).
Figure 1 shows the distribution of patients according to age: 32% were under 60 years and 26% over 70 years. Since only 1% were under 40 years, the disease is relatively rare in this age group. The average age of all patients is 62.2 years. Figure 1 also gives the distribution of patients according to sex; the sex ratio is 55 males to 45 females. Average age did not differ significantly according to sex (median survival is 63.5 years for females and 60.7 years for males).

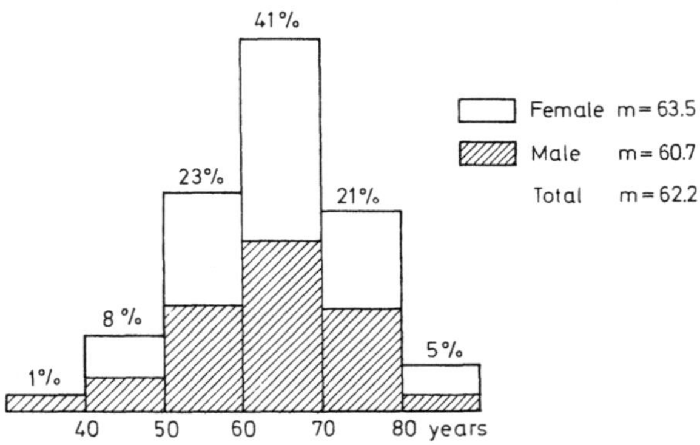

Fig. 1. Distribution of the 120 patients according to age and sex

Figure 2 classifies patients according to the length of the period between the appearance of the first symptoms and diagnosis. In over 50% of cases, the disease has been diagnosed less than 6 months after the first symptom(s) appeared. In some cases, however, the prediagnostic period lasted more than 1 year.

Staging Classification

Patients have been classified according to the criteria of DURIE and SALMON [21] as shown in Table 3. Fourteen cases (11.5%) were considered stage I, 54 (45%) stage II, and 52 (43.5%) stage III. Seventy-nine patients (66%) with creatinemia below 20 mg/ml were classified in group A and 41 (34%) with creatinemia above 20 mg/ml in group B.

Cyclic Sequential Chemohormonotherapy Trial

1. Twenty patients with stage II or III myeloma have been treated in a phase 22 trial according

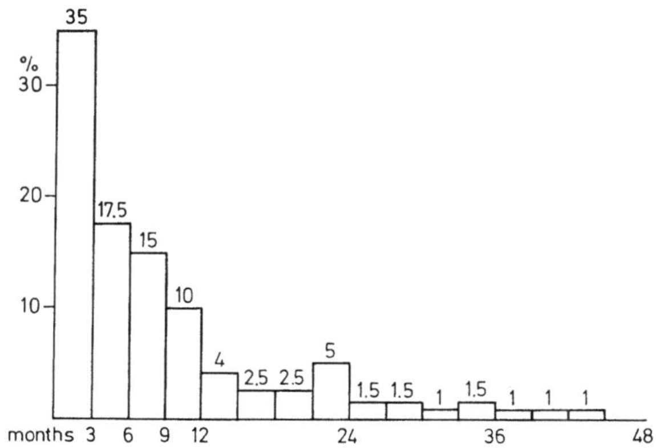

Fig. 2. Distribution of the 120 patients according to prediagnosis period

Table 3. Multiple myeloma staging system[a]

			Measured myeloma cell mass
Stage I:	Hb $\geqslant$ 10 g/100 ml $Ca^2 \leqslant$ 120 mg/liter IgG $\leqslant$ 50 g/liter of IgA 30 g/liter B.J. $\leqslant$ 4 g/24 h R.X. not more than 1 lytic lesion	All of the criteria	$0.6 \times 10^{12}/m^2$
Stage II:	Fitting neither stage I nor stage III (intermediate)		$0.6–1.2 \times 10^{12}/m^2$
Stage III:	Hb $\leqslant$ 8.5 g/100 ml $Ca^2 \geqslant$ 120 mg/liter IgG $\geqslant$ 70 g/liter or IgA 50 g/liter B.J. $\geqslant$ 10 g/24 h R.X. disseminated lesions	One or more criteria	$1.2 \times 10^{12}/m^2$

[a] DURIE and SALMON [21].

to regimen A, which consists of the administration of monthly cycles of chemohormonotherapy, each cycle comprising four sequences of 7 days. The first sequence includes a daily dose of 4 mg/m^2 melphalan, the second a daily dose of 40 mg/m^2 prednisone, the third a daily dose of 75 mg/m^2 cyclophosphamide, and the fourth exactly the same daily dose of prednisone as the first. Each cycle was repeated in identical fashion every 4 weeks, i.e., the drugs were administered in the order just indicated: melphalan, prednisone, cyclophosphamide, prednisone (Table 4).

2. In the present analysis, the survival of the 20 patients undergoing regimen A is compared to the survival of 81 control patients having "comparable" stage II or III multiple myeloma (Table 4). Thirty-eight of the 81 patients were treated according to regimen B, which consists of continuous chemohormonotherapy combining a daily dose of 20 mg/m^2 prednisone and an initial daily dose of 60 mg/m^2 cyclophosphamide administered up to maximum hematologic tolerance (2500 WBC). This was followed by intermittent chemotherapy in which the rate of cyclophosphamide administration was secondarily adapted to hematologic tolerance. Twenty-seven patients were treated according to regimen C which consists of continuous chemohormonotherapy combining the same previous daily dose of 20 mg/m^2 prednisone, with an initial daily dose of 3 mg/m^2 melphalan up to maximum hematologic tolerance (2500 WBC). This was

Table 4. Chemotherapy regimens

Protocol	Melphalan (MPH)	Cyclophosphamide (CPM)	Prednisone (PDN)	No. of alkylating agents	Administration
A	4 mg/m^2 per day × 7	60 mg/m^2 per day × 7	40 mg/m^2 per day × 7	2	Sequential[a]
B		60 mg/m^2 per day	20 mg/m^2 per day	1	Continuous[b]
C	4 mg/m^2 per day		20 mg/m^2 per day	1	Continuous[b]
D			40 mg/m^2 per day × 7	0	Historical control

[a] Sequential "PAPE" regimen with cycles of CPM × 7/day, MPH × 7/day, PDN × 7/day.
[b] Until hematologic toxicity.

followed, as previously, by intermittent chemotherapy in which melphalan administration was secondarily adapted to hematologic toxicity.

3. Finally, 16 cases were treated with prednisone alone, in daily doses of 20 mg/m^2, administered intermittently, depending on the clinical symptoms (regimen D) (see Table 4). Whenever necessary, regimen A patients as well as control patients (regimens B, C, and D) underwent sharply focalized irradiation of bone localizations which were either painful or involved a risk of mechanical complications (paraglegia) at the onset or in the course of their disease.

Expression of Results

Results are expressed as survival curves, using the direct method.

Results

Need to Classify Multiple Myeloma According to Prognosis Before Attemping Therapeutic Trial—Prognostic Factors

Immunologic Types

Figure 3 shows survival curves for the different groups of patients, classified according to the type of myeloma. Prognosis is better for the IgG than the IgA type of myeloma, since the survival median is 48 months for the IgG type out of only 11 months for the IgA type. In both cases, however, the disease is characterized by a certain degree of stabilization after about 20 months. Curves tend to describe a pseudoplateau at around 45% for IgG type myeloma and at only 20% for IgA type myeloma. On the other hand, prognosis for nonexcreting myeloma seems better, since six out of the eight patients in our study are still alive, and in five of these six cases, more than 36 months have elapsed since the beginning of the disease.

Although only a few patients died during the 1st year, κ and λ light chains myeloma have been found to be associated with a poor prognosis after 1 year, since only 2 patients out of 13 in our study are still living after 36 months. Most patients died of gradually increasing renal insufficiency often with amyloidosis. For the Bence Jones type myelomas included in the present study, the survival median is 33 months.

Tumor Size

Figure 4 shows the survival curve for the different groups of patients, classified according to the initial clinical stage of myeloma.

For stage I myeloma patients, median survival is still not reached after a 60-month follow-up. There were no deaths in the stage I group before the 30th month. On the other hand, the prognosis for stage III myeloma patients is significantly less favorable: the median survival is only 7 months and the survival curve has no tendency to reach a plateau even after a 36-month follow-up. However, for stage II multiple myeloma patients, the prognosis is better than for stage III patients but not as good as for stage I patients, since the survival curve lies somewhere between the curves for stages I and II. For stage II myeloma patients, the survival median is 28 months. After 36 months, there are seven survivors, and three patients had died.

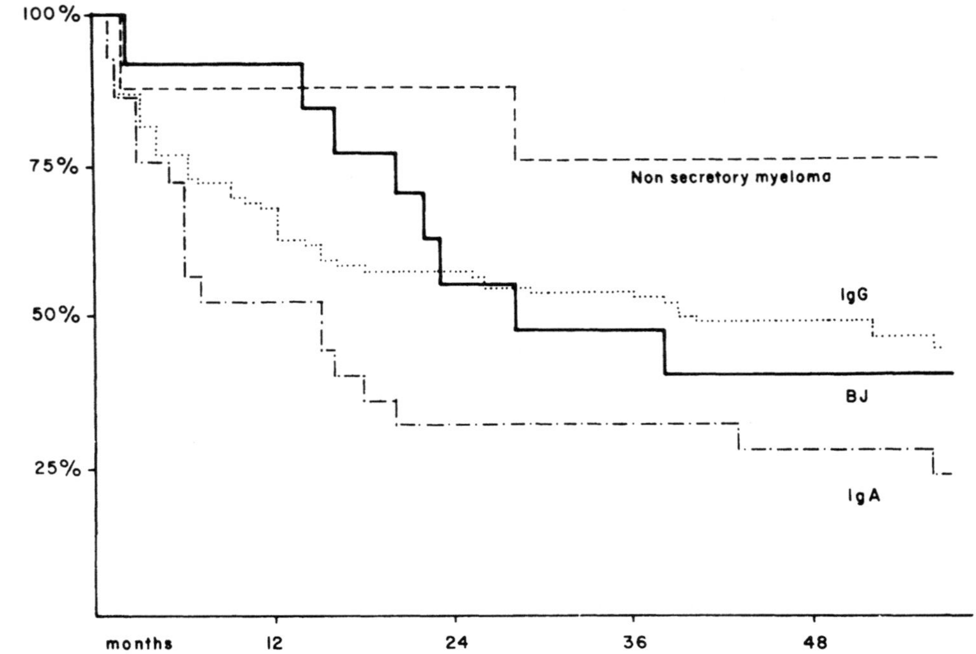

Fig. 3. Survival of the 120 patients according to immunologic types of myeloma

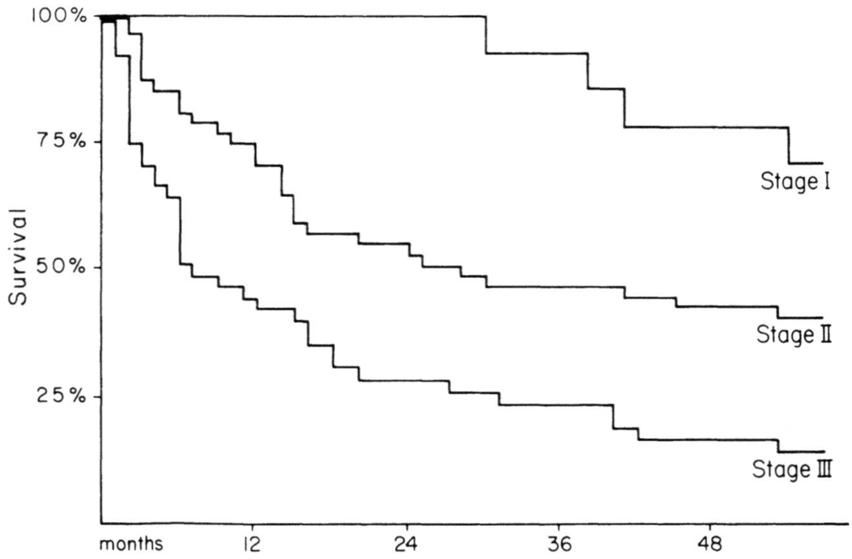

Fig. 4. Survival of the 120 patients according to the staging classification proposed by DURIE and SALMON [21]

Degree of Renal Insufficiency

Figure 5 shows the survival curves for the two groups of patients, classified according to their creatinemia level at the time of diagnosis. For patients with creatinemia above 20 mg/m² (group B), the median survival is 12 months, whereas this median is still not reached for patients with creatinemia below 20 mg/m² (group A).

Other Prognostic Factors

Since 90% of the patients of our series were over 50 (Fig. 1), the question arises as to whether general pathologic complaints associated with myeloma may not affect the mortality rate. Table 5 shows that in our series 10% of patients died of a cause not directly related to myeloma.

Cyclic Sequential Chemohormonotherapy in Stage II and III Myeloma Patients

General and Hematologic Tolerance

Hematologic tolerance of cyclic sequential chemohormonotherapy (regimen A) was satisfactory in all 20 stage II and III myeloma patients, even in those with bone localizations who had required complementary local irradiation. In all 20 cases, general tolerance was good enough, so that patients could be treated as outpatients.

Comparison of Different Series

Prognosis for the 20 patients treated by cyclic sequential chemohormonotherapy was compared to that for patients of the three other series (Table 4). The four series were considered

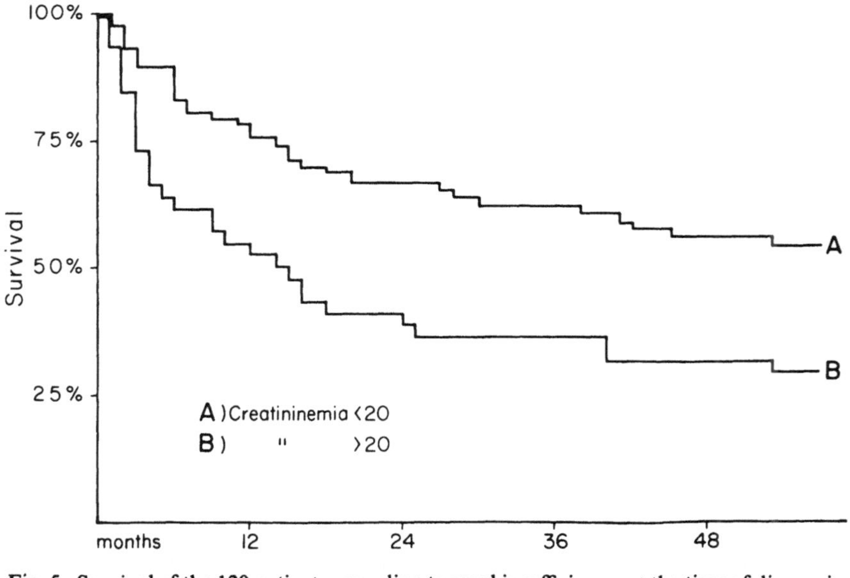

Fig. 5. Survival of the 120 patients according to renal insufficiency, at the time of diagnosis

Table 5. Cause of death in patients with multiple myeloma

Cause	No. of patients	Percentage		
Renal failure and/or hypercalcemia	26	34%		
Bone marrow aplasia (infectious and hemorrhage)	12	16%		
Not determined	12	16%		
Medullar compression syndrome	9	12%		
Cause unrelated to myeloma	7	9%	Ethyl cirrhosis	(1)
			Pulmonary embolism	(1)
			Cardiac failure	(2)
			Myocardial infarction	(1)
			Gastric ulcus	(1)
			Cerebral softening	(1)
Amyloidosis	6	8%		
Plasmocytic leukemia	3	4%		
Intestinal hemorrhage	1	1%		
Total	76	100%		

Table 6. Search for risk factors in groups of stage II and III myeloma patients submitted to regimens

Groups	No. of patients	% of stage III	% of stage B
Protocol A (MPH, CPM, PDN)	20	68%	36%
Protocol B (CPM, PDN)	38	48%	35%
Protocol C (MPH, PDN)	27	47%	36%
Protocol D (historical control)	16	43%	43%
Total	101		

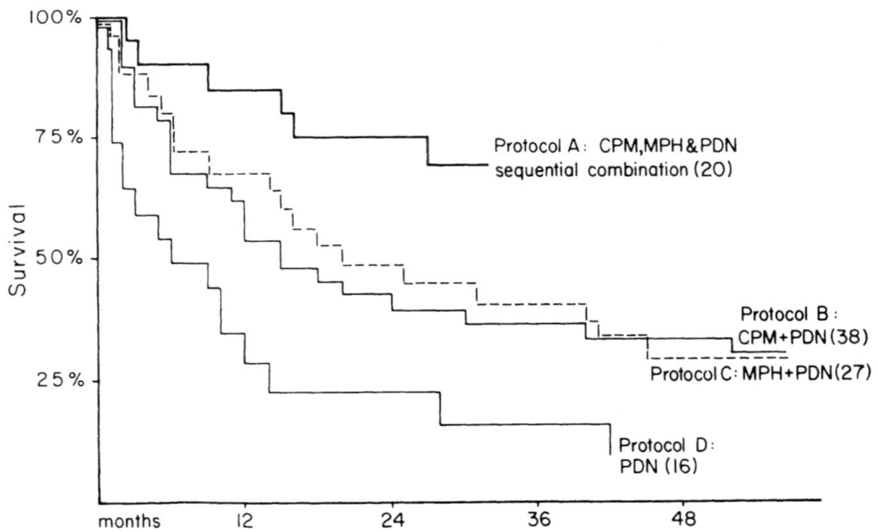

Fig. 6. Survival of 101 stage II or III myeloma patients according to different therapeutic protocols (direct survival curves)

comparable because there was no significant difference between them as regards the percentage of patients in stages II and III and in the A and B prognostic groups, respectively (Table 6).

Results

Figure 6 gives the survival curves for the different series classified according to the regimen applied. For what may be termed the historical group, which was given prednisone only (regimen D), the survival median was 8 months. Results were appreciably better for patients treated with a combination of either prednisone and cyclophosphamide (regimen B) or prednisone and melphalan (regimen C), since survival medians were 22 and 15 months respectively. Although the results argue in favor of replacing melphalan by cyclophosphamide in this type of monochemohormonotherapy, the difference is not, in fact, significant. On the other hand, survival was longer for the protocol A group treated by cyclic sequential chemohormonotherapy directly combining prednisone with the two alkylating agents, since the median was still not reached at 30 months. Here, the difference between this group and the others included in the trial is significant.

Discussion

Little progress has been recorded in multiple myeloma treatment since the introduction of melphalan, irrespective of whether this alkylating drug is administered alone or in combination with prednisone [16] or whether this drug is given continuously or intermittently at low or high dose regimens [4, 24, 25, 34] (Table 1). The results of the present work confirm the prognostic value of various parameters applying to Kahler's disease, such as the immunologic type of myeloma, tumor size and the degree of renal insufficiency [5, 13]. These data also confirm the prognostic value of DURIE and SALMON'S three-stage classification of the disease [21]. From the methodologic point of view, the existence of these different prognosis parameters must certainly be considered important, and failure to take them into account probably explains certain contradictory results in the literature.

From the therapeutic point of view, our data suggest that for stage II and III multiple myeloma better results are obtained in terms of survival when cyclophosphamide and melphalan are administered sequentially in combination with prednisone. Although these findings only cover a type II trial including 20 patients and must necessarily be considered preliminary, they are, nevertheless, encouraging, the more so as the survival curves obtained for our control groups (prednisone only, prednisone + cyclophosphamide, or prednisone + melphalan) are comparable to those reported in the literature [16, 23, 29, 38, 43]. The excellent hematologic and general tolerance of our intermittent cyclic sequential regimen is also a factor that should be taken into account, particularly in view of the advanced age of most of the patients treated.

Although better prognosis classification is now possible and there is hope of improving survival by direct sequential use of an melphalan-cyclophosphamide combination, much remains to be done in treating this disease, for which the prognosis is still poor. Several ways of improving treatment may be suggested:

1. In stage III patients, better use of intensive care, particularly extrarenal dialysis, in cases of severe renal insufficiency [14, 31], more widespread use of hematologic reanimation (transfusions of red or white blood cells or platelets) to cover uncompensated medullary insufficiency, and the development of more effective anti-infectious treatments for these potentially infected patients.
2. Establishment of more effective chemotherapy combinations in stage II and III cases

using, in addition to alkylating drugs, adriamycine [1, 2] or certain nitrosoures [6, 30]. Such combinations should be based firstly on myeloma tumor proliferation kinetics [19, 44, 45, 47] and secondly on the possible existence of interdrug pharmacodynamic potentialization [11, 18, 53].

3. Various immunostimulants such as BCG (administered, for instance, between chemotherapy cycles) should also be used since there is a considerable immunodepression induced by tumor proliferation and aggravated by chemotherapy [37].

Finally, from a general point of view, the present work emphasizes the need for cooperation between rheumatologists, hematologists, and nephrologists in studying a disease characterized by several different facets, and above all, the need for an overall coordinated therapeutic attitude in a disease for which the prognosis is still in many cases extremely guarded.

Summary

1. A type 2 therapeutic trial consisting of the administration of monthly cycles of chemohormonotherapy, each cycle combining weekly sequences of mephalan, prednisone, cyclophosphamide, and prednisone, has been achieved in 20 stage II or III myeloma patients. Tolerance of this regimen in treated out-patients was found to be excellent. Preliminary data indicate that the better survival rate in patients treated by this regimen is still not reached at a 30-month follow-up examination by three other nonrandomized control groups of patients receiving continuous therapy with prednisone alone, prednisone + cyclophosphamide, or prednisone + melphalan.

2. Analysis of the main prognostic factors of the four trials indicates that a) IgG-type myelomas are associated with a better prognosis than IgA type; nonexcreting myelomas are associated with the best prognosis, while Bence Jones myelomas are associated with a prognosis as poor as that of the IgA type; b) tumor volume as well as renal insufficiency, at the time of diagnosis, are also prognosis factors; this study confirms the prognostic value of the recently proposed clinical staging system based on these parameters but outlines that 10% of the patients died from a cause not directly related to myeloma plasmocyte proliferation.

3. In conclusion, these results point out: a) the possible advantage of using two alkylating agents instead of one at the beginning of the disease; b) the need to classify multiple myeloma according to prognosis before attempting therapeutic trials.

References

1. Alberts, D. S., Salmon, S. E.: Adriamycin (NSC-12127) in the treatment of alkylator-resistant multiple myeloma: a pilot study. Cancer Chemother. Rep. *59*, 345–350 (1975)
2. Alberts, D. S., Durie, B. G. M., Salmon, S. E.: Doxorubicin/BCNU chemotherapy for multiple myeloma in relapse. Lancet *1976 I*, 926–928
3. Alexanian, R., Bergsagel, D., Migliore, P., Vaughan, W., Howe, C. D.: Melphalan therapy for plasma cell myeloma. Blood *31*, 1 (1968)
4. Alexanian, R., Haut, A., Khan, A. V., Lane, M., McKelvey, E. M., Migliore, P. J., Stuckey, W. J., Wilson, H. E.: Treatment for multiple myeloma: combination chemotherapy with different melphalan dose regimens. J.A.M.A. *208*, 1680–1685 (1969)
5. Alexanian, R., Balarzak, S., Boneet, J. D., Gehan, E. A., Haut, A., Hewlett, J. S., Monto, R. W.: Prognostic factors in multiple myeloma. Cancer *36*, 1192–1201 (1975)
6. Azam, L., Delamore, I. W.: Combination therapy for myelomatosis. Br. Med J. *1974, IV*, 560–564
7. Bergsagel, D. E.: Evaluation of new chemotherapeutic agent in the treatment of multiple myeloma. IV. Phenylalanine mustard (NSC 8806). Cancer Chemother. Rep. *21*, 87–99 (1962)

8. BERGSAGEL, D. E.: Myeloma proteins and the clinical response to melphalan therapy. Science *148*, 367–377 (1965)
9. BERNARD, J., SELIGMANN, M., DANON, F.: Essai de traitement de 21 malades atteints de myelome ou de macroglobulinémie par le pdi 2 chloréthylaminolphenyl alanine (Melphalan). Nouv. Rev. Fr. Hematol. *2*, 611–616 (1962)
10. BONTOUX, D., CHENEBIT, D., DELBARRE, F.: Essai dêtude comparative du melphalan et de la cyclophosphamide dans le traitement de la maladie de Kahler. Rev. Rhum. *37*, 817–824 (1970)
11. BROCK, N., HOHORST, A. J.: Metabolism of cyclophosphamide. Cancer *20*, 900–904 (1967)
12. CAGGIANO, V., CUTTNER, J., SALOMON, A.: Myeloma proteins. Bence Jones proteins and normal immunoglobulins in multiple myeloma. Blood *30*, 265–287 (1967)
13. CARBONE, P. P., KELLERHOUSE, L. E., GEHAN, E. A.: Plasmocytic myeloma: a study of the relationship of survival to various clinical manifestations and anomalous protein type in 112 patients. Am. J. Med. *42*, 937–949
14. CHAVAZ, A., MIGNON, F., KANFER, A., RICHET, G.: Traitement de l'insuffisance rénale du myelome multiple par l'hémodialyse chronique. A propos de 4 cas. Nouv. Presse Med. *5*, 565–569 (1975)
15. COSTA, G.: An assessment of L phenylalanine mustard in human multiple myeloma. Proc. Am. Assoc. Cancer Res. *4*, 12 (1963)
16. COSTA, G., ENGLE, R. L., SCHILLING, A., CARBONNE, P., KOCHWA, S., NACHMAN, R. L., GLIDEWELL, O.: Melphalan and prednisone: an effective combination for the treatment of multiple myeloma. Am. J. Med. *54*, 589–599 (1973)
17. DELBARRE, F., SIGUIER, F., GODEAU, P., SAPORTA, L., SELIGMAN, M., HUREZ, D.: La maladie de Kahler à plasmocytes non excrétants. Ann. Med. Interne. (Paris) *121*, 537–544 (1970)
18. DE VITA, V. T., SCHEIN, P. S.: The use of drugs in combination for the treatment of cancer: rationale and results. N. Engl. J. Med. *288*, 998 (1973)
19. DREWINKO, M., BROWN, B. W., HUMPHREY, R., ALEXANIAN, R.: effect of chemotherapy on the labelling index of myeloma cells. Cancer *34*, 526 (1974)
20. DRIVSHOLM, A., VIDEBACK, A.: Alkeran (melphalan) in the treatment of myelomatosis. Acta Med. Scand. *179*. (Suppl. 445), 187–193 (1966)
21. DURIE, G. M., SALMON, S. E.: A clinical staging for multiple myeloma. Correlation of measured myeloma cell mass with presenting clinical features. Response to treatment and survival. Cancer *36*, 842–854 (1975)
22. FAHEY, J. L., SCOGGINS, R. S., UTZ, J. P., SZWED, C.: Infection, antibody response and gammaglobulin components in multiple myeloma and macroglobulinemia. Amer. J. Med. *35*, 698–707 (1963)
23. FEINLEIB, M., MACMAHON, B.: Duration or survival in multiple myeloma. J.N.C.I. *24*, 1259–1269 (1960)
24. GEORGE, R. P., POTH, J. L., GORDON, D., SCHRIER, S. L.: Multiple myeloma intermittent combination chemotherapy compared to continuous therapy. Cancer *29*, 1665–1670 (1972)
25. HOOGSTRATEN, B., COSTA, J.: Intermittent melphalan therapy in multiple myeloma. J.A.M.A. *209*, 251–253 (1967)
26. JONES, H. B.: On a new substance occurring in the urine of a patient with urollitics ossium. Philos, Trans. R. Soc. Lond. (Biol. Sci.) 55–62 (1848)
27. KAHLER, O.: Zur Symptomatologik des multiplen Myeloms: Beobachtung von Albumosurie. Prag. Med. (Wochenscht.) *14*, 33–35 (1889)
28. KORST, D. R., WILSON, H. E., FOWLER, W. M., WILL, J. R., CLIFFORD, G. O., LOUIS, J.: Treatment of multiple myeloma. An analysis of cyclophosphamide (cytoxan) therapy in 170 patients. J. LAb. Clin. Med. *62* 990 (1963)
29. KORST, D. R., CLIFFORD, G. O., FOWLER, W. M., LOUIS, J., WILL, J., WILSON, H. E.: Multiple myeloma. II. Analysis of cyclophosphamide therapy in 165 Patients. J.A.M.A. *189*, 758–762 (1964)
30. LEE, B. J., SAHAKIAN, G., CLARKSON, B. D., KRAKOFF, I. H.: Combination chemotherapy of multiple myeloma with alkeran, cytoxan, vincristine, prednisone and BCNU. Cancer *33*, 533–538 (1974)
31. LEE, S. H., POLESKY, H. F., SHAPIRO, F. L.: Chronic hemodialysis in myelomatosis. Ann. Intern. Med. *77*, 239–242 (1972)
32. MANNIK, M., KUNKEL, H. G.: Classification of myeloma proteins, Bence Jones proteins and macroglobulins into two groups on the basis of common antigenic characters. J. Exp. Med. *116*, 859–877 (1962)
33. MAVLIGIT, G. M., GUTTERMAN, J. U., HERSH, E. M., ALEXANIAN, R.: Cell mediated immunity to plasma cell myeloma: specific inhibition by a serum factor adhering to effector lymphocytes (38382). Proc. Soc. Exp. Biol. Med. *147*, 537–540 (1974)
34. MCARTHUR, J. R., ATHENS, J. W., WINTROB, M. M., CARTWRIGHT, G. E.: Melphalan and myeloma. Experience with a low-dose continuous regimen. Ann. Intern. Med. *72*, 665–670 (1970)
35. Medical Research Council, London W1N 4AL: Report of the medical research council's working party for therapeutic trials in leukemia. Myelomatosis: comparison of melphalan and cyclophosphamide therapy. Br. Med. J. *1971 I*, 640–641

36. Meshak, G., Seligman, M., Jacquillat, C., Basch, A., Bernard, J.: Le traitement du myelome multiple par le melphalan. Presse Med. *75*, 2301–2306 (1967)
37. Nauts, H. C.: Multiple Myeloma: Beneficial Effects of Acute Infectious or Immunotherapy (Bacterial Vaccines). Monograph 13. New York: Cancer Research Institute Inc. 1975
38. Osgood, E. E.: The survival time of patients with plasmocytic myeloma. Cancer Chemother. Rep. *9*, 1–10 (1960)
39. Paraskevas, F., Heremans, J., Waldenstrom, J.: Cytology and electrophoretic pattern in γ1A (β2A) myeloma. Acta Med. Scand. *170*, 575–589 (1961)
40. Rivers, S. L., Patno, M.E.: Cyclophosphamide vs melphalan in treatment of plasma cell myeloma. J.A.M.A. *207*, 1328–1334 (1969)
41. Rivers, S. L., Whittington, R. M., Patno, M. E.: Cyclophosphamide in treatment of multiple myeloma. Cancer Chemother. Rep. *29*, 115–119 (1963)
42. Rivers, S. L., Whittington, R. M., Patno, M. E.: Comparison of effect of cyclophosphamide and a placebo in treatment of multiple myeloma. Cancer Chemother. Rep. *29*, 115–119 (1963)
43. Saporta, L., Hugon, C., Rondier, J., Bontoux, D., Delbarre, F.: Pronostic de la maladie de Kalher chez des patients traités ou non par les agents alkylants (à propos de 45 cas). rev. Rhum. *39*, 11–18 (1972)
44. Salmon, S. E.: Expansion of the growth fraction in multiple myeloma with alkylating agents. Blood *45*, 119–129 (1975)
45. Salmon, S. E., Smith, B. A.: Immunoglobulin synthesis and total body tumor cell number in IgG multiple myeloma. J. Clin. Invest. *49*, 1114–1121 (1970)
46. Salmon, S. E., Smith, B. A.: Sandwich solid phase radioimmunoassays for the characterization of human immunoglobulins synthesized in vitro. J. Immunol. *104*, 665 (1970)
47. Salmon, S. E., Smith, B. A.: Induction of tumor susceptibility to cycle active agents in IgG multiple myeloma. Clin. Res. *20*, 570 (1972)
48. Salomon, A., Fahey, J. L., Malmgren, R. A.: Immunohistologic localization of gamma 1 macroglobulins Beta 2A myeloma proteins 6.6S gamma-myeloma proteins and Bence-Jones protein. Blood *21*, 403–423 (1963)
49. Speed, D. E., Galton, D. A. G., Swan, A.: Melphalan in the treatment of myelomatosis. Br. Med. J. *1964 I*, 1664
50. Sullivan, P. W., Salmon, S. E.: Kinetics of tumor growth and regression in IgG multiple myeloma. J. Clin. Invest. *51*, 1697–1708 (1972)
51. Rustizky, J. von: Multiple myelom. Dtsch. Chir. *3*, 162–172 (1873)
52. Waldenstrom, J.: Melphalan therapy in myelomatosis. Br. Med. J. *1964 I*, 859–865
53. Wheller, G. P.: Studies related to mechanisms of resistance to biological alkylating agents. Cancer Res. *23*, 1334 (1963)
54. Zinneman, H. H., Hall, W. H.: Recurrent pneumonia in multiple myeloma and some observations on immunologic response. Ann. Intern. Med. *41*, 1152–1163 (1954)

Pathological Staging in Adult Previously Untreated Non-Hodgkin's Lymphomas

G. Bonadonna, R. Castellani, C. Narduzzi, P. Spinelli, and F. Rilke

During the past 15 years, different efforts were made to properly stage malignant lymphomas [12, 16]. The intent was always that of improving the selection between patients suitable for curative radiotherapy and those who are candidate for a systemic treatment program. Over the years, lymphography, needle marrow biopsy, laparotomy, and laparoscopy have become important steps in the clinical accuracy for staging both adults and children.

The systematic use of available procedures to determine the anatomic extent of disease led first to the Rye and then to the Ann Arbor international staging classifications for Hodgkin's disease. This latter staging system [6] has also been adopted for the group of non-Hodgkin's lymphomas. The adoption of the Ann Arbor classification implies a dual system of stage designation: according to clinical staging (CS) only and according to pathological staging (PS). CS rests on the history, physical examination, initial diagnostic biopsy, laboratory tests, and radiographic evidence. PS adds definitive additional histopathologic information obtained through biopsy of strategic sites (e.g., marrow, liver, spleen, and abdominal lymph nodes) as well as of other clinically involved tissues (e.g., skin, lung, etc.).

During the past decade, staging laparotomy has been extensively used to detect occult abdominal disease both in Hodgkin's [12] and non-Hodgkin's lymphomas [3, 11, 16]. In consideration of the more extensive use of chemotherapy for the intermediate stages of Hodgkin's disease as well as for the initial stages of non-Hodgkin's lymphomas, staging laparotomy became the subject of clinical reevaluation as a routine staging procedure for patients with no overt extranodal lymphoma [2, 9]. Therefore, some centers began to replace laparotomy with laparoscopy especially in those patients in whom the assessment of splenic status was not crucial to modify the treatment program [2, 4, 8, 17].

This paper describes the current approach for PS of previously untreated non-Hodgkin's lymphomas in adults as carried out at the Istituto Nazionale Tumori of Milan. The paper will also report the patterns of occult disease in some histopathologic subgroups of the Rappaport classification.

Staging Procedures

Table 1 outlines the procedures deemed necessary in our institute to carry out correct CS and PS. Due to the high incidence of primary site in Waldeyer's ring [3], physical examination includes a systematic exploration of the pharynx with biopsy of any evident or suspicious growth. Extranodal involvement of accessible sites is always subjected to biopsy. Since about 20% of patients with lesions in the Waldeyer's ring also show a concomitant involvement of the stomach either at the time of initial presentation or within 2 years of diagnosis [3], gastroscopy is performed in cases with pharyngeal lymphoma. Bilateral lower extremity lymphography is carried out in all instances, regardless of the presence of nodal or extranodal extension. Since November, 1975, Jamshidi needle biopsy was carried out on both posterior iliac crests, and

Table 1. Necessary procedures for staging non-Hodgkin's lymphomas currently employed at the Istituto Nazionale Tumori of Milan

1.	Detailed history and physical examination to include Waldeyer's ring
2. a)	Excisional biopsy of one or more superficial lymph nodes
b)	Mediastinoscopy with node biopsy if only mediastinal/hilar adenopathy is present
c)	Punch biopsy of any evident or suspicious growth within the Waldeyer's ring
d)	Biopsy of any other accessible lesion (e.g., skin, breast, stomach, rectum, testicle, thyroid, lung, pleura)
3.	Complete blood count, ESR, BSP at 45 min, serum alkaline phosphatase, uric acid, electrophoresis
4.	Chest roentgenogram (PA and lateral); mediastinal/hilar tomography in the presence of adenopathy
5.	Gastrointestinal series; gastroscopy in the presence of Waldeyer's ring involvement
6.	Bilateral lower extremity lymphography
7.	Skeletal survey to include the base of skull in the presence of Waldeyer's ring involvement
8.	Bilateral Jamshidi needle marrow biopsy; bone marrow aspiration in the presence of extrinsic cells in the peripheral blood
9.	Lumbar puncture in children and in adults with diffuse histology
10.	Laparoscopy with multiple biopsies of liver and, whenever feasible, of spleen

Table 2. Ancillary procedures required under certain conditions

1.	Intravenous pyelography and/or inferior cavography to supplement equivocal lymphographic findings
2.	Skeletal scintigram in the presence of persisting bone pain with a negative roentgenogram
3.	Hepatic and splenic scintigrams in the presence of palpable organs and when laparoscopy or laparotomy is not feasible
4.	Gallium or bleomycin scans when the results of other conventional diagnostic procedures are not conclusive
5.	Laparotomy in the presence of gastrointestinal involvement, especially if lesions are bleeding

lumbar puncture was performed in all adults with diffuse histology. Since November, 1973, laparoscopy was systematically utilized in the surgical abdominal exploration. Staging laparotomy, which was introduced in our institute in September, 1970, was still performed from November, 1973–June, 1976 only in patients showing negative histologic findings in the liver on laparoscopy and in the bone marrow on needle biopsy.

Table 2 presents some ancillary procedures which may be required under certain clinical conditions. In our institute, we abandoned the routine use of hepatic and splenic scintigrams in November, 1973. At present, these scans are utilized only when it is thought that they can add further information to define CS more accurately. In our institute, exploratory laparotomy for staging purposes is performed only in very selected patients (e.g., in the presence of gastric or intestinal involvement, especially when associated to occult blood in stools).

Staging Laparoscopy

The technique and the advantages of staging laparoscopy, as derived from our initial experience [2, 4, 7, 15] as well as from that of other investigators [8, 17] are summarized in Table 3. Whenever technically feasible, spleen is also subjected to one or more needle biopsies during laparoscopy. Although we have found splenic biopsy practically devoid of major

Table 3. Technique and advantages of laparoscopy

Technique
1. Sedation with diazepam and local anesthesia with Xylocaine
2. Insertion of a Verress needle into the left lower quadrant of the abdomen and creation of pneumoperitoneum (2–3 liters CO_2)
3. Insertion of trocar 1–2 cm above the umbilicus in the midline. In patients with prior abdominal surgery, the trocar is placed laterally on the right
4. Examination through Wolf cold light endoscope
5. Liver biopsies (four to six) with Tru-cut needle. Biopsy of liver edge carried out with Palmer forceps
6. Spleen biopsies (one to three) with Tru-cut needle

Advantages
1. Detects liver involvement in most patients with hepatic infiltration
2. Detects spleen involvement in approximately one-third of patients with splenic infiltration, especially when tumor nodules are present on the surface
3. Can be easily repeated to assess the status of remission when liver is involved before chemotherapy
4. Can be performed under local anesthesia; operating room is not required; the procedure is usually completed in 20–30 min
5. Produces minimal morbidity, and recovery is rapid (12–48 h)
6. Reduces costs and hospital stay

complications [2, 4, 7, 15], it is not recommended as a routine procedure in staging laparoscopy. When there are no tumor nodules on the surface, blind biopsies of both liver and spleen are performed.

Results of Combined Laparoscopy and Needle Marrow Biopsy

From November, 1973–April 30, 1977, a total of 241 previously untreated adults with histologic diagnosis of non-Hodgkin's lymphoma were subjected to PS by combining laparoscopy plus needle (Jamshidi) marrow biopsy. They are consecutive with reference to no prior treatment, age above 15 and below 73 years, absence of lymphoma cells in the peripheral blood, and performance status above 60.

Table 4 presents the distribution of patients according to the histologic subgroups of the Rappaport classification. Due to either poor quality of slides made in other hospitals or because of the small size of specimens (e.g., from Waldeyer's ring) or because the initial biopsy

Table 4. Distribution of 241 previously untreated patients according to histologic subgroups (Rappaport classification)

Subgroups	Total		Nodular		Diffuse		Uncertain	
	No.	%	No.	%	No.	%	No.	%
Lymphocytic well-differentiated (LWD)	2	1	0	—	2	100	—	—
Lymphocytic poorly differentiated (LPD)	97	40	31	32	56	58	10	10
Histiocytic (H)	63	26	3	5	58	92	2	3
Mixed type (M)	47	20	15	32	32	68	0	—
Undifferentiated (DU)	6	2	—	—	6	100	—	—
Unclassified (U)	26	11	—	—	—	—	—	—
Total	241	100	49	20	154	64	12	5

was taken from extranodal sites (e.g., Waldeyer's ring, skin), a total of 26 patients (11%) could not be correctly classified according to the cytologic subgroups of the RAPPAPORT classification, and in 12 patients (5%), the histologic pattern could not be defined with certainty. Cases showing nodular and diffuse pattern, even if nodularity was focal, were classified as nodular. As already shown in previous series studied in our institute [3, 4, 14], diffuse lymphomas (64%) were much more often observed than nodular lymphomas (20%), and diffuse histiocytic (DH) lymphoma represented the single largest subgroup (58 of 241 patients or 24%) followed by diffuse lymphocytic poorly differentiated (DLPD) lymphoma (56 patients or 23%). The reason for the predominance of unfavorable histology in our series remains unknown.

The positive histologic findings by combined laparoscopy and needle marrow biopsy in the whole series of 241 patients are recorded in Table 5. Laparoscopy was performed 1–3 days after Jamshidi biopsy and, therefore, without knowing the results of the bone marrow histology. CS IV includes two subgroups. The first consisted of 14 patients who could be diagnosed as having

Table 5. Positive findings by combined laparoscopy and needle marrow biopsy in 241 patients

CS	Patients	Liver		Spleen		Other sites		Marrow	
		No.	%	No.	%	No.	%	No.	%
I-IE	64	6	9	4/47	9	2[d]	3	4/62 (3)	6
II-IIE	57	4	7	7/51	14	0		6/57 (5)	11
III-IIIE-IIIS	70	24	34	25/53	47	0		18/70 (6)	26
IV: For liver[a]	14	3	21	3/11	27			3/14 (3)	21
For other sites[b]	36	10	28	7/31	23	1[e]	3	7/36 (1)	19
Total	241	47	20	46/193[c]	24	3	1.2	38/239(18)	16

[a] Ann Arbor criteria.
[b] Skin (10), bone (3), lung (3), pleura (2), breast (1), rectum (1), thyroid (1), intestine (1), multiple sites (14).
[c] Patients with adequate sample.
[d] Peritoneum (multiple nodules).
[e] Abdominal mass.
The number of patients with a positive marrow in the absence of positive liver are in parentheses.

liver involvement according to the criteria adopted at Ann Arbor [6]. In this group, laparoscopy was performed to verify the accuracy of clinical criteria. The second subgroup included 36 cases for whom the diagnosis of stage IV disease was already established by histologic and/or clinical evidence of lymphoma in one or more extranodal sites. In these patients, laparoscopy plus bone marrow biopsy was performed to document a possible correlation between the involvement of liver and marrow and the involvement of other extranodal sites. Furthermore, a complete PS was also carried out to document all extranodal sites of disease which could be subjected to a restaging biopsy should the patients achieve a clinical complete remission after combination chemotherapy. Liver, spleen, and marrow were found infiltrated in all clinical stages of the disease, but the yield of positive findings was higher in patients with abnormal lymphography. Spleen was positive in 46 of 193 patients (24%) in whom the biopsy was feasible and the specimen adequate for histologic examination. It is interesting to note that in two patients with CS I, laparoscopy revealed the presence of tumor nodules scattered throughout the peritoneum as the only apparent site of disease below the diaphragm. In another patient, laparoscopy documented the presence of an abdominal mass which was not palpable on physical examination. The correlation between liver and marrow involvement is presented in Table 6.

Table 7 confirms the observation of BRUNNING et al. [5], i.e., that in all histologic patterns and types two needle biopsies can document a higher incidence of bone marrow involvement (23%) than in patients in whom only one Jamshidi biopsy is performed (13%). It is noteworthy that

Table 6. Correlation between liver and bone marrow involvement in 65 patients with documented infiltration by laparoscopy plus needle marrow biopsy

	No.	(%)
Liver + marrow −	27	41
Liver − marrow +	18	28
Liver + marrow +	20	31

Table 7. Yield of unilateral versus bilateral needle marrow biopsy

	1 biopsy		2 biopsies	
	+	%	+	%
Pattern				
Nodular	1/34	3	3/15	20
Diffuse	19/115	17	11/38	29
Uncertain	1/8	13	0/4	—
Type				
LPD	13/65	20	9/32	28
LWD	1/1	—	0/1	—
H	1/48	2	2/14	14
M	4/36	11	3/11	.27
DU	2/6	33	—	—
Unclassified	2/18	11	1/7	14
Total[a]	23/175	13	15/64	23

[a] In 2 patients needle marrow biopsy was not adequate. Subsequent laparotomy plus open marrow biopsy yielded negative specimens.
LPD: lymphocytic poorly differentiated; LWD: lymphocytic well-differentiated; H: histiocytic; M: mixed type; DU: diffuse undifferentiated.

marrow infiltration was more often observed in patients with diffuse (20%) than with nodular pattern (8%). Furthermore, histiocytic lymphoma was the subgroup with the lowest risk for occult positive marrow (5%).

Table 8 shows the incidence of PS IV in 205 patients in whom the presence of occult extranodal disease was detected only by laparoscopy and needle marrow biopsy. The low yield of occult lymphoma (27%) compared with other series [8] is probably due to the high incidence of DH lymphoma present in our series. As will be shown later, DH is associated with a very low incidence of both liver and marrow involvement at the time of initial diagnosis compared with other histologic subgroups.

Table 8. Pathologic stage IV documented through laparoscopy plus needle marrow biopsy in 205 patients

CS	No.	PS	IV
		No.	%
I-IE	64	11	17
II-IIE	57	9	16
III-IIIE-IIIS	70	30	43
IV (liver)	14	6	43
Total	205	56	27

Laparoscopy vs. Laparotomy and Needle vs. Open Marrow Biopsy

To verify the accuracy of laparoscopy plus needle marrow biopsy in the detection of occult liver and marrow infiltration, a sequential study utilizing two surgical procedures was performed in 122 of 241 patients. Those with negative histologic findings in the liver on laparoscopy and in the bone marrow on needle biopsy were subjected to the classic staging laparotomy with unilateral open marrow biopsy. The results are summarized in Table 9. After the first combined procedure, 32% of the patients were classified as PS IV. Of the remaining 83 patients with negative extranodal findings, the second combined surgical procedure detected six additional patients with lymphoma infiltration in the liver, marrow, or both. Therefore, laparotomy modified the stage in 7% of the patients because of occult extralymphatic involvement. In particular, there were five false negative findings in the liver (two in stage I) and two in the bone marrow (both patients had unilateral Jamshidi biopsy). Thus, of 45 patients with documented PS IV, 39 (87%) were detected through a less traumatic procedure. On the contrary, staging laparotomy documented the presence of other additional occult lesions (spleen: eight patients; para-aortic nodes: five; other abdominal nodes mostly mesenteric: 19; small intestine: three). In particular, the intestine was found to be infiltrated in the absence of clinical symptoms and positive or suspicious roentgenologic examination in two patients with stage II and in one patient with stage III. The presence of positive additional lymphatic sites at laparotomy produced a stage modification in 15 of 83 patients (18%).

Clinical vs. Pathologic Staging in Specific Subgroups

Table 10 presents the final comparison between CS and PS for the numerically consistent subgroups of the present series. In short, DH lymphoma was the subgroup with the highest incidence of PS I and II (29%), while DLPD lymphoma was the subgroup with more patients classified as PS IV (49%).

Tables 11–15 present the final PS IV related to nodal and extranodal presentation for five major histologic subgroups initially classified as CS I-II-III. PS IV due to occult involvement of liver, marrow, or both occurred more often in patients with nodal compared to extranodal presentation in nodular mixed (NM) (33% vs. 0%), and DLPD (67% vs. 30%), while the opposite finding was observed in diffuse mixed (DM) (27% vs. 35%). In DH (12% vs. 14%) and in nodular lymphocytic poorly differentiated (NLPD) (25% vs. 25%), there was an equal proportion of nodal and extranodal presentation. Among patients with extranodal presentation, those with Waldeyer's ring involvement showed the lowest risk of occult extranodal sites if they were classified as DH (8%) and the highest risk when classified as DLPD lymphoma (40%). It is important to note that in this particular series Waldeyer's ring and stomach involvement, a well-known clinical association [3], showed liver and/or marrow infiltration in 67% of the patients.

Conclusions

In non-Hodgkin's lymphomas scientific and practical controversies abound. In addition, there is controversy in the area of histopathology where lack of a universally accepted classification system, which is both scientifically accurate and clinically relevant, prevents clinicians from

Table 9. Sequential laparoscopy plus needle marrow biopsy and laparotomy plus open marrow biopsy

CS	No.	PS IV by laparoscopy					PS	No.	PS IV by laparotomy				
		No.	%	L	M	L + M			No.	%	L	M	L + M
I-IE	38	9	24	5(+2)[a]	1	1	I-IE	29	2	7	2	0	0
II-IIE	31	4	13	2	2	0	II-IIE-IIS	26	0	—	—	—	—
III-IIIE-IIIS	43	20	47	8	4	8	III-IIIE-IIIS	28	4	14	2	1	1
IV (liver)	10	6	60	3	3	0							
Total	122	39	32	18(+2)[a]	10	9	Total	83	6	7	4	1	1

[a] Peritoneum: 2 patients.
L: liver; M: marrow.

Table 10. Clinical vs. pathologic staging in five histologic subgroups

	Stage I-IE				Stage II-IIE				Stage III-IIIE-IIIS				Stage IV			
	CS		PS		CS		PS		CS		PS		CS[a]		PS	
	No.	%	No.	%	No.	%	No.	%	No.	%	No.	%	No.	%	No.	%
DH (49)	18	37	14	29	18	37	14	29	12	24	14	29	1	2	7	14
DLPD (49)	13	27	8	16.5	10	20	7	14.5	21	43	10	20	5	10	24	49
NLPD (29)	8	28	7	24	8	28	6	21	12	41	9	31	1	3	7	24
DM (28)	5	18	2	7	12	43	10	36	8	28	6	21	3	11	10	36
NM (15)	5	33	4	27	2	13	2	13	7	47	5	33	1	7	4	27
Total (170)	49	29	35	21	50	30	39	23	60	35	44	26	11	6	52	30

[a] For liver (Ann Arbor criteria).

Table 11. Diffuse histiocytic lymphoma with clinical stage (CS) I-II-III. Final pathologic stage (PS) IV related to patterns of clinical presentation (results are in percentages)

	I (18)	II (18)	III (12)	Total PS IV (6)	L (3)	M (3)
CS → PS IV	17	6	17	12.5	50	50
Nodal presentation	18	11	0	12		
Extranodal presentation	14	0	33	14		
Waldeyer's ring				8		
Gastrointestinal				20		
Other sites				33		

L: liver; M: marrow. The number of patients are in brackets.

Table 12. Diffuse lymphocytic poorly differentiated lymphoma with clinical stage (CS) I-II-III. Final pathologic stage (PS) IV related to patterns of clinical presentation (results are in percentages)

	I (13)	II (10)	III (21)	Total PS IV (20)	L (6)	M (5)	L + M (9)
CS → PS IV	23	30	67	45	30	25	45
Nodal presentation	60	50	78	67			
Extranodal presentation	0	17	58	30			
Waldeyer's ring				40			
Waldeyer's ring + stomach				67			
Gastrointestinal				20			
Skin				33			

L: liver; M: marrow. The number of patients are in brackets.

Table 13. Nodular lymphocytic poorly differentiated lymphoma with clinical stage (CS) I-II-III. Final pathologic stage (PS) IV related to patterns of clinical presentation (results are in percentages)

	I (8)	II (8)	III (12)	Total PS IV (7)	L (4)	M (2)	L + M (1)
CS → PS IV	25	12.5	33	25	57	29	14
Nodal presentation	25	17	30	25			
Extranodal presentation	—	0	50	25			
Waldeyer's ring				25			

L: liver; M: marrow. The number of patients are in brackets.

Table 14. Diffuse mixed lymphoma with clinical stage (CS) I-II-III. Final pathologic stage (PS) IV related to patterns of clinical presentation (results are in percentages)

	I (5)	II (12)	III (8)	Total PS IV (8)	L (4)	M (3)	L + M (1)
CS → PS IV	40	17	50	32	50	37.5	12.5
Nodal presentation	25	0	40	27			
Extranodal presentation	100	20	67	35			
Waldeyer's ring				20			
Gastrointestinal				100			
Bone				100			
Skin				100			

L: liver; M: marrow. The number of patients are in brackets.

Table 15. Nodular mixed lymphoma with clinical stage (CS) I-II-III. Final pathologic stage (PS) IV related to clinical presentation (results are in percentages)

	I (5)	II (2)	III (7)	Total PS IV (3)	L (3)	M (0)
CS → PS IV	0	50	29	21	100	
Nodal presentation	0	50	40	33		
Extranodal presentation	0	—	0	0		

L: liver; M: marrow. The number of patients are in brackets.

correlating their data with the histopathologic scheme. From the practical point of view, research clinicians are still inclined to utilize the Rappaport classification until the superiority of any of the newer systems is convincingly established. In fact, the Rappaport scheme provides a clinically useful major distinction in prognosis between nodular and diffuse lymphoma. Another controversial area is that concerning the optimal use of radiotherapy and chemotherapy in initial and intermediate stages of the disease. Although extensive irradiation alone is unable to provide a satisfactory control in a consistent fraction of patients [10, 16], it is also true that the initial controlled studies with adjuvant chemotherapy have so far failed to make a significant impact on the overall survival of patients with stage I-II disease [10, 13].
How extensively should a patient with non-Hodgkin's lymphoma be staged? This also could be the subject of controversy. The systematic use of lymphography, bone marrow biopsy, and more recently, of staging laparotomy have markedly improved our knowledge on the preferential sites of tumor involvement. As exemplified by the results obtained with two marrow biopsies, the more extensively a patient is studied, the higher the incidence of occult findings. With the exception of diffuse histiocytic lymphoma, the occurrence of occult findings in some extranodal sites such as liver or bone marrow is considerably high. Therefore, the major efforts in the pathologic staging should be directed toward accurately exploring these strategic extranodal sites. Our past [4, 7] and present findings as well as those of Chabner et al. [8], indicate that staging laparoscopy can represent a valid alternative to staging laparotomy in the detection of liver involvement. The more widespread use of new chemotherapeutic regimens in combination with radiotherapy for the treatment of early stages is probably a sufficient clinical reason for abandoning the use of laparotomy in favor of laparoscopy. Laparoscopy is a safer (Table 16) and quicker diagnostic procedure and can be successfully used to elucidate the patterns of relapse and to verify the completeness of an apparent complete remission [1]. The same concepts apply to the use of bilateral Jamshidi marrow biopsies versus the open surgical technique.
We have probably reached a point in the knowledge of anatomic extent as well as the natural history of non-Hodgkin's lymphomas where pathologic staging for therapeutic purposes should remain accurate but must be concentrated on rapid procedures which should limit the hospital stay to a minimum. A major task will be how to reinterpret the large body of adequate clinical data collected in several research institutions by utilizing the new functional histopathologic

Table 16. Morbidity from laparoscopy in 241 patients

None	234 (97%)
Abdominal bleeding	4 (1.7%)
From spleen	2
From liver	1
Site unknown	1
Acute hypotension	1
Hepatitis (probably traumatic)	1
Choliperitoneum	1

classifications, should one or more of them prove to be reproducible among hemopathologists. In short, non-Hodgkin's lymphomas represent a complex group of diseases whose clinical presentation differs in many aspects from that of Hodgkin's disease (e.g., higher incidence of primary and occult extranodal involvement, lower incidence of mediastinal adenopathy as well as of systemic symptoms). Accurate pathologic staging remains an important step not only for planning proper treatment but documenting the completeness of remission. Since in the large majority of patients primary treatment includes chemotherapy, staging procedures should be simple in consideration of the frequent rapid progression of the disease.

References

1. Anderson, T., Rosenoff, S., Bender, R., et al.: Peritoneoscopy: A useful tool in restaging lymphoma patients. Proc. Am. Assoc. Cancer Res. *17*, 268 (1976)
2. Beretta, G., Spinelli, P., Rilke, F., Tancini, G., Canetta, R., Gennari, L., Bonadonna, G.: Sequential laparoscopy and laparotomy combined with bone marrow biopsy in staging Hodgkin's disease. Cancer Treat. Rep. *60*, 1231–1237 (1976)
3. Bonadonna, G., Pizzetti, F., Musumeci, R., Valagussa, P., Banfi, A., Veronesi, U.: Staging laparotomy in non-Hodgkin's lymphomata. Br. J. Cancer (suppl. II) *31*, 252–260 (1975)
4. Bonadonna, G., Beretta, G., Castellani, R., Canetta, R., Spinelli, P., Gennari, L., Rilke, F., Veronesi, U.: Current views on surgical staging in planning the treatment of malignant lymphomas. In: Recent Advances in Cancer Treatment. Tagnon, H. J., Staquet, M. J. (eds) New York: Raven Press 1977, p. 55
5. Brunning, R. D., Bloomfield, C. D., McKenna, R. W., Peterson, L.: Bilateral trephine bone marrow biopsies in lymphoma and other neoplastic diseases. Ann. Intern. Med. *82*, 365–366 (1975)
6. Carbone, P. P., Kaplan, H. S., Musshoff, K., Smithers, D. W., Tubiana, M.: Report of the Committee on Hodgkin's Staging Classification. Cancer Res. *31*, 1860–1861 (1971)
7. Castellani, R., Bonadonna, G., Spinelli, P., Bajetta, E., Galante, E., Rilke, F.: Sequential pathologic staging of untreated non-Hodgkin's lymphomas by laparoscopy and laparotomy combined with marrow biopsy. Cancer *40*, 2322–2328 (1977)
8. Chabner, B. A., Johnson, R. E., Young, R. C., Canellos, G. P., Hubbard, S. P., Johnson, S. K., De Vita, V. T., Jr: Sequential nonsurgical and surgical staging of non-Hodgkin's lymphoma. Ann. Intern. Med. *85*, 149–154 (1976)
9. De Vita, V. T., Jr., Bagley, C. M., Jr., Goodell, B., O'Kieffe, D. A., Trujillo, N. P.: Peritoneoscopy in the staging of Hodgkin's disease. Cancer Res. *31*, 1746–1750 (1971)
10. Glatstein, E., Donaldson, S. S., Rosenberg, S. A., Kaplan, H. S.: The potential for combined modality therapy in malignant lymphomas (in press)
11. Goffinet, D. R., Castellino, R. A., Kim, H., Dorfman, R. F., Fuks, Z., Rosenberg, S. A., Nelsen, T., Kaplan, H. S.: Staging laparotomies in unselected previously untreated patients with non-Hodgkin's lymphomas. Cancer *32*, 672–681 (1973)
12. Kaplan, H. S., Dorfman, R. S., O'Conor, G. T., et al. (Organizing Committee): International Symposium on Hodgkin's Disease. Natl. Cancer Inst. Monogr. *36*, 1–587 (1973)
13. Monfardini, S., Lattuada, A., Milani, F., Banfi, A., Bonadonna, G.: Controlled study with radiotherapy (RT) vs RT plus CVP in stage I-II non-Hodgkin's lymphomas. Proc. Am. Assoc. Cancer Res. and ASCO *18*, 283 (1977)
14. Monfardini, S., Tancini, G., De Lena, M., Villa, E., Valagussa, P., Bonadonna, G.: Cyclophosphamide, vincristine, and prednisone (CVP) versus adriamycin, bleomycin, and prednisone (ABP) in stage IV non-Hodgkin's lymphomas. Med. Pediatr. Oncol. *3*, 67–74 (1977)
15. Spinelli, P., Beretta, G., Bajetta, E., Tancini, G., Castellani, R., Rilke, F., Bonadonna, G.: Laparoscopy and laparotomy combined with bone marrow biopsy in staging Hodgkin's disease. Br. Med. J. *1975 IV*, 554–556
16. Symposium on non-Hodgkin's Lymphomata: Br. J. Cancer *31* (suppl. II) (1975)
17. Vinciguerra, V., Coleman, M., Degnan, T. J., Lightdale, C. J., Goldstein, M., Silver, T.: Comparison of peritoneoscopy and laparotomy in the staging of Hodgkin's disease. Proc. Am. Ass. Cancer Res. and ASCO *16*, 269 (1975)

Staging in Adult Non-Hodgkin's Lymphomas

S. A. Rosenberg, M. Ribas-Mundo, D. R. Goffinet, and H. S. Kaplan

Introduction

Since June, 1971, staging laparotomies have been performed at Stanford Medical Center for patients with non-Hodgkin's lymphomas. The procedure was performed for these patients as part of a study on the value of the diagnostic surgical procedure in an overall treatment program. An early analysis of the information obtained from staging laparotomies in 69 patients was published in 1973 [4]. This report presents selected analyses of the Stanford material by Ribas-Mundo of 200 consecutive patients accrued to the formal treatment regimens, including 107 staging laparotomies, and from a larger series published by Goffinet of 423 consecutive untreated patients, including 197 staging laparotomies [5].

Materials and Methods

The two series of patients covered the same time period, between June, 1971 and June, 1976. All patients were previously untreated, with biopsy confirmation at Stanford of non-Hodgkin's lymphoma. The Rappaport classification was used, as previously described [7]. Diagnostic procedures were as previously reported [4, 5]. Needle bone marrow biopsy was obtained in all patients, usually with a Jamshidi needle [9].

Staging laparotomy and splenectomy were performed on patients who did not demonstrate bone marrow or other stage IV involvement, who had no medical contraindication, and who were between the ages of 15 and 65. Selected patients younger and older than these ages were occasionally subjected to the surgical procedure.

The details of the surgical staging procedure have appeared in previous reports [5]. Needle and wedge biopsies of the liver were obtained. Splenectomy was performed routinely. The surgeon attempted to remove the most abnormal retroperitoneal lymph nodes demonstrated by lymphography. Mesenteric lymph nodes were removed in most patients, even if they were of normal size. The bone marrow was sampled by means of an open iliac crest biopsy in all patients. In the larger Goffinet series of 423 patients, 15 patients with previously demonstrated bone marrow involvement were studied with diagnostic laparotomy. For other details of staging designations, regimen eligibility, patient selection, diagnostic procedures, and surgical technique, previous publications from the Stanford group should be consulted [4, 5, 9, 2].

Selected Results

Selected information attained from these series of patients will be described. The operative morbidity was 11%, with one fatal complication in a patient who developed pancreatitis.

Bone Marrow Involvement

In the series of 200 patients, 114 had nodular lymphomas and 86 were diffuse. As seen in Table 1, a total of 60% of the nodular patients and 24% of the diffuse patients had bone marrow involvement after the complete diagnostic study. In the nodular lymphocytic poorly differentiated type (NLPD), 76% had bone marrow involvement. In this common subtype, 65% can be shown to have bone marrow involvement with a single needle iliac crest biopsy, obviating the need for diagnostic laparotomy. However, even after one negative needle bone marrow biopsy, the larger open marrow biopsies demonstrated lymphoma involvement in 32% of the remaining patients. For all subtypes, the needle biopsy demonstrated 71, or 35.5% of the patients, to have bone marrow involvement. An additional 20 patients were shown to have involved bone marrows at laparotomy, i.e., 16% of the group who had had a prior negative single needle biopsy.

Table 1. Results of needle and open biopsy of the bone marrow in 200 consecutive patients with non-Hodgkin's lymphomas

Subtype	Needle biopsy	Open biopsy	Total	Percentage
		Nodular		
NLPD	47/72[a]	8/25	55/72	76
NM	8/30	3/22	11/30	36
NH	1/12	1/11	2/12	17
		Diffuse		
DLWD	5/6	1/1	6/6	100
DLPD	0/13	2/13	2/13	15
DM	6/9	1/3	7/9	78
DH	3/56	4/53	7/56	13
DU	0/2	0/2	0/2	—

[a] Number positive/number studied.
NLPD: nodular, lymphocytic poorly differentiated; NM: nodular, mixed lymphocytic and histiocytic; NH: nodular, histiocytic; DLWD: diffuse, lymphocytic well-differentiated; DLPD: diffuse, lymphocytic poorly differentiated; DM: diffuse, mixed lymphocytic and histiocytic; DH: diffuse histiocytic; DU: diffuse, undifferentiated.

The frequency of bone marrow involvement after sequential bone marrow biopsy and diagnostic laparotomy is correlated with the clinical stage of disease but is different for the various histologic subtypes.

Figure 1 shows the percentage of those patients eventually shown to have bone marrow involvement in the various major subtypes. It can be seen that over 60% of clinical stage III and 100% of clinical stage IV nodular patients can be shown to have bone marrow involvement. This is very different from those with diffuse histiocytic (DH) lymphoma, where 24% and 10% have bone marrow involvement of clinical stage III and IV, respectively. It can be seen that patients with other diffuse subtypes have very frequent bone marrow involvement in the presence of clinical stages III and IV disease.

Figure 2 demonstrates the differences in the frequency of bone marrow involvement in the three different nodular subtypes. More than 80% of the clinical stage III NLPD patients can be shown to have a positive bone marrow, and 33% of those with clinical stage I or II disease have, in fact, stage IV disease due to bone marrow involvement. Peripheral blood counts do not give an indication of bone marrow involvement in these patients, the great majority being normal. In contrast to patients with Hodgkin's disease [8], the serum alkaline phosphatase is not an indicator of bone marrow involvement by non-Hodgkin's lymphoma. Table 2 shows that less than 10% of patients have an elevated serum alkaline phosphatase, whether or not they can be shown to have lymphoma in the marrow.

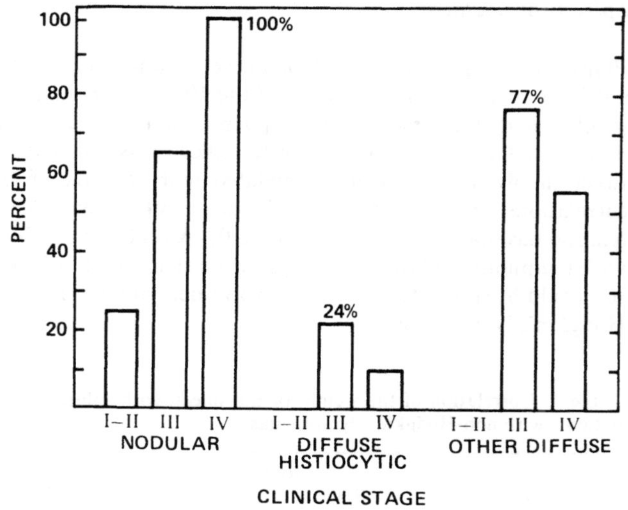

Fig. 1. The percentage of patients with bone marrow involvement according to clinical stage prior to bone marrow biopsy in non-Hodgkin's lymphomas

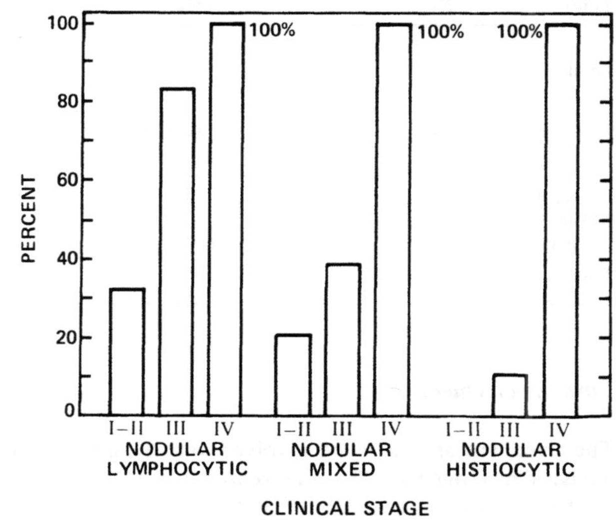

Fig. 2. The percentage of patients with bone marrow involvement according to clinical stage prior to bone marrow biopsy in patients with nodular non-Hodgkin's lymphomas

Table 2. Serum alkaline phosphatase levels in 200 consecutive patients with non-Hodgkin's lymphomas with or without bone marrow involvement

Biopsy	No.	Serum alkaline phosphatase Elevated	Borderline	Normal
Uninvolved	110	8%	16%	76%
Involved	90	4%	9%	87%

Spleen Involvement

Five of the 197 patients in the Goffinet series who underwent laparotomy in other hospitals did not have their spleens removed. Of the 192 patients undergoing splenectomy, 78 (41%) had involvement of the spleen with lymphoma. In the RIBAS-MUNDO series of 107 patients taken to diagnostic laparotomy, the size of the spleen was correlated to involvement with lymphoma. Liver involvement was also correlated with the size of the spleen. Table 3 shows these correlations. It can be seen that involvement of the spleen was more frequent in nodular lymphomas than diffuse, 52% versus 29%. All spleens weighing more than 400 g were involved with lymphoma in both subgroups. More than two-thirds of the patients with spleens of this size could be shown to have liver involvement at laparotomy, in both nodular and diffuse non-Hodgkin's lymphomas.

Table 3. Correlation of the weight of the spleen with spleen and liver involvement in 107 consecutive patients with non-Hodgkin's lymphomas

Spleen weight	Nodular			Diffuse		
	No.	Spleen involved	Liver involved	No.	Spleen involved	Liver involved
<200 g	40	40%	10%	34	15%	3%
200–400 g	10	70%	20%	10	30%	10%
>400 g	6	100%	67%	7	100%	71%
Total	56	52%	18%	51	29%	14%

Total

Spleen weight	No.	Spleen involved	Liver involved
<200 g	74	35%	7%
200–400 g	20	50%	15%
>400 g	13	100%	69%
Total	107	41%	16%

Liver Involvement

The liver was shown to be involved with lymphoma in 14% of 197 laparotomy patients analyzed by GOFFINET. This represents only 5.2% of the total group of 423 patients in the series. In the RIBAS-MUNDO series, 12 of 19 patients (63%) with liver involvement also had bone marrow involvement. Of 27 patients with bone marrow involvement who had liver biopsies, 12 (44%) also had positive bone marrows. The majority of the patients with bone marrow involvement did not have pathologic studies performed on their liver because percutaneous liver needle biopsies and laparoscopies were not performed in this series. There are no important differences for the various histologic subtypes in these correlations.

Lymph Node Involvement

GOFFINET's analyses showed that the lymphogram was accurate in 87% of the patients at laparotomy, when the appropriate para-aortic lymph nodes were removed for histologic

examination. This was equally true for positive or negative interpretations by the diagnostic radiologists.
However, mesenteric lymph nodes were frequently involved. In 71% of the nodular patients and 27% of the diffuse patients, mesenteric involvement was demonstrated. When the lymphogram was positive in the nodular lymphomas, 79% had involved mesenteric lymph nodes. However, even when the lymphogram was interpreted as normal, 9 of 19 (47%) patients with nodular lymphomas had mesenteric involvement. In patients with diffuse lymphomas, 52% with positive lymphograms had mesenteric tumor but this was found in only 9% of those with negative lymphograms.

Change in Stage

As seen in Table 4, from the GOFFINET series of 197 laparotomy patients, 15 (8%) were downstaged and 62 (31%) were upstaged as a result of laparotomy. Of those with nodular lymphomas, 41% had advancement of their stage, whereas only 4 of 108 patients had a lower pathologic than clinical stage. Fewer patients with diffuse lymphomas had a change in their clinical stage as a result of laparotomy, 20% were increased and 12% decreased.
The final distribution of pathologic stage in the RIBAS-MUNDO series of 200 consecutive patients, studied with sequential bone marrow biopsy and diagnostic laparotomy, is shown in Fig. 3. It is evident that the frequency of the various stages is quite different for the RAPPAPORT histologic subtypes and all of the groups are different from the distribution of similarly studied patients with Hodgkin's disease [6].

Table 4. Correlation of clinical stage (CS) and pathologic stage (PS) in 197 consecutive patients with non-Hodgkin's lymphomas after diagnostic laparotomy and splenectomy

		Nodular—108 patients				
		PS				
		I	II	III	IV	Total
CS	I	8	1	2	3	14
	II	3	13	9	2	27
	III	1	—	37	27	65
	IV	—	—	—	2	2
Total		12	14	48	34	108
		Diffuse—89 patients				
		PS				
		I	II	III	IV	Total
CS	I	17	2	—	—	19
	II	1	28	2	1	32
	III	2	7	10	13	32
	IV	—	1	—	5	6
Total		20	38	12	19	89

Downstaged 15/197 (8%). Upstaged 62/197 (31%).

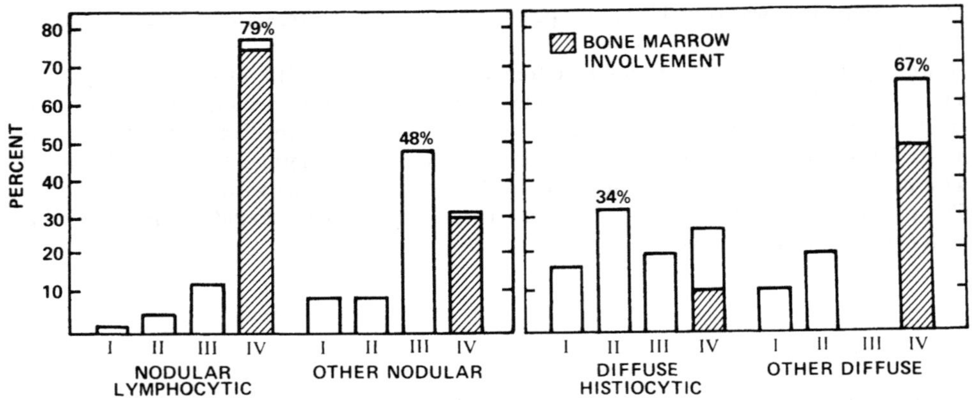

Fig. 3. Distribution of pathologic stages in 200 consecutive adult patients with non-Hodgkin's lymphomas

Conclusions

It is evident from the experience at Stanford and from the studies of others [10, 3] that patients with non-Hodgkin's lymphomas have more widespread disease than is clinically evident. The sequential use of bone marrow biopsy and laparotomy with splenectomy is valuable in identifying the site of involvement and more accurately staging the patient. The Stanford series does not provide information on the relative value of multiple needle bone marrow biopsies [1] nor the role of routine sequential percutaneous needle liver biopsy and laparoscopy [3].

The final distribution of disease extent is quite distinct for the various histologic subtypes. It seems reasonable that treatment programs can be more logically selected and studied as a result of the greater accuracy and insights provided by the staging procedures described. However, no data are yet available from the Stanford experience nor from other centers to indicate that improvement in survival and cure rates has, in fact, resulted from these aggressive staging procedures. Until such evidence becomes available, exploratory laparotomy for patients with non-Hodgkin's lymphomas should still be reserved for selected patients or for patients in clinical studies designed to test the value of the procedure.

Acknowledgements

The studies reported herein were supported, in part, by Grants CA-05838 and CA-08122 from the National Cancer Institute, N.I.H. Dr. Ribas-Mundo was supported by a grant from the Commission of Cultural Exchange between Spain and the United States.

References

1. Brunning, R. D., Bloomfield, C. D., McKenna, R. W., Peterson, L.: Bilateral Trephine Bone Marrow Biopsies in Lymphoma and Other Neoplastic Diseases. Ann. Intern. Med. *82*, 365–366 (1975)
2. Carbone, P. P., Kaplan, H. S., Musshoff, K., Smithers, D. W., Tubiana, M.: Report of the Committee on Hodgkin's disease staging classification. Cancer Res. *31*, 1860–1861 (1971)

3. Chabner, B. A., Johnson, R. E., Chretian, P. B., Schein, P. S., Young, R. C., Canellos, G. P., Hubbard, S. H., Anderson, T., Rosenoff, S. H., DeVita, V. T.: Percutaneous Liver Biopsy, Peritoneoscopy and Laparotomy: An assessment of relative merits in the lymphomata. Br. J. Cancer *31*, 242–247 (1975)
4. Goffinet, D. R., Castellino, R. A., Kim, H., Dorfman, R. F., Fuks, Z., Rosenberg, S. A., Nelsen, T., Kaplan, H. S.: Staging Laparotomies in Unselected Previously Untreated Patients with Non-Hodgkin's Lymphomas. Cancer *32*, 672–681 (1973)
5. Goffinet, D. R., Warnke, R., Dunnick, N. R., Castellino, R., Glatstein, E. J., Nelsen, T. S., Dorfman, R. F., Rosenberg, S. A., Kaplan, H. S.: Clinical and Surgical (Laparotomy) Evaluation of Patients with Non-Hodgkin's Lymphomas. Cancer Treat. Rep. (in press)
6. Kaplan, H. S., Dorfman, R. F., Nelsen, T. S., Rosenberg, S. A.: Staging laparotomy and splenectomy in Hodgkin's disease—Analysis of indications and patterns of involvement in 285 consecutive, unselected patients. Natl. Cancer Inst. Monogr. *36*, 291–310 (1973)
7. Rappaport, H., Winter, W. J., Hicks, E. B.: Follicular Lymphoma. A re-evaluation of its position in the scheme of malignant lymphoma, based on survey of 253 cases. Cancer *9*, 792 (1956)
8. Rosenberg, S. A.: Hodgkin's Disease of the Bone Marrow. Cancer Res. *31*, 1733–1736 (1971)
9. Rosenberg, S. A., Dorfman, R. F., Kaplan, H. S.: The Value of Sequential Bone Marrow Biopsy and Laparotomy and Splenectomy in a Series of 127 Consecutive Untreated Patients with Non-Hodgkin's Lymphoma. Br. J. Cancer *31*, 221–227 (1975)
10. Veronesi, U., Musumeci, R., Pizzetti, F., Gennari, L., Bonadonna, G.: The Value of Staging Laparotomy in Non-Hodgkin's Lymphomas. Cancer *33*, 446–459 (1974)

Invasion of the Upper Respiratory and Digestive Tract in Adult Lymphoid Neoplasias

J. BRUGERE, J. DUMONT, C. JAULERRY, and G. SCHWAAB

For many years, non-Hodgkin's malignant lymphomas (NHML) of the upper respiratory and digestive tract (URDT) were treated and followed up only by radiotherapists and ENT specialists, when they were confined to the head and neck. Concerted studies on these patients during the last 15 years have yielded a better analysis of the results obtained by a locoregional irradiation and led to a better approach to the treatment.

Importance of NHML of URDT in Oncology of Head and Neck

The head and neck specialist is involved in the diagnosis of lymphoid neoplasias in these locations in three different ways:

1. When symptoms arise in the URDT
2. By discovering asymptomatic involvement of the air or food passages by an ENT examination, which was indicated by the presence of cervical nodes
3. Occasionally in a generalized disease

The URDT is involved in about 20% of the patients suffering from these neoplasias. They are mainly located in the Waldeyer's ring, especially in the tonsil. One or more lymphoid regions of this ring may be involved at the same time. Invasion of the nasal and paranasal cavities is not uncommon. The distributions of the locations are similar in the three important series published [1, 3, 6] (Table 1).

In adults, NHML of the URDT makes up only 3% of the cancers seen by the head and neck oncologist but represent 12% of the nasopharyngeal malignancies and 8% of the cancers of the tonsil. The sex ratio is very different from that of carcinomas, particularly for the base of the tongue and the tonsil (Table 2). The highest incidence is in the 5th and 6th decades of life, but many patients are aged 16–39 years (19%) and 18% are over 70 years of age [1, 3] (Fig. 1).

Table 1. Non-Hodgkin's malignant lymphomas of the upper respiratory and digestive tract

	Fondation Curie Paris (1919–1973)	Institut Gustave Roussy Villejuif (1958–1972)	Instituto dei Tumori Milan (1950–1971)	Total	
Tonsil	208	98	108	414	48%
Nasopharynx	83	42	106	231	26%
Base of tongue	26	18	15	59	7%
Miscellaneous	44	60	63	167	19%
Total	361	218	292	871	—

Table 2. Malignancies of the upper respiratory and digestive tract[a]
Sex ratio

	NHML	Carcinomas
Tonsil	1.8	13
Nasopharynx	1.5	3
Base of tongue	0.5	32
Paranasal cavities	1	1.8
Total	1.5	10

[a] Data from Institut Gustave Roussy.
NHML: non-Hodgkin's malignant lymphomas.

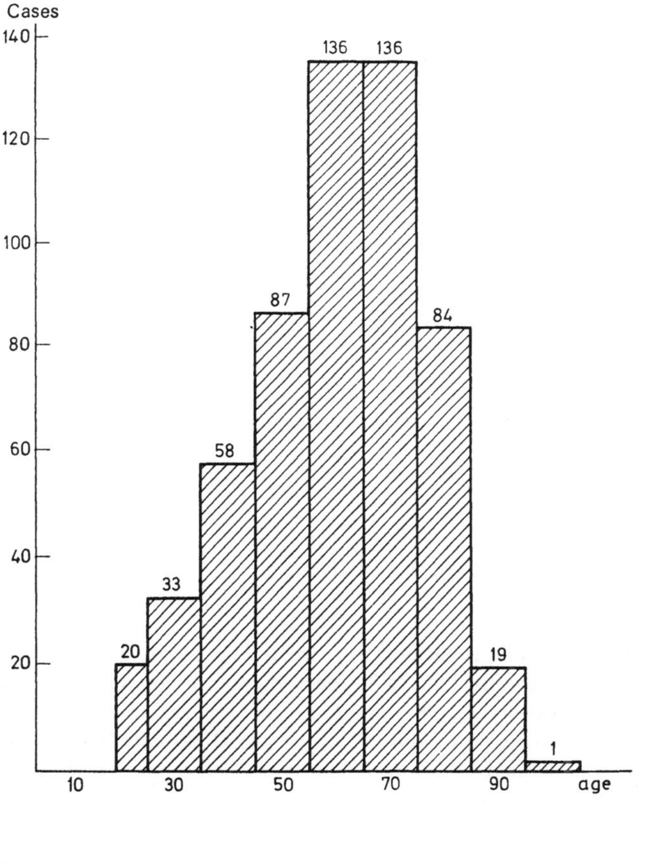

Fig. 1. Non-Hodgkin's malignant lymphomas of the upper respiratory and digestive tract in adults. Age distribution of 574 cases. (Fondation Curie—Institut Gustave Roussy)

Clinical Aspects

The involvement of the cervical nodes is frequent at the first presentation; the same rate (65%) is found in two series (Fondation Curie 233/361; Institut Gustave Roussy: 142/218). Invaded nodes are more frequent in the lymphoid neoplasias of the Waldeyer's ring (120/158: 76%) than in those of the paranasal cavities (16/4: 33%) [3]. The three series referred to earlier [1, 3, 6] concern many patients seen over long periods. These studies analyze the patients who were accurately explored and correctly staged in recent years together with the patients who had not had lymphography or bone examination in the past. For example, only 94 patients had lymphography among the 218 reported by Institut Gustave Roussy [3]. We must point out this bias because lymphography performed in patients who clinically looked to be in stages I or II revealed more than 35% abnormalities. These results depend on the location and are more frequent in cases of involvement of the Waldeyer's ring (30/76: 39%) than of paranasal cavities (3/18: 15%) [3].

The modification of the clinical staging after lymphography is presented in Table 3; 17 patients of 94 evaluated as stages I or II before lymphography were upstaged to stage III [3]. If a comparable rate of erroneous downstaging (18%) is observed in the other former patients analyzed in this series [3], the results of the treatment cannot be read without reservation. This comment also applies to the other retrospective series [1, 6]. This defect must be kept in mind for the analysis of the clinical staging at the first presentation: about 60%–70% of the patients belong to stages I or II [1, 3], 15%–20% to stage III, and 10%–15% to stage IV.

In the retrospective studies, pathologic classification was according to the RAPPAPORT system and generally showed 90%–95% of the cases to be diffuse lymphomas and revealed a predominance of the histiocytic type.

Table 3. Non-Hodgkin's malignant lymphomas of the upper respiratory and digestive tract: modifications of clinical staging after lymphography[a]

Before lymphography	Staging	After lymphography
26	I	23
45	II	31
12	III	29
11	IV	11

[a] Data from Institut Gustave Roussy, 1973.

Treatment and Evolution

All stage I and II patients were treated by radiation therapy to the primary site and the bilateral cervical regions. During 30 years, the tumor dose has increased from 3000 to 5000 rad over 3.5 weeks. Boosts of 1000–2000 rad were delivered to bulky tumors and/or residual nodes.

The initial response of all 152 stage I and II patients was evaluated in the Gustave Roussy series. It was defined as the disappearance of all clinically detectable disease, for at least 2 months following completion of the radiotherapy. Despite additional treatment for residual disease, local control was not achieved in all patients [2]. Disappearance of the primary tumor was achieved in 131/152 (86%); nine of the 21 failures were among the 103 small tumors and 12 were among the 49 big tumors (two or more regions or with contiguous bone involvement). The common primary sites which were not initially controlled with irradiation were nasopharynx, with involvement of the base of the tongue (seven cases), bulky tonsillar tumors (seven cases), and advanced paranasal sinus tumors (four cases). Failure in cervical nodes was more unusual; among 89 stage II patients, only four bulky involvements of the neck were not controlled. In short, 2 months after completion of the irradiation of URDT and neck, 85% of the stage I and II patients were free of disease (129/152); no difference has been noticed according to the pathologic type.

A first relapse was observed in 66 of the 129 initially responding patients (51%). Most of them occurred in the 1st year following the radiation therapy (50/66: 76%), seven during the 2nd year, and nine up until the 6th year after treatment. It consisted of a recurrence in a previously treated area in 18 patients: 11 at the site of the primary tumor, especially in the paranasal sinuses (8/11), and seven in the cervical nodes. Involvement of lymphoid areas distant from head and neck is less frequent than involvement of extralymphoid regions. Ten patients had such invasion (inguinal nodes: three cases, retroperitoneal nodes: two, mediastinum: three, and spleen: two). The mediastinum is rarely involved, as reported in other studies [7, 8]. Extranodal dissemination was the most frequent modality of relapse (36 patients). Secondary involvement of the gastrointestinal tract was observed in 13 patients. This frequency has already been noted by BANFI et al. [1]. The other sites of distant relapse were bone (eight cases), skin (five cases), liver (five cases), and lungs (five cases). Only two patients had a leukemic conversion. The prognosis of the first relapse is poor: among 66 patients, a subsequent remission was noted in only 11; it was obtained in 7 of these 11 patients by a second treatment of the local recurrence.

The 5-year survival rates observed are all about 40% for stage I and II patients in the three main studies (Table 4). For a group of true stage I and II patients correctly staged before treatment, a locoregional irradiation confined to head and neck is probably able to increase the 5-year control rate of survival in 50% of the patients. The prognostic features have been studied from a retrospective point of view; thus, many inconsistencies can be pointed out concerning age, sex, local and cervical extension, and site and classic pathologic types [5].

Table 4. Non-Hodgkin's malignant lymphomas of the upper respiratory and digestive tract: survival rates in stage I and II patients

	3 years	5 years
Fondation Curie (Paris)		36%
Institut Gustave Roussy (Villejuif)	45%	38%
Instituto dei Tumori (Milan)	57%	42%

New Concepts of Treatment

For many years, NHML were compared, on the one hand, by hematologists and radiotherapists with Hodgkin's disease and, on the other hand, by ENT specialists with epidermoid carcinomas of the URDT. The latter pointed out the common features; as with carcinomas, NHML gradually involve the structures of the URDT and the cervical nodes, they may affect one or several sites, can be cured by locoregional treatment, and may recur or relapse in distant sites [4]. However, the progression of the disease is now well-documented. For example, in 136 deceased patients from Institut Gustave Roussy series, 92 had distant involvement and only 11 died with locoregional disease and without distant involvement. The frequency of distant dissemination in stage I and II patients is evidence of the need for a new approach to treatment. Prior to external radiotherapy, systemic chemotherapy may be used according to the pathologic findings. After radiotherapy, long-term chemotherapy is used for 2 years, according to pathologic types and the age of the patient.

References

1. Banfi, A., Bonadonna, G., Ricci, S., Milani, F., Molinari, R., Monfardini, S., Zucareli, R.: Malignant lymphomas of Waldeyer's Ring: natural history and survival after radiotherapy. Br. Med. J. *1972 III*, 140–143
2. Brugere, J., Cachin, Y., Gerard-Marchant, R., Pierquin, B., Richard, J.: Lymphosarcomes et réticulosarcomes des voies aéro-digestives supérieures. Bull. Cancer (Paris) *61*, 79–92 (1974)
3. Brugere, J., Schlienger, M., Gerard-Marchant, R., Tubiana, M., Pouillart, P., Cachin, Y.: Non-Hodgkin's Malignant Lymphoma of upper digestive and respiratory tract. Br. J. Cancer *31*, 435–440 (1975)
4. Cachin, Y., Misset, J. L.: Les Lymphosarcomes et Réticulosarcomes des Voies Aéro-Digestives Supérieures. Paris: exposés annuels d'ORL Arnette ed. (in press) (1975)
5. Ennuyer, A.: Radiothérapie des Lymphomes non Hodgkiniens des Voies Aéro-Digestives Supérieures aux Stades I et II. A paraitre dans Encycl. allemande de Radiothérapie Springer, ed.
6. Ennuyer, A., Bataini, P.: Les lymphosarcomes des voies aéro-digestives supérieures (361 cas). Nouv. Presse Med. *2*, 175–178 (1973)
7. Jones, S., Fuks, Z., Bull, M., Kadin, M., Dorfman, R., Kaplan, H. S., Rosenberg, S., Kim, B.: Non Hodgkin's lymphomas: clinicopathologic correlation in 405 cases. Cancer *31*, 806–823 (1973)
8. Van Der Werf Messing, B.: Reticulum cell sarcoma and lymphosarcoma. A retrospective study of potential survival in loco regional disease. Eur. J. Cancer *4*, 549–558 (1968)

Non-Hodgkin's Lymphoma of the Upper Digestive and Respiratory Tract: Histopathology and Implications for Treatment

J. Dumont, A. Mazabraud, A. Ennuyer, P. Bataini, and J. Brugere

For many years at the Curie Foundation, non-Hodgkin's lymphomas localized in the upper digestive and respiratory tract (UDRT) have been treated by locoregional irradiation, and the disappearance of the tumor has been achieved in more than 80% of the patients [3, 5]. Nevertheless, only 36% of the patients were alive at 5 years, and it appears necessary to try to improve the prognosis by other means of treatment. Chemotherapy may be one of the most useful, and in order to select a new therapeutic regimen, we reviewed some data which may have prognostic significance, particularly the histopathologic pattern of the biopsies which had permitted the diagnosis.

Material and Methods

We analyzed histopathologic material from 128 patients. The biopsies were performed before any treatment, and as they were usually rather small and immediately fixed, the technical results were quite valuable. We eliminated all the material which was not sufficient for good classification (14 cases) and all the biopsies which did not finally permit the diagnosis of the so-called "non-Hodgkin's malignant lymphomas" (18 cases).

The biopsies were reviewed independently without any clinical information by two histopathologists and were classified according to the most important categories of the Lukes' classification [7], which seemed to us the most appropriate for getting new information about these tumors.

We employed the following terms: follicular center cell lymphoma (nodular or diffuse), with some predominant cells: small cleaved, large cleaved, mixed, noncleaved cells, with or without nucleoli which were more or less frequent and seemed to correlate with the degree of maturity of the tumor; immunoblastic cell lymphoma; "true" histiocytic cell lymphoma; and mycosis fungoides. Furthermore, we had to introduce the term "lymphoblastic" cell lymphoma, which is not used by Lukes but by Lennert, who included in this group the convoluted cell lymphoma, the undifferentiated types, and Burkitt's cell types.

The different histologic patterns defined several groups of patients, and correlation was made with their mean and median survival and the percentage of 5-year survivors. Indeed, most of the patients were followed for more than 5 years, and as many of them were old patients, another disease had frequently to be taken into account as the cause of the death.

Results

Histologic Results

The results from 96 biopsies retained for analysis are summarized in Table 1. Corresponding patients were 35–75 years old, except two of them who were 12 and 13. There were 43 females

Table 1. Histologic classification of 96 cases

Follicular center cells (nodular: 3, diffuse: 76)		79
Small cleaved cells	14	
Large cleaved cells	12	
Mixed cells	13	
Noncleaved cells	40	
Immunoblastic cells		7
Undifferentiated cells (lymphoblastic?)		5
True histiocytic cells		2
Mycosis fungoides cells		3
Total		96

and 53 males. As has been already described, we found very few biopsies with a nodular pattern: 3 out of 96 biopsies. Most of them showed a diffuse pattern, and most of them seemed to be composed of cells resembling transformed follicular center cells of lymph nodes [7]. We found 79 biopsies with this aspect, 14 of which were composed of predominant small cleaved cells, 12 of predominant large cleaved cells, 40 of predominant noncleaved and nucleolated cells, and 13 of mixed cells.

Seventeen biopsies were not classified as follicular center cell lymphomas: two of them could be included in the group of the so-called "true histiocytic" lymphomas with a very important condensation of reticulin fibers making a pericellular frame very easy to see with argentic staining. In 12 cases, we observed a rather monomorphic aspect, with round or oval cells constituting the entire population of the tumor. In some cases, these cells were large, with prominent nucleoli and extensive cytoplasm, and coexisted with a few plasmacytoid features. These lymphomas were called "immunoblastic," according to the LUKES classification. In other cases, the cells were smaller, round, and with or without visible nucleoli and a thin cytoplasm. We called them "lymphoblastic" cells, and they would probably have been classified by LUKES as "undifferentiated" or "non-Burkitt's" lymphoma. The so-called "convoluted" pattern was only seen in one case in this subgroup. In three cases, we found the peculiar aspect of "mycosis fungoides:" epitheliotropism and microabscesses of Darier and Pautrier, with some special big cells [8,10]; one of these patients developed skin lesions which confirmed the diagnosis.

Correlation of Results

In the most important group of 79 patients with follicular center cell lymphomas, we tried to find a correlation between the prognosis and the degree of maturity of the tumor cells (Fig. 1). We were unable to find any valid difference between the four subgroups.

About 40% of the patients survived to 5 years. The mean survival was around 60 months. However, the median survival was longer in the large cleaved (27 months) and mainly mixed (42 months) cell groups than in the nucleolated (20 months) and small cleaved (19 months) cell groups. The survival of patients with the so-called lymphoblastic pattern was very short: the mean duration of the disease was ca. 6 months. There were no survivors after 1 year. The prognosis of the immunoblastic group seemed to be better (mean survival: 41 months), but in fact there was no survivor after 5 years. In the two other groups, the prognosis seemed to be poor, but it was not really evaluable because of the very small number of patients.

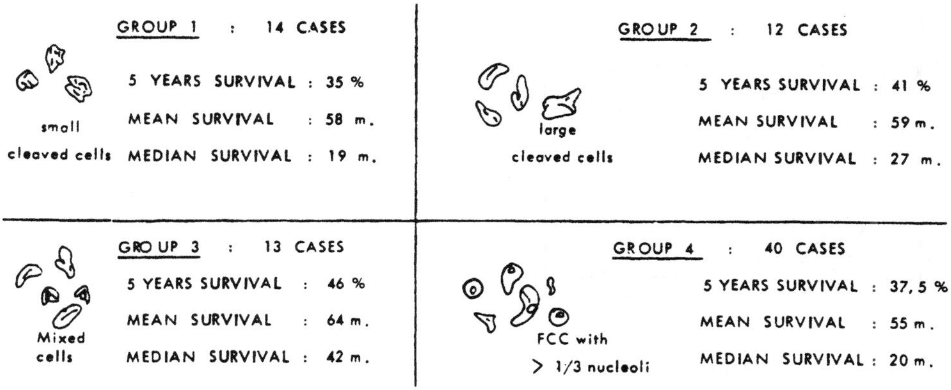

Fig. 1. Follicular center cell lymphomas (79 cases). Survey according to the predominant cell type (four groups)

Discussion

It was shown some years ago that the histologic picture of the lymph nodes correlates with the favorability of the prognosis [6, 9, 10]. It seems that even if the disease is initially disseminated, the prognosis could be favorable if the histologic pattern is nodular and/or composed of differentiated cells [2, 4, 6, 9]. On the contrary, it seems very difficult for some unfavorable histologic forms to be totally cured, even if the disease is localized [11].

UDRT lymphomas are generally considered to have a good prognosis, but it is unknown whether these localizations have exactly the same histologic pattern as nodal localizations. In previously published series on this kind of lymphoma, the histologic data were reported either very briefly [1, 3] or according to the Rappaport classification [2, 10]. The emergence of new classifications and the almost complete disappearance of the previous category "reticulosarcoma" or "histiocytic malignant lymphoma" induced us to undertake this histologic review of the large series of the Curie Foundation.

After the survey of almost 100 cases, we were surprised to note that the great majority of them had to be classified as "follicular center cell" lymphoma, always with a composite population among which a predominant cell type permitted us to define some subgroups. Cleaved cells are very easy to recognize on histologic preparations and to separate from monomorphous immature cells of undifferentiated lymphomas. Furthermore, in this category of follicular center cell lymphomas, we found only adult patients (we had only two children in our series, one of them was in the lymphoblastic group and the other in the immunoblastic group). There was an equal distribution between male and female patients, as in nodular lymphoma, but unlike other groups of non-Hodgkin's lymphomas of the UDRT and carcinoma, where male patients are predominant. The whole group had almost the same prognosis, not as good as expected, but not too bad if the fact is taken into account that they were diffuse histologic lymphomas and that radiotherapy was the only treatment at that time. In another series of *nodal* non-Hodgkin's lymphomas, we found that diffuse follicular center cell lymphomas retain, at least during the initial years, a prognosis as good as lymphocytic well-differentiated and intermediate cell lymphomas (Fig. 2). In contrast, lymphoblastic or immunoblastic cell lymphomas retain a very poor prognosis, and it is strongly recommended that chemotherapy be associated to radiotherapy in order to improve the therapeutic results.

The treatment of UDRT non-Hodgkin's lymphomas could probably be conceived on the same

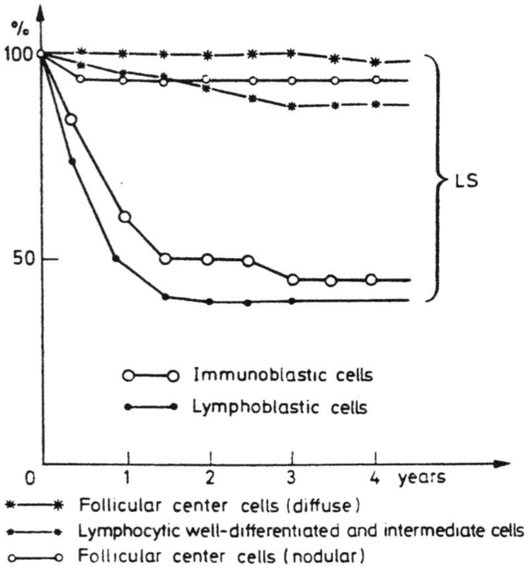

Fig. 2. Survival rate, related to morphologic pattern of lymph nodes (actuarial curve) in a group of 63 patients

principles as applied to lymph node lymphomas, and if so, it may be very important to define the degree of malignancy of each histologic group of these tumors. The choice of the products and of the length of chemotherapy could depend on this classification. This is the reason why we think it important to work in this field and to try to acquire greater experience with the new proposed classifications.

References

1. BANFI, A., BONADONNA, G., RICCI, S. B., MILANI, F., MOLINARI, R., MONFARDINI, S. ZUCALI, R.: Malignant lymphomas of Waldeyer's ring: natural history and survival after radiotherapy. Br. J. Med. *3*, 140 (1972)
2. BROWN, T. C., PETERS, M. V., BERGSAGEL, D. E., REID, J.: A retrospective analysis of the clinical results in relation to the Rappaport histological classification. Br. J. Cancer *31*, 174 (1975)
3. BRUGERE, J., SCHLIENGER, M., GERARD-MARCHANT, R., TUBIANA, M., POUILLART, P., CACHIN, Y.: Non-Hodgkin's malignant lymphomata of upper digestive and respiratory tract: natural history and results of radiotherapy. Br. J. Cancer *31*, 435 (1975)
4. DUMONT, J., DUFFILLOT, C., FLANDRIN, G., CHELLOUL, N., TRISTANT, H., BERNARD, J.: Non Hodgkin's lymphomata: clinical and immunological data in relation to histology. Br. J. Cancer *31*, 187 (1975)
5. ENNUYER, A., BATAINI, P.: Les lymphosarcomes des voies aéro-digestives supérieures. Traitement radiothérapique. A propos de 361 cas formes généralisées exceptées. Nouv. Presse Med. *2*, 175 (1973)
6. JONES, S. E., FUKS, Z., BULL, M., KADIN, M. E., DORFMAN, R. F., KAPLAN, H. S., ROSENBERG, S. A., KIM, H.: Non-Hodgkin's lymphomas. IV. Clinicopathologic correlation in 405 cases. Cancer *31*, 806 (1973)
7. LUKES, R. J., COLLINS, R. D.: New approaches to the classification of the lymphomata. Br. J. Cancer *31*, 1 (1975)
8. RAPPAPORT, H.: Tumors of Hematopoietic System. Washington D.C.: Armed Forces Institute of Pathology 1966, p. 91

9. RAPPAPORT, H., THOMAS, L. B.: Mycosis fungoides: the pathology of extra cutaneous involvement. Cancer *34*, 1198 (1974)
10. RAPPAPORT, H., WINTER, W. J., HICKS, E. B.: Follicular lymphoma: a re-evaluation of its position in the scheme of malignant lymphoma, based on a survey of 253 cases. Cancer *9*, 792 (1956)
11. ROSENBERG, S. A., KAPLAN, H. S.: Clinical trials in the Non-Hodgkin's lymphomata of Stanford University: Experimental design and preliminary results. Br. J. Cancer *31*, 456 (1975)

Staging in Childhood Non-Hodgkin's Lymphoma What Are Its Benefits? How Extensive Should It Be?

N. Jaffe

Introduction

Although childhood non-Hodgkin's lymphoma represents a conglomerate of histologic subtypes, it is generally agreed that most forms of the disease, if untreated, will convert to acute lymphoblastic leukemia. In recent years, this has led to the adoption of chemotherapy as a major therapeutic approach. As a result, a small but significant number of children with localized disease and the potential for cure by surgery and/or radiation therapy will be exposed unnecessarily to the deleterious effects of chemotherapy. Alternatively, radiation therapy with its delayed consequences might be recommended for eradication of localized surgically curable disease. These factors have led to the adoption of staging for the planning of rational treatment. However, the extent to which careful pretreatment evaluation should be implemented and the benefits which might accrue have not been defined. This study was undertaken in an effort to elicit such information.

Materials and Methods

A review of reports of the management of childhood non-Hodgkin's lymphoma published during the past decade was undertaken. Information was extracted principally from studies where a staging system had been utilized with a view to defining the utility and practical application of the system. To simplify the analysis, the histologic subtypes were classified as a single entity, and it was assumed that each treatment carried an equal potential for cure. It was recognized that this could produce erroneous results, but the premise was advanced that there was probably a common distribution of subtypes and that treatment was optimum in the major centers from which the reports emanated. In each communication, an attempt was made to evaluate the influence on staging of the following factors:

1. Primary site;
2. Lymphangiography;
3. Laparotomy;
4. Bone marrow aspirate;
5. Bone marrow biopsy;
6. Biochemical investigations;
7. Lumbar puncture;
8. Miscellaneous investigations.

Results

Information for staging was derived from one or more of the following procedures: clinical examination, hemogram, bone marrow aspirate and/or biopsy, radiographs of the chest, liver function studies, and specific studies, as dictated by the mode of presentation. Patients with abdominal lymphoma were usually evaluated by laparotomy.

The majority of publications employed a modification of the Ann Arbor staging system involving omission of laparotomy [1, 2, 3, 9, 11, 13, 15]. The latter, however, was employed in selected institutions [7, 17]. The staging systems utilized by MURPHY and WOLLNER are outlined in Tables 1 and 2 [10, 19]. Generally, extensive extranodal involvement was designated stage IV. An alternative classification for Burkitt's lymphoma was devised by ZIEGLER [21] (Table 3); patients with minimal tumor were designated stages A or B, those with single or multiple extra-abdominal sites, stage AR, and those with gross intra-abdominal tumor with or without extra-abdominal, central nervous system, or marrow involvement, stages C or D.

Examination of the spinal fluid did not constitute a routine staging procedure. In the series reported by JAFFE, MURPHY, ZIEGLER, and WOLLNER and their respective co-workers, clinical staging included lumbar puncture with cytocentrifuge examination of the cerebrospinal fluid

Table 1. Staging system [MURPHY et al., 10]

Stage I
- A single tumor (extranodal) or single anatomic area (nodal), with the exclusion of mediastinum or abdomen

Stage II
- A single tumor (extranodal) with regional node involvement
- Two or more nodal areas on the same side of the diaphragm
- Two single (extranodal) tumors with or without regional node involvement on the same side of the diaphragm
- A primary gastrointestinal tract tumor, usually in the ileocecal area, with or without involvement of associated mesenteric nodes only

Stage III
- Two single tumors (extranodal) on opposite sides of the diaphragm
- Two or more nodal areas above and below the diaphragm
- All the primary intrathoracic tumors (mediastinal, pleural, thymic)
- All extensive primary intra-abdominal disease

Stage IV
- Any of the above with initial CNS and/or bone marrow involvement

Table 2. [WOLLNER et al. 19] Staging of nodal and extranodal disease in non-Hodgkin's lymphoma in children

Nodal	Stage	Extranodal
One site	I	One site
Two or more sites either above or below diaphragm	II	One site + regional node Two sites + regional nodes either above or below diaphragm
Two or more sites above and below diaphragm: extensive intrathoracic; extensive intra-abdominal	III	Two or more sites above and below diaphragm; extensive intrathoracic; extensive intra-abdominal
Central nervous system and/or bone marrow involvement	IV	Central nervous system and/or bone marrow involvement

Table 3. [ZIEGLER et al. 21] Clinical staging of Burkitt's lymphoma

Stage	Extent of tumor
A	Single extra-abdominal site
B	Multiple extra-abdominal sites
C	Intra-abdominal tumor with involvement of one or more extra-abdominal sites
AR	Stage C but with >90% of tumor surgically resected

[5, 11, 19, 21]. Most other investigators, however, indicated that a lumbar puncture would be performed if bone marrow conversion to acute leukemia were demonstrated.

Bilateral lower extremity lymphangiography did not constitute a routine staging procedure. It was employed with greater frequency by GLATSTEIN et. al. and LEMERLE et al. [2, 9], but its utility was not defined. In the series reported by JOHNSON et al. [7], which included five patients under 20 years of age, the investigation upstaged 15 stage I–II cases to stage III. During the past 10 years, it was employed in a fair number of patients at the Sidney Farber Cancer Institute. However, as experience accumulated and the frequency of positive results diminished, particularly in patients with clinically localized stage I disease (usually of the head and neck), enthusiasm for the procedure waned [4, Unpublished data]. In the series reported by WOLLNER et al., lymphangiography was performed provided there was no massive mediastinal lesion or pleural effusion [19]. There appeared to be a greater tendency for patients with disseminated disease or primary lesions in the abdomen or inguinal areas to be associated with a positive result [13; unpublished data]

Staging laparotomy and splenectomy were performed with reasonable consistency by GLATSTEIN and his co-workers in a limited number of children [2]. Several patients in the series reported by JOHNSON et al. [7] and VERONESI et al. [17] were also subjected to this investigation. The procedure together with other studies (bone marrow biopsy and closed liver biopsy) progressively increased the incidence of defined extranodal dissemination in JOHNSON's studies [7]. Most investigators, however, did not adopt laparotomy as a routine therapeutic or staging maneuver except in children with abdominal lymphomas. In such cases, it was recommended that biopsies of the para-aortic and mesenteric lymph nodes and liver be performed. Several workers also recommended a "second-look" surgical procedure for resection of residual disease or determination of the efficacy of treatment following a defined period [19]. Restaging was performed by ZIEGLER and his co-workers before starting new treatment in relapsed patients [21].

Needle or other bone marrow biopsies were performed by STEIN et al. [14] and JONES et al. [8]. They demonstrated the superiority of this procedure in comparison to bone marrow aspirate. It appeared to offer early identification of marrow involvement which correlated with advanced stage, cellular composition of the lymphoma and, in the nodular lymphomas, splenomegaly and constitutional symptoms. In the series reported by WOLLNER et al., marrow biopsy was performed when aspiration was suspicious but not diagnostic [19]. There was no correlation between hemogram, biochemical studies, and the various stages. Gross abnormalities, however, including hyperuricemia, were more consistent with advanced disease. Other studies reported in the reviews included radionucleotide bone scanning and ultrasound [19, 20]. It appeared that additional experience would be required before the utility of these investigations is determined.

Assessment of Results

Staging appeared to be of major benefit in predicting prognosis. Thus, survival was superior in patients with localized or stage I and II disease [2, 4, 9, 19]. Those with an advanced stage did poorly and were also at risk of developing central nervous system disease.

In terms of primary site, staging permitted verification of the extent of the tumor and areas of high risk. Patients with limited abdominal disease (regional or stages I and II) had an excellent prognosis. Those with advanced unresectable abdominal tumor had a poor prognosis with death occurring within 6 months [5, 6, 11]. Survival was also diminished when there was serosal involvement, tumor at the surgical margins, mesenteric and para-aortic node invasion, or abdominal fluid or blood at surgery [12]. The prognosis in patients with localized head and neck lymphoma was also good [16].

Staging also demonstrated that patients with primary mediastinal involvement and American Burkitt's lymphoma frequently developed central nervous system disease [3, 10, 20]. It was also noted in patients with advanced disease usually after bone marrow relapse [18]. In contrast, the risk appeared less in patients with localized surgically resectable non-Hodgkin's lymphoma of the abdomen, head and neck, and elsewhere [3, 12, 16].

Unfortunately, staging did not permit a firm identification of patients who apparently could be cured solely by surgery, radiation therapy, or chemotherapy. Possibly, such information will be obtained with the use of functional classifications and tumor markers in the future.

The reviews did not specify the minimum number of procedures to be performed, and differences in extent of pretreatment evaluation were noteworthy. Of significance was the observation that identical stages defined by variable procedures frequently exhibited the same end results. Thus, major invasive procedures do not appear indicated for all cases. Jaffe et al. noted that a reasonable assessment of disease could be obtained by means of physical examination, chest radiograph, and bone marrow studies [4]. This was particularly applicable to tumors of the head and neck [16].

Current concepts in the treatment of childhood non-Hodgkin's lymphoma would also suggest that a compulsive search for clinically undetected disease appears unwarranted. Such disease will be exposed to systemic chemotherapy. However, to some extent, staging might assist in the identification of bulk disease for treatment with radiation therapy [1, 2, 4]. Ideally, then, each patient should receive individual consideration. Diagnostic evaluation should consist of a series of tests, sequentially performed and interrupted whenever sufficient information has been assembled for institution of therapy. Such tests should range from the minimally hazardous to the more invasive and should be planned with minimum delay.

Summary

A review of published reports of the management of childhood non-Hodgkin's lymphoma was undertaken to determine the extent to which a staging procedure should be implemented and the benefits which could be derived. A variety of clinical, radiographic, surgical, and laboratory investigations were performed by different investigators. Overall, similar results were obtained for the different stages. The utility of the individual studies was not defined in any single review. However, it appeared that bone marrow biopsy was superior to bone marrow aspirates, staging laparotomy was generally not required, and lymphangiography did not constitute a routine staging procedure. Staging permitted identification of patients with primary sites at high risk for the development of central nervous system disease or failure. The reviews did not specify the minimum number of procedures to be performed. It is concluded that each patient should receive individual consideration, and diagnostic evaluation should consist of a series of tests sequentially performed and interrupted whenever sufficient information has been assembled for institution of therapy.

Acknowledgements

This work was supported in part by a research grant (CA06516) from the National Cancer Institute and by a grant (RR-05526) from the Division of Research, National Institutes of Health.

References

1. Aur, R. J. A., Hustu, H. O., Simone, J. V., Pratt, C. B., Pinkel, D.: Therapy of localized and regional lymphosarcoma of childhood. Cancer *27*, 1328–1351 (1971)
2. Glatstein, E., Kim, H., Donaldson, S., Dorfman, R. J., Gribble, T. J., Wilbur, J. R., Rosenberg, S. A., Kaplan, H. S.: Non-Hodgkin's lymphomas. VI. Results of treatment in childhood. Cancer *34*, 204–211 (1974)
3. Hutter, J. J., Favara, B. E., Nelson, M., Holton, C. P.: Non-Hodgkin's lymphoma in children. Correlation of CNS disease with initial presentation. Cancer *36*, 2132–2137 (1975)
4. Jaffe, N., Buell, D., Cassady, J. R., Traggis, D., Weinstein, H.: The role of staging in childhood non-Hodgkin's lymphoma. Cancer Treat. Rep. *61*, 1001–1007 (1977)
5. Jenkin, R. D. T.: The management of malignant lymphoma in childhood. In: Modern Radiotherapy—Malignant Disease in Children. Deeley, T. J. (ed.) London: Butterworths 1974, pp. 341–359
6. Jenkin, R. D. T., Sonley, M. J., Stephens, C. A., Darte, J. M. M., Peters, M. V.: Primary gastrointestinal tract lymphoma in childhood. Radiology *92*, 736–767 (1969)
7. Johnson, R. E., Chretien, P. B., O'Conor, G. T., Devita, V. T., Thomas, L. B.: Radiotherapeutic implications of prospective staging in non-Hodgkin's lymphoma. Radiology *110*, 655–657 (1974)
8. Jones, S. E., Rosenberg, S. A., Kaplan, H. S.: Non-Hodgkin's lymphomas. I. bone marrow involvement. Cancer *29*, 954–960 (1972)
9. Lemerle, M., Gerard-Marchant, R., Sarrazin, D., Sancho, H., Tchernia, G., Flamant, F., Lemerle, J., Schweisguth, O.: Lymphosarcoma and reticulum cell sarcoma in children. Retrospective study of 172 cases. Cancer *32*, 1499–1507 (1973)
10. Murphy, S. B.: The management of childhood non-Hodgkin's lymphoma. Cancer Treat. Rep. *61*, 1161–1173 (1977)
11. Murphy, S. B., Frizerra, G., Evans, A. E.: A Study of childhood non-Hodgkin's lymphoma. Cancer *36*, 1499–1507 (1973)
12. Nelson, D. F., Cassady, J. R., Traggis, D., Baez-Giangreco, A., Vawter, G. F., Jaffe, N., Filler, R. M.: The role of radiation therapy in localized resectable intestinal non-Hodgkin's lymphoma in children. Cancer *39*, 89–97 (1977)
13. Pinkel, D., Johnson, W., Aur, R. J. A.: Non-Hodgkin's lymphoma in children. Br. J. Cancer *31* (suppl. II), 298–323 (1975)
14. Stein, R. S., Ultmann, J. E., Byrne, G. E., Jr., Moran, E. M., Golomb, H. M., Oetzel, N.: Bone marrow involvement in non-Hodgkin's lymphoma. Implications for staging and therapy. Cancer *37*, 629–636 (1976)
15. Sullivan, M. P.: Non-Hodgkin's lymphoma in childhood. In: Clinical Pediatric Oncology. Sutow, W. W., Vietti, T. J., Fernbach, D. J. (eds.) St. Louis: C. V. Mosby 1973, Vol. XIV, pp. 313–336
16. Traggis, D., Jaffe, N., Vawter, G., Baez-Giangreco, A.: Non-Hodgkin's lymphoma of the head and neck in childhood. J. Pediatr. *87*, 933–936 (1975)
17. Veronsei, U., Musumeci, R., Pizzetti, F., Gennari, L., Bonadonna, G.: The value of staging laparotomy in non-Hodgkin's lymphomas. (With emphasis on the histiocytic type). Cancer *33*, 446–459 (1974)
18. Watanabe, A., Sullivan, M. P., Sutow, W. W., Wilbur, J. R.: Undifferentiated lymphoma, non-Burkitt's type. Meningeal and bone marrow involvement in children. Am. J. Dis. Child. *125*, 57–61 (1973)
19. Wollner, N., Burchenal, J. H., Lieberman, P. H., Exelby, P. R., d'Angio, G. J., Murphy, M. L.: Non-Hodgkin's lymphoma in children Med. Pediatr. Oncol. *1*, 235–263 (1975)
20. Ziegler, J. L., Bluming, A. Z., Morrow, R. H., Fass, L., Carbone, P. P.: Central nervous system involvement in Burkitt's lymphoma. Blood *36*, 718–728 (1970)
21. Ziegler, J. L., Devita, V. T., Graw, R. G., Jr., Herzig, G., Leventhal, B. G., Levine, A. S., Pomeroy, T. C.: Combined modality treatment of American Burkitt's lymphoma. Cancer *38*, 2225–2231 (1976)

Systematic Restaging in Non-Hodgkin's Lymphoma: The Need to Define Complete Remission

T. S. HERMAN and S. E. JONES

Introduction

Improved treatment programs for lymphoma have led to the hope of cure for many patients [5, 7, 17]. In the past, treatment was often palliative, and the need to rigorously define the quality of response was small. Now, however, the majority of patients experience the disappearance of clinical symptoms and signs of disease, and accordingly a strong need has emerged to define the "completeness" of remission as an endpoint to treatment (with prognostic value) and as a basis for comparing the relative efficacy of various therapeutic programs. Accordingly, a plan for systematic and thorough reevaluation of all patients in apparent complete remission was incorporated into the latest Southwest Oncology Group (SWOG) trial of induction therapy for patients with advanced stages of non-Hodgkin's lymphoma (NHL). We have previously reported the initial findings of "systematic restaging" for assessing the completeness of response in these patients [11]. This paper will extend these observations to a larger number of patients with NHL who have been restaged and will also examine the impact of restaging upon their ensuing course.

Patients and Methods

In October, 1974, the SWOG began a new clinical trial of combination chemotherapy for patients with advanced non-Hodgkin's lymphomas designed to define the minimum treatment necessary to induce sustained remissions of disease (SWOG study 7426/7427). The specifics of this trial have been previously reported [11], and the most recent update of its results appears in this monograph (S. E. Jones: Chemoimmunotherapy Versus Chemotherapy for Remission Induction in Patients With Non-Hodgkin's Lymphoma. Progress Report of a Southwest Oncology Group Study.)

Briefly, remission induction therapy for responding patients consisted of eight courses of treatment given at 3–4-week intervals followed by systematic restaging (as outlined in Table 1) if all clinical signs and symptoms of lymphoma had disappeared. Patients considered to be free of disease after restaging were then assigned at random to receive either no further therapy or BCG by scarification at monthly intervals for 18 months with close follow-up for signs of relapse. Those patients with residual disease detected at restaging were to receive three additional courses of the same chemotherapy followed by a second restaging evaluation if there was no clinical evidence of disease. A schematic representation of the study is presented in Fig. 1.

The records of the first 140 patients who achieved an apparent complete remission after eight courses of therapy and then underwent systematic restaging were reviewed in detail and the results of restaging analyzed with regard to the clinical features of the patients, histologic type,

Table 1. Procedures to be used in restaging patients in apparent complete remission

Careful physical examination
Biopsy of any residual enlarged lymph nodes, particularly if region was involved initially
Routine laboratory tests: CBC, liver function studies, etc.
Chest x-ray (with whole lung tomograms if initially abnormal)
Bone marrow core biopsy
Repeat other initially abnormal studies:
Lymphangiogram (or follow-up abdominal x-ray if dye persists)
Liver-spleen scan
Liver biopsy
Tumor scans (^{67}Ga citrate or ^{111}In bleomycin)
Laparoscopy
Consider exploratory laparotomy, mediastinoscopy, and thoracotomy in selected patients

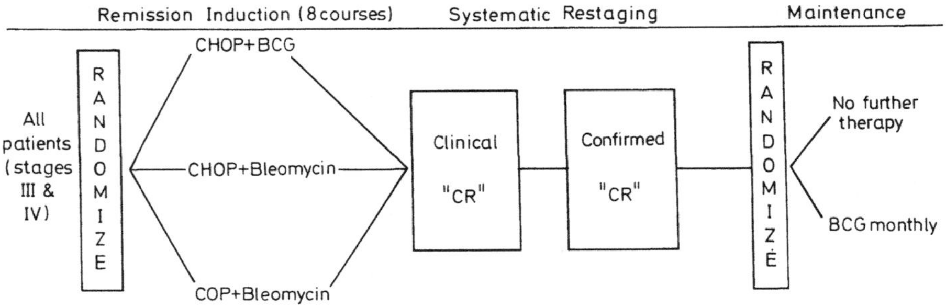

Fig. 1. Schematic representation of the treatment plan in the SWOG study 7426/7427 for patients with advanced non-Hodgkin's lymphoma (October, 1974–July, 1977)

initial sites of involvement, and treatment. The subsequent course of patients with residual disease detected after eight courses of therapy and the patterns of relapse in the group of patients with no detectable disease at restaging after either 8 or 11 courses of therapy were also analyzed. Time to relapse was calculated from the date of completion of restaging.

Results

Thirty-four (24%) of the 140 patients believed to be in complete remission by clinical criteria were found to have persistent disease during systematic restaging. The clinical characteristics of these patients and of the patients in whom no disease was detected at restaging are presented in Table 2. There were no significant differences between these groups with respect to age, sex, histologic type of lymphoma, induction treatment, or the presence of constitutional symptoms at initial presentation. The patients found to have persistent disease, however, more often had stage IV disease at the outset than those with confirmed complete remissions (74% vs. 55%).
A summary of the results of tests done at systematic restaging is presented in Table 3. In general, lymphography and bone marrow biopsy proved to be the most useful procedures for restaging. Bone marrow biopsy detected disease in 17 (13%) of 129 patients at restaging and lymphography (or follow-up abdominal radiography) revealed disease in 14 (12%) of 119 patients. Chest radiography was the least helpful study, revealing disease in only 1 of the 140 patients reexamined.

Table 2. Systematic restaging in NHL: clinical features and results in 140 patients restaged after eight courses of therapy

	Total group (140)	Residual disease (34 patients—24%)	No evidence of disease (106 patients—76%)
Mean age (range)	52 (19–79)	52	52
Male/female	77/63	17/17	60/46
Histology[a]			
Diffuse	47	10	37
Nodular	93 (66%)	24 (70%)	69 (65%)
Pathologic stage[b]			
II_E	6	0	6
III	51	6	42
IV	83 (59%)	25 (74%)	58 (55%)
B symptoms	44 (31%)	13 (38%)	31(29%)
Induction treatment[c]			
COP-Bleo	52 (38%)	16 (47%)	36 (33%)
CHOP-Bleo	44	10	34
CHOP-BCG	44	8	36

[a] Classification of Rappaport [16].
[b] Criteria of the Ann Arbor Conference [3].
[c] COP: cyclophosphamide, vincristine, and prednisone; CHOP: cyclophosphamide, adriamycin, vincristine, and prednisone; bleo: bleomycin; BCG: Calmette-Guérin.

Table 3. Systematic restaging in NHL: diagnostic yield of various restaging procedures employed after eight courses of therapy (No. abnormal/No. performed [%])

Nonsurgical procedures

Chest x-ray	Lymphangiogram	Liver-spleen scan
1/140 (1%)	14/119 (12%)	3/88 (3%)

Surgical procedures

Peripheral lymph node biopsy	Bone marrow biopsy	Liver biopsy	Laparotomy and splenectomy
1/4 (25%)	17/129 (13%)	2/45 (4%)	3/5 (60%)

Radionuclide liver-spleen scans were interpreted as abnormal in 3 (3%) of 88 patients at restaging, but in only one of these cases was lymphomatous involvement actually documented histologically. (This occurred in a patient with splenomegaly on scan who subsequently underwent laparotomy and splenectomy and was found to have splenic involvement.) At reevaluation, liver biopsy revealed lymphoma in 2 (4%) of 45 patients. Neither patient had undergone liver scanning prior to biopsy. Four patients underwent biopsy of residually enlarged peripheral lymph nodes, but in only one patient was histologic evidence of persisting lymphoma found. One of the three patients with negative biopsies at restaging, however, subsequently relapsed in the same region. Five patients had an exploratory laparotomy at restaging and in three, persistent lymphoma was demonstrated. Two of these patients were found to have splenic involvement, and the third patient was found to have para-aortic node involvement. Repetition of tests with abnormal results at initial staging clearly had the most clinical utility in terms of detecting lymphoma at restaging. Continuing abnormalities indicative of lymphoma were found in 15 (24%) of 61 repeat bone marrow core biopsies, 11 (16%) of 68 repeat lymphangiograms, 3 (15%) of 20 repeat liver-spleen scans, and 2 (10%) of 20 repeat liver biopsies. In contrast, repetition of initially normal studies was much less useful, detecting only

2 (3%) positive bone marrow biopsies in 68 patients with initially normal results of bone marrow examinations and 1 abnormal lymphangiogram in 47 patients with initially normal results of studies.

The sites of persisting lymphoma found at restaging are shown in Table 4. Since restaging was often terminated when one site of lymphoma was discovered, it was not possible to determine the total number of patients who may have had persistent disease in multiple sites. At least three patients, however, did have multiple sites of involvement demonstrated at restaging. Abdominal lymph nodes (14 patients) and bone marrow (17 patients) were by far the major sites of residual disease. When the sites of disease found at restaging were compared with the sites of disease at initial staging, we found that in 88% of the patients with nodular lymphoma and in 75% of the patients with diffuse lymphoma, lymphoma persisted in sites previously known to be involved. At least 11 (79%) of 14 patients with abdominal lymph node involvement at restaging had had involvement in the same area at staging (two patients had not had initial lymphangiograms performed), and 15 (88%) of 17 patients with bone marrow involvement at restaging had had initial bone marrow involvement as well.

Of the thirty-four patients with residual lymphoma detected, 21 received three additional courses of the same chemotherapy and underwent a second restaging. Thirteen patients did not undergo a second restaging because of progressive disease while on therapy (four patients), refusal of further therapy (two patients), loss to follow-up (two patients), and treatment which has not yet been completed (five patients). Residual disease was identified in 8 (38%) of 21 patients at the second restaging. The patients with residual disease detected after 11 courses were not different from patients free of disease at restaging when analyzed for age, sex ratio, histology. As in patients restaged after eight courses, patients with residual lymphoma after 11 courses more often had stage IV disease (89% vs. 69%) than patients without persistent disease. At the time of the second restaging, in four of eight patients with residual disease, it was detected in bone marrow and in the other four in abdominal lymph nodes. One additional patient had biopsy-proven lymphoma in a peripheral lymph node and another patient had biopsy-proven persistent liver involvement as well. Two patients had two sites involved. The correlation between sites of disease at second restaging and sites of disease detected at both initial staging and at first restaging was 100%. Of the 13 patients without disease detected at the time of second restaging, five have relapsed with a mean time to relapse of 5 months. The mean time of observation for patients who have not relapsed is 7 months.

Table 4. Systematic restaging in NHL: sites of disease at restaging (34 patients) and correlation with original sites of involvement

Site	No. positive at restaging	No. positive at initial staging	Percentage correlation
Nodal			
Abdominal	14[a]	11	79
Peripheral	1	1	100
Extranodal			
Bone marrow	17	15	88
Liver	2	2	100
Lung[b]	1	1	100
Spleen	2	1[c]	50
Total	37[d]	31	84[e]

[a] Two patients had no initial lymphogram.
[b] Biopsy proven.
[c] Based on positive radionuclide scan.
[d] Three patients had two sites of disease identified at restaging.
[e] Correlation by histology, nodular: 88%; diffuse: 75%.

The 119 patients considered to be in complete remission following restaging after either 8 (106 patients) or 11 courses (13 patients) of chemotherapy have been followed for evidence of relapse. As of June, 1977, 35 (29%) of these patients experienced recurrence of lymphoma with a mean time to relapse of 6 months (range 1–13 months) calculated from the completion of restaging. The mean time of observation for the patients remaining continuously in remission is 14 months. The clinical and pathologic features of the patients who have relapsed and those who have remained continuously free of disease were analyzed, and there were no significant differences between the two groups. At this time, relapse has been independent of the type of initial induction treatment and the use of BCG for maintenance.

The sites of relapse for the 35 relapsing patients are shown in Table 5. The predominant sites of relapse were peripheral nodes (22 patients) and skin (seven patients). The correlation between sites of disease at relapse and those identified at initial staging is 55% overall. If, however, the correlation between sites of relapse and initial involvement is analyzed for the time to recurrence following restaging, a definite pattern emerges (Table 6). Patients with early relapse (less than 8 months) had recurrence in initially involved sites in 71% of instances, whereas only 17% of those who relapsed later than 8 months after restaging had recurrence in originally involved sites ($p = 0.01$).

Discussion

This study demonstrates the importance of careful evaluation of patients for evidence of persisting lymphoma even though all signs and symptoms of the disease may have disappeared.

Table 5. Systematic restaging in NHL: sites of disease at relapse (35 patients) and correlation with original sites of involvement

Site	No. positive at relapse	No. positive at initial staging	Percentage correlation
Nodal			
Abdominal	6	4	67%
Peripheral	22	12	55
Extranodal			
Bone marrow	3	2	67%
Skin	7	3	43
Liver	1	1	100
Spleen	1	0	0
Total	40[a]	22	55[b]

[a] Five patients had two sites of involvement at relapse.
[b] Correlation by histology; nodular: 60%; diffuse: 47%.

Table 6. Systematic restaging in NHL: patterns of relapse and relationship to initial sites of disease

Type of relapse	No. of patients[a]	No. of sites at relapse	Correlation with original sites of disease[b]
Early ($\leq$ 8 months)	25 (21%)	28	71%
Late (> 8 months)	10 (8%)	12	17%

[a] Based on 119 patients with negative restaging after 8 or 11 courses.
[b] $p = 0.01$.

Thirty-four of 140 patients with clinical resolution of disease were found to have residual lymphoma when they underwent systematic restaging (Table 1). These results have considerable implications for the definition of "complete response" as used in current clinical trials, since they indicate that without rigorous restaging, complete remission rates may be grossly overestimated.

In addition, several reports have suggested that documentation of complete response is important prognostically in both Hodgkin's disease and the non-Hodgkin's lymphomas [5, 11, 17, 18, 19]. For example, in one recent investigation of combination chemotherapy for patients with diffuse histiocytic lymphoma, 6 of 18 patients undergoing restaging were found to have residual lymphoma. The 12 patients who had no evidence of disease after careful restaging have remained continuously free of disease (with a median duration of unmaintained remission of 12+ months), whereas the patients with residual disease discovered at restaging have not survived significantly longer than partial responders or even nonresponders [18].

The clinical characteristics and sites of disease for the 34 patients with residual disease found at restaging and for the 25 patients who relapsed early after the completion of restaging (within 8 months) were quite similar, with the most frequently involved sites being lymph nodes, bone marrow, and, in relapsing patients, the skin. In both groups, the sites of persistent lymphoma at restaging and recurrent disease at relapse closely reflected the pattern of initial involvement (84% correlation at restaging and 71% at early relapse). In patients experiencing late relapse (more than 8 months after negative restaging), sites of relapse were frequently quite different from the pattern of initial involvement. The similarities between the early relapsing patients and those with residual disease at restaging suggest that these two groups of patients are probably the same, i.e., patients with incomplete remissions, and that for the patients who relapsed early, residual lymphoma went undetected at restaging. Indeed, it appeared to us that more thorough restaging might have prevented at least half of the early relapses because additional treatment, even with the same combination of agents, seems to be of value in patients with minimal persistent disease detected by restaging. For example, 13 (52%) of 25 patients with persistent disease after eight courses of treatment achieved a pathologically documented complete remission after a total of 11 courses of treatment. Five of these patients subsequently relapsed but eight (32%) remain in continuous unmaintained remission.

Many of the early relapses in this series appear to be due to inadequate restaging evaluations, but the thoroughness of restaging has seemingly improved as individual investigators of the Southwest Oncology Group become more familiar with the concept and with some of our earlier observations on restaging [11]. Indeed, in our first analysis, we reported that 18% of 100 patients were found to harbor foci of lymphoma at restaging; in this analysis, the overall rate of detection is now 24%. Finally, this analysis has prompted us to formulate some guidelines for improving the accuracy of systematic restaging:

1. A thorough pretreatment diagnostic evaluation [4, 12] is essential for clear identification of all potential sites of disease, since residual disease at restaging will be found in these locations.
2. Restaging should be sufficiently individualized to emphasize comprehensive reevaluation of all previously known sites of disease. For example, in a patient with known liver involvement, liver-spleen scanning, percutaneous liver biopsy, laparoscopy with biopsy, or even laparotomy with open biopsy might be required to document a complete remission in that particular organ [4, 18]. Multiple bone marrow core biopsies might be helpful, even for patients without initial involvement [2]. Repeat lymphography should be performed in patients with initial retroperitoneal lymph node involvement [6].
3. Serious consideration must be given to the use of laparoscopy [1] in selected patients and even laparotomy with splenectomy [9] in cases where retroperitoneal, hepatic, or splenic disease was initially present or is suspected at restaging. In this study, three of five laparotomies detected residual lymphoma.
4. Multiple skin biopsies of previously affected areas and examination of the specimens with electron microscopy might be useful in those patients with initial skin involvement by

lymphoma. In this series, three of the seven patients who relapsed in the skin had had skin involvement originally.

5. Although there are serious drawbacks to the use of currently available tumor-imaging agents like ^{67}Ga citrate and ^{111}In bleomycin for defining minimal residual disease [13, 15], other new imaging techniques such as computerized axial tomography show great promise [14], and it is likely that we will come to rely more heavily on these methods in the future. In addition, research in the area of tumor markers, cell sorting, and in vitro assays of tumor stem cells may provide new means of assessing the presence of minimal residual disease [8, 10].

It is clear that systematic restaging of patients with non-Hodgkin's lymphoma who have achieved clinical disappearance of disease should be mandatory in all cases where discontinuation of therapy is being considered. Moreover, modern lymphoma treatment trials must incorporate rigorous restaging into the design of these studies in order to derive accurate and reproducible results.

Summary

One hundred and forty patients with advanced non-Hodgkin's lymphoma in apparent clinical remission after eight courses of combination chemotherapy underwent systematic restaging to assess the completeness of response. Thirty-four (24%) of these patients were found to have residual disease—predominantly in bone marrow (17 patients) and lymph nodes (15 patients). The sites of disease detected at restaging were predictable; in 88% of the patients with nodular lymphoma and in 75% of those with diffuse lymphoma, disease was found in sites originally involved by lymphoma. Twenty-five patients with disease detected after eight courses of therapy have received additional courses of the same chemotherapy and 13 (52%) have achieved pathologically documented complete remissions. Thirty-five (29%) of the 119 patients without demonstrable disease after either 8 or 11 courses have relapsed. Predominant sites of relapse were lymph nodes (28 patients) and skin (seven patients). Two patterns of relapse were identified. Patients who relapsed within 8 months of restaging did so predominantly in areas of previous involvement (71%), while those relapsing after 8 months infrequently relapsed in sites of disease identified at initial staging (17%, $p < 0.01$). Systematic restaging emphasizing a thorough reevaluation of all sites of disease determined at initial staging should be an objective of all lymphoma trials in order to standardize the definition of complete remission. In addition, careful restaging should be performed in clinical practice before stopping treatment since a significant proportion of patients with occult lymphoma detected at restaging can achieve a complete remission with additional therapy.

Acknowledgements

This work was supported in part by Public Health Service grants CA-13612 and CA-19892 from the National Cancer Institute, National Institutes of Health, Department of Health, Education, and Welfare.

References

1. Anderson, T., Rosenoff, S., Bender, R. et al.: Peritoneoscopy: a useful tool in restaging lymphoma patients. (abstr C-125). Proceedings of ASCO/AACR *17*, 268 (1976)

2. Brunning, R. D., Bloomfield, C. D., McKenna, R. W., et al.: Bilateral trephine bone marrow biopsies in lymphoma and other neoplastic diseases. Ann. Intern. Med. *82*, 365–366 (1975)
3. Carbone, P. P., Kaplan, H. S., Musshoff, K. et al: Report of the Committee on Hodgkin's Disease Staging Classification. Cancer Res. *31*, 1860–1861 (1971)
4. Chabner, B. A., Johnson, R. E., Young, R. C. et al.: Sequential nonsurgical and surgical staging of non-Hodgkin's lymphoma. Ann. Intern. Med. *85*, 149–154 (1976)
5. DeVita, V. T., Canellos, G. P., Chabner, B. A. et al.: Advanced diffuse histiocytic lymphoma, a potentially curable disease. Lancet. I, 248–251 (1975)
6. Dunnick, N. R., Fuks, Z., Castellino, R. A.: Repeat lymphography in non-Hodgkin's lymphoma. Radiology *115*, 349–354 (1975)
7. Frei, E. III, Luce, J. K., Gamble, J. F. et al.: Combination chemotherapy in advanced Hodgkin's disease. Ann. Intern. Med. *79*, 376–382 (1973)
8. Frei, E. III, Schlossman, S., Israel, M.: New approaches to the treatment of non-Hodgkin's lymphoma. Cancer Treat. Rep. *61*, 1209–1217 (1977)
9. Goffinet, D. R., Castellino, R. A., Kim, H., et al.: Staging laparotomies in unselected patients with non-Hodgkin's lymphomas. Cancer *32*, 672–681 (1972)
10. Hamburger, A. W., Salmon, S. E.: Primary bioassay of human tumor stem cells. Science *197*, 461–463 (1977)
11. Herman, T. S., Jones, S. E.: Systematic restaging in the management of non-Hodgkin's lymphomas. Cancer Treat. Rep. *61*, 1009–1015 (1977)
12. Jones, S. E.: Non-Hodgkin lymphomas. J. Am. Med. Assoc. *234*, 633–638 (1975)
13. Jones, S. E., Lilien, D. L., O'Mara, R. E. et al.: Indium-111 bleomycin tumor scanning in lymphoma. Med. Pediatr. Oncol. *1*, 11–21 (1975)
14. Jones, S. E., Tobias, D. A., Waldman, R. S.: Computed tomographic scanning in patients with lymphoma. Cancer *41*, 480–486 (1978)
15. Kay, D. N., McCready, V. R.: Clinical isotope scanning using ^{67}Ga citrate in the management of Hodgkin's disease. Br. J. Radiol. *45*, 437–442 (1972)
16. Rappaport, H., Winter, W. J., Hicks, E. B.: Follicular lymphoma: A reevaluation of its position in the scheme of malignant lymphoma, based on a survey of 253 cases. Cancer *9*, 792–821 (1956)
17. Schein, P. S., Chabner, B. A., Canellos, G. P. et al.: Potential for prolonged disease-free survival following combination chemotherapy of non-Hodgkin's lymphoma. Blood *43*, 181–189 (1974)
18. Schein, P. S., DeVita, V. T., Jr., Hubbard, S. et al.: Bleomycin, adriamycin, cyclophosphamide, vincristine, and prednisone (BACOP) combination chemotherapy in the treatment of advanced diffuse histiocytic lymphoma. Ann. Intern. Med. *85*, 417–422 (1976)
19. Young, R. C., Chabner, B. A., Canellos, G. P. et al.: Maintenance chemotherapy for advanced Hodgkin's disease in remission. Lancet, *I*, 1339–1342 (1973)

Involvement of the Nervous System in Non-Hodgkin's Lymphomas

B. LONGPRE, J. LAMARCHE, M. ROCHON, and M. LEPINE

Introduction

Nervous system involvement in non-Hodgkin's lymphoma (NHL) is a well-recognized form of neurologic disease. In the past 6 years, we have observed 26 cases of nervous system involvement in our medical center. They were: primary lymphomatous tumor of the central nervous system (CNS) [2], lymphomatous meningitis [14], peripheral nerve and spinal cord compression [4], paraneoplastic polyneuropathy [3], and cranial bone neoplasic lesions and proptosis [3]. Our presentation will be concerned only with primary and secondary lymphomas of the CNS.

Materials and Methods

This is a retrospective study of 138 patients who were admitted to the Centre Hospitalier Universitaire de Sherbrooke from 1970–1976. The Ann Arbor classification [3] for the clinical staging of extent of the patients' lymphomas was used; routine laparotomy was not part of the regimen. The lymph nodes and bone marrow biopsies were reviewed by two pathologists. The lymphomas were classified histologically according to the criteria proposed by RAPPAPORT [13]. The neurologic involvement was confirmed either by the presence of malignant cells in the cerebrospinal fluid (CSF) during life or at the time of autopsy. The patients were treated by a modification of the MOPP, the CVPP regimen [11]; they received, whenever possible, six or more cycles.

Ten patients received intrathecal methotrexate twice a week until disappearance of the malignant cells, which was then followed by a weekly administration of this drug. Two patients also received radiotherapy (2400 rad). The autopsy material was examined both by a pathologist and a neuropathologist. It included specimens from the brain, spinal cord, meninges, and cranial nerves.

Results

Primary Malignant Lymphoma of the CNS

There were two patients, one male and one female (both 55 years of age). They both had personality changes along with symptoms and signs of increased intracranial pressure. The type of tumor was a histiocytic lymphoma. In one patient, it was localized in the cerebellum and in the other patient, it was localized in the frontal lobe with extension to the corpus callosum (Fig. 1 and 2). Both patients died within weeks and had no opportunity of receiving any radiotherapy or chemotherapy. Autopsies showed minimal lymphomatous infiltration of the kidneys in one patient.

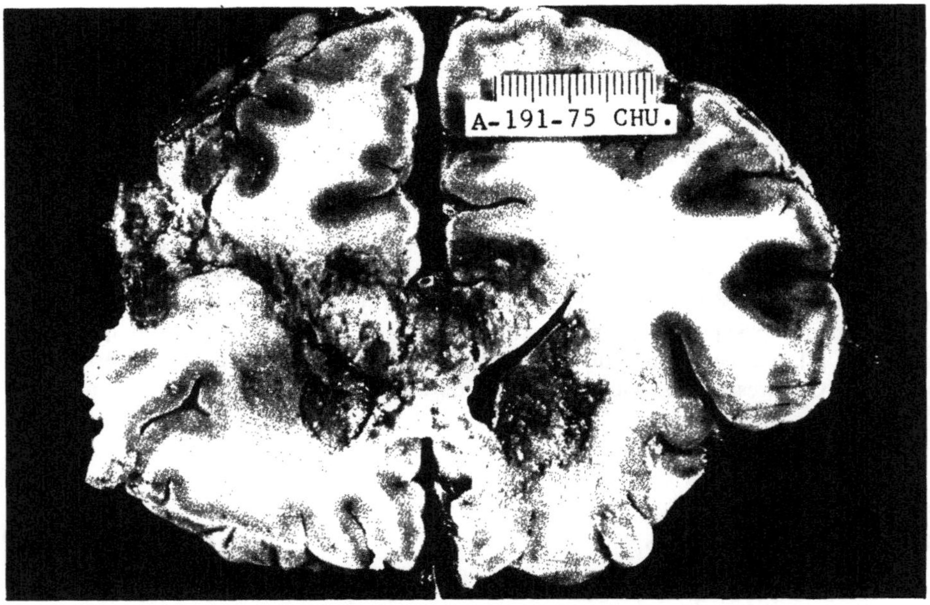

Fig. 1. Infiltration of the corpus callosum and basal ganglia by primary histiocytic lymphoma

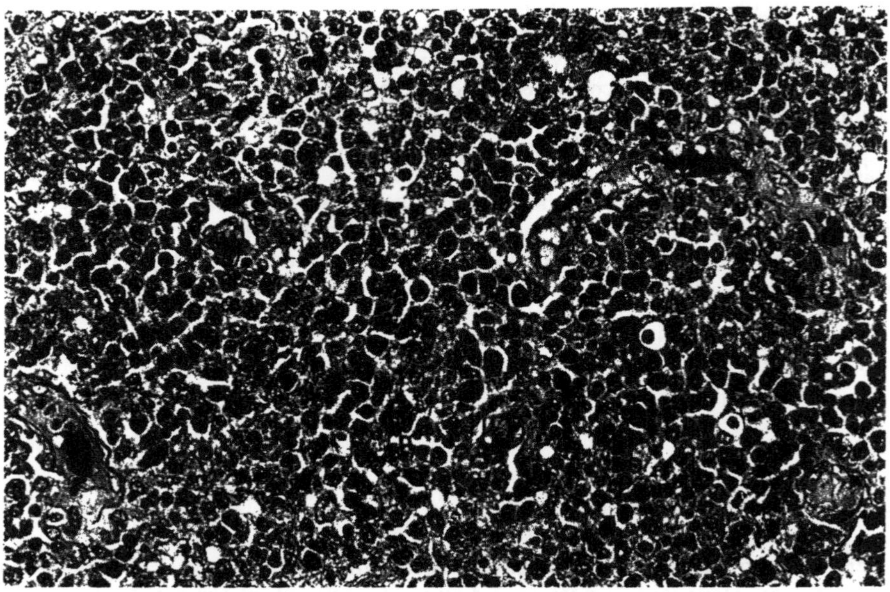

Fig. 2. Primary histiocytic lymphoma of the brain (H & E × 750)

Lymphomatous Meningitis (LM)

There were 14 patients, seven males and seven females, with an age distribution that was the same as for the whole group (Fig. 3). The incidence of LM was 10% and of the more malignant variety, 16%. Thirteen patients were at stage III or IV at the time of diagnosis; of these patients, two had leukemia at the onset, the remaining patient was at stage I, 4 years prior to the occurrence of the neurologic complication. The types of primary lymphomas found were as follows: poorly differentiated nodular lymphocytic lymphoma, [1]; histiocytic lymphoma, [9]; poorly differentiated lymphocytic lymphoma, [2]; and undifferentiated lymphoma, [2]. Seven patients had gross or microscopic localized neoplasic infiltration of the cranial dura. This dural infiltration, which was found at autopsy, was the only evidence of nervous system involvement in three of the cases. In the other four patients, the dural involvement was associated with an infiltration of the leptomeninges and the cranial nerves; the nervous parenchyma together with the choroid plexus were implicated in half of these patients (Figs. 4, 5, and 6). The bone marrow was infiltrated from the onset in five patients; also simultaneously with the lymphomatous meningitis in four patients. The neurologic involvement occurred early in four of the patients, later during the course of the disease in six, with an average of 5 months after the onset. It was found at autopsy in four additional patients.

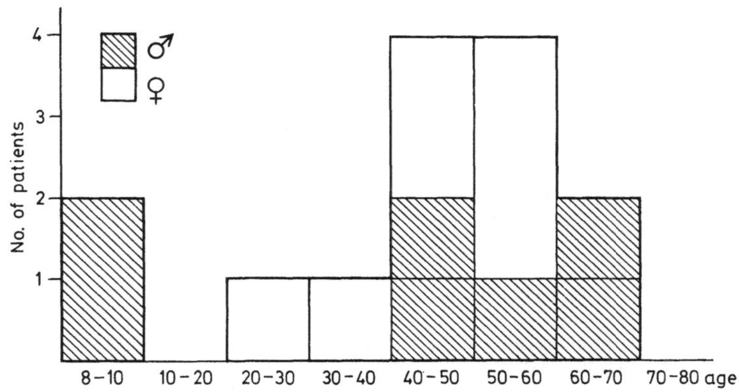

Fig. 3. Age and sex distribution in 14 patients with lymphamatous meningitis

Initial symptoms and signs included the following: cranial nerve palsy (II, VI, VII) (six patients), meningismus (five patients), increased intracranial pressure syndrome (four patients), and ataxia (one patient). Some patients had more than one of these parameters. The examination of the CSF with the cytocentrifuge permitted visualization of the malignant cells in all cases when the neurologic involvement was suspected: either clinically, when the electroencephalogram showed bilateral, diffuse, slow sinusoidal waves, or when the echoencephalogram showed a displacement of the third ventricle.

Treatment was usually followed by a regression of most symptoms and signs and by disappearance of the malignant cells from the CSF. However, this improvement was usually shortlived. Eight patients died with an average survival time of 6 months. Two patients are still alive. One patient, after 5 months, is showing persistent signs of systemic and CNS disease, and the other patient, after 12 months, is asymptomatic without systemic or CNS disease. In six patients (50%), the neurologic complications were thought to be a direct cause of death.

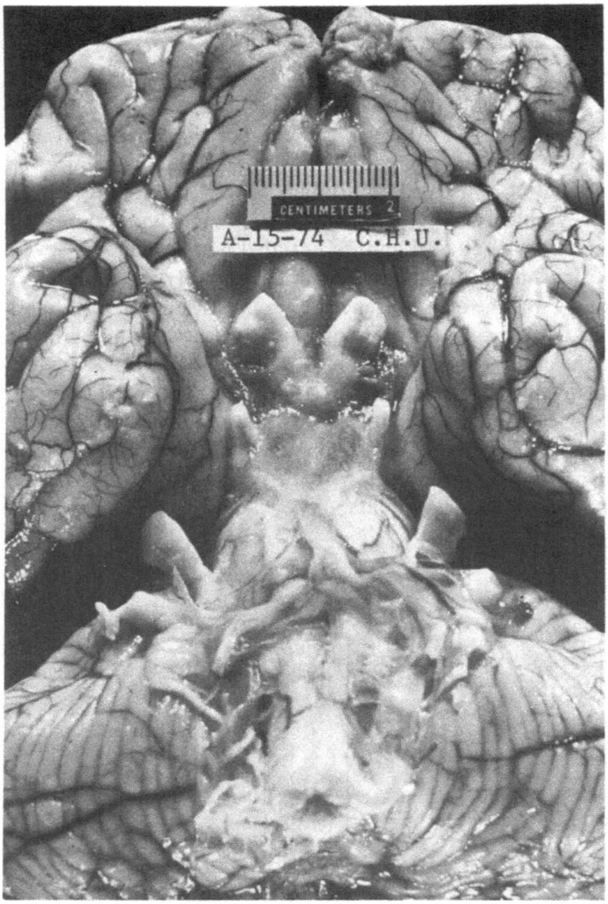

Fig. 4. Note the cloudening of the leptomeninges and the thickening of the cranial nerves produced by the lymphomatous infiltration

Discussion

Primary lymphoma of the CNS is rare. The largest series to date is that of HENRY et al. who reported 83 cases in 1974 [7]; these authors proposed that the common origin for the primitive cells located in the perivascular area of both peripheral organs and CNS could best explain the histologic similarity between CNS and peripheral malignant lymphoma. Six of the 83 cases showed visceral lesions at autopsy that were not suspected during life of the patient. Survival time [15], with or without treatment, is brief. Only the occasional patient lives more than 5 years. Our study appears to be similar to that of Henry et al.

Meningeal infiltration by lymphoma was considered uncommon until recently. At autopsy, JOHN and NABARRO found 2 examples in 93 patients [8] and SPARLING et al. found 1 in 118 [16]. However, GRIFFIN et al., in 140 autopsies 6 years ago, reported 15 histologically confirmed cases [6]. The incidence in our series was 10% and 16% of the more malignant variety. This figure increases in the series published where the lymphoma is undifferentiated [2], in children [1], in adolescents with mediastinal localization [10], and in one instance where the patient had achieved complete remission [2].

Lymphomatous meningitis bears some clinical and pathologic similarities to leukemic meningitis. The presentation in both situations can be insidious and the histologic picture is generally similar. This complication, however, is more frequent in acute leukemia [12]. While it occurs during remission in the leukemias [12], it has been reported only once in the

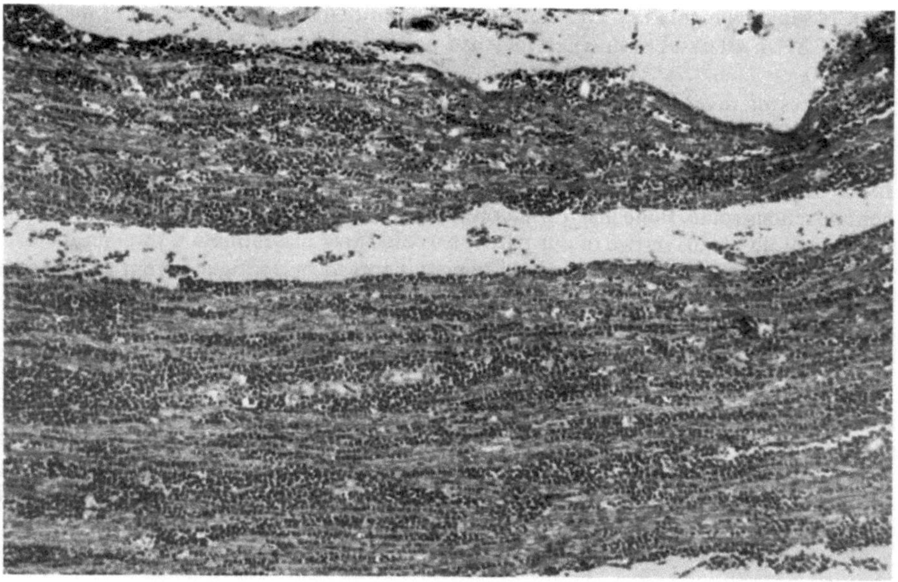

Fig. 5. Facial nerve with extensive secondary lymphocytic lymphomatous infiltration (H & E × 300)

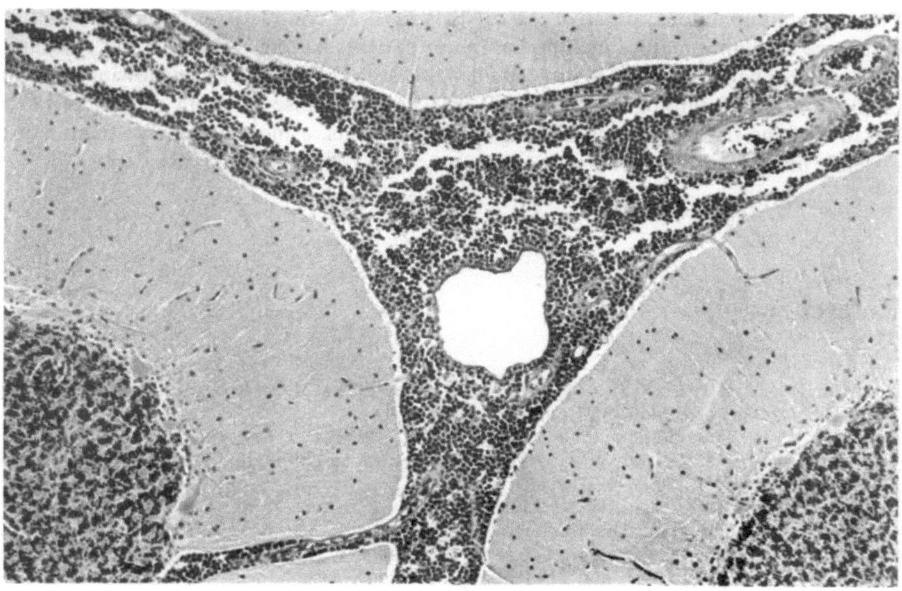

Fig. 6. Cerebellar leptomeninges densely infiltrated by secondary lymphocytic lymphoma (H & E × 300)

lymphomas [2]. Cranial nerve palsy appears to be more common in the lymphomas [9]. Finally, the anatomic lesion is widespread in the leukemias, while it may be localized in the lymphomas [6].

The high frequency of histiocytic lymphoma in this series suggests that the CSF should be examined routinely in patients with stage IV disease, especially if the bone marrow is infiltrated. It was infiltrated in nine of our patients; in four instances, it was simultaneous with the CNS involvement. The cytocentrifuge [5] permitted the demonstration of malignant cells in the CSF in all cases even when they had not been detected by routine examination (three patients).

The routes of invasion of the CNS by lymphoma have not been clearly established. The lymphomas that involve the retroperitoneal or mediastinal lymph nodes have a tendency to disseminate into the epidural space and the spinal cord through the draining lymphatics of the spinal canal. It is also probable that some lymphoma cells spread to the nervous system via the hematogenous route. Bone marrow involvement is frequent [8, 12], and the striking infiltration of the choroid plexus in two of our patients would favor dissemination through the CSF. The finding of solitary dural nodules could suggest a spread by contiguity from an adjacent bone marrow lesion [2, 6].

Survival time of our patients was brief and is comparable with other studies [2, 6]. More aggressive treatment [2, 4, 14] of the underlying disease with multiple drug combinations that should include adriamycin and bleomycin is now recommended because of the present poor results, perhaps a prophylactic treatment of the CNS with methotrexate, and possibly other drugs, should be carried out in those patients having a more malignant variety of lymphoma with systemic disease, or as found in lymphomas in children, adolescents with mediastinal localization and T-lymphocytes, and perhaps in those that have achieved a complete remission.

Conclusion

Primary lymphomatous tumor of the CNS is rare. In contrast, we observed a rather high incidence of lymphomatous meningitis. In our patients having lymphomatous meningitis, 13 of 14 patients had disseminated disease when first seen with the majority showing bone marrow infiltration. The neurologic involvement was a direct cause of death in 50% of our cases. Because of the poor prognosis in this group of patients, a more aggressive treatment of the systemic disease and a prophylactic treatment of the CNS should be considered.

References

1. Aur, R. J. A., Hustu, O., Simone, J. V., Pratt, C. B., Pinkel, D.: Therapy of Localized and Regional lymphosarcoma of Childhood. Cancer *27*, 1328 (1971)
2. Bunn, P. A., Jr., Schein, P. S., Banks, P. M., DeVita, V. T., Jr.: Central Nervous System Complications in Patients With Diffuse Histiocytic and Undifferentiated Lymphoma: Leukemia Revisited. Blood *47* (1), 3, (1976)
3. Carbone, R. P., Kaplan, H. S., Musshoff, K., Smithers, D. W., Tubiana, M.: Report of the Committee on Hodgkin's Disease Staging Classification. Cancer Res. *31*, 1860 (1971)
4. DeVita, V. T., Canellos, G. P., Chabner, B., Schein, P., Hubbard, S., Young, R. C.: Advanced Diffuse Histiocytic Lymphoma, a Potentially Curable Disease. Lancet *1975 I*, 248
5. Evans, D., O'Rourke, C., Morris-Jones, P.: Cerebrospinal Fluid in Acute Leukemia of Childhood Studies with the Cytocentrifuge. J. Clin. Pathol. *27*, 226 (1974)

6. Griffin, J. W., Thompson, R. W., Mitchinson, M. J., Kiewiet, J. C., de, Welland, F. H.: Lymphomatous leptomeningitis. Am. J. Med. *51*, 200 (1971)
7. Henry, J. M., Heffner, R. R., Jr., Dillard, S. H., Earle, K. M., Davis, R. L.: Primary Malignant Lymphomas of the Central Nervous System. Cancer *34*, 1293 (1974)
8. John, H. T., Nabarro, J. D. N.: Intracranial Manifestations of Malignant Lymphoma. Br. J. Cancer *9* (3), 386 (1955)
9. Law, I. P., Dick, F. R., Bloom, J., Bergevin, P. R.: Involvement of the Central Nervous System in Non-Hodgkin Lymphoma. Cancer *36* (1), 225 (1975)
10. Nathwani N., Kim, H., Rappaport, H.: Malignant Lymphoma, Lymphoblastic. Cancer *8* (2), 964 (1976)
11. Nicholson, W. M., Beard, M. E. J., Crother, D., Stanfield, A. G., Vartan, C. P., Malpas, J. S., Fairley, G., Hamilton, R. B. Scott: Combination Chemotherapy in generalised Hodgkin's Disease. Br. Med. J. *1970 III*, 7
12. Nyman, C. B., Bogle, J. M., Brubaker, C. A., Williams, H., Hammond, D.: Central Nervous System Involvement in Children. Blood *25*, 1 (1968)
13. Rappaport, H.: Tumors of the Hemopoietic System. Atlas of Tumor Pathology, Sect. 3, Fasc. 8. Washington, DC: Armed forces Institute of Pathology 1966
14. Rodriguez, V., Cabanillas, F., Burgess, M. A., McKelvey, E. M., Valdivieso, M., Bodey, G. P., Freireich, E. J.: Combination Chemotherapy ("CHOP-Bleo") in Advanced (Non-Hodgkin) Malignant Lymphoma. Blood *49* (3) 325 (1977)
15. Schaumburg, H. H., Plank, C. R., Adams, R. D.: The Reticulum Cell Sarcoma—Microglioma Group of Brain tumors. Brain *95* 199, (1972)
16. Sparling, H. L., Adams, R. D., Parker, F., Jr.: Involvement of the Nervous System by Malignant Lymphoma. Medicine *26*, 285 (1947)

Leukemic (or Stage V) Lymphosarcoma

G. Mathé, J. L. Misset, M. Gil-Delgado, M. Delgado, and F. De Vassal

There are two possible involvements of the bone marrow (Table 1) by a lymphosarcoma (LS): 1. the first, which characterizes a *stage IV* LS, consists of nodules of lymphosarcoma cells which appear at histologic examination circumscribed, with preservation of fat cells (Fig. 1). No more than 10% LS cells are found on the smears of the bone marrow taken by aspiration in one site, and most sites are normal when bone marrow is taken up by aspiration on several sites. Finally, there is no bone marrow insufficiency, no anemia, no neutropenia, and no thrombocytopenia.

2. The other involvement, which could be called "*stage V*", is *leukemic*: the infiltration of the marrow appears diffuse and most often regular, with disappearance of fat cells (Fig. 1). One finds more than 10% LS cells on *all* smears of bone marrow taken up in several sites. There are manifestations of bone marrow insufficiency, anemia, and/or thrombopenia. These are the two different stages to which two different kinds of treatments are usually applied, as will be seen later. We will also see later that there are intermediate conditions. It is no less important to distinguish two kinds of leukemic LS: 1) *the leukemic, secondarily converted LS*, in which there is a time gap between the nonleukemic phase and the leukemic phase, and 2) *the LS which is leukemic at the outset* ("*d'emblée*" *leukemic LS*) (the diagnosis will be discussed later) and complicated by leukemic infiltration of the marrow from the very beginning.

All histopathologic types of LS may be converted into a leukemic stage as shown in Table 2, in which the WHO categorization is used [20]. The following will not be discussed in this paper:

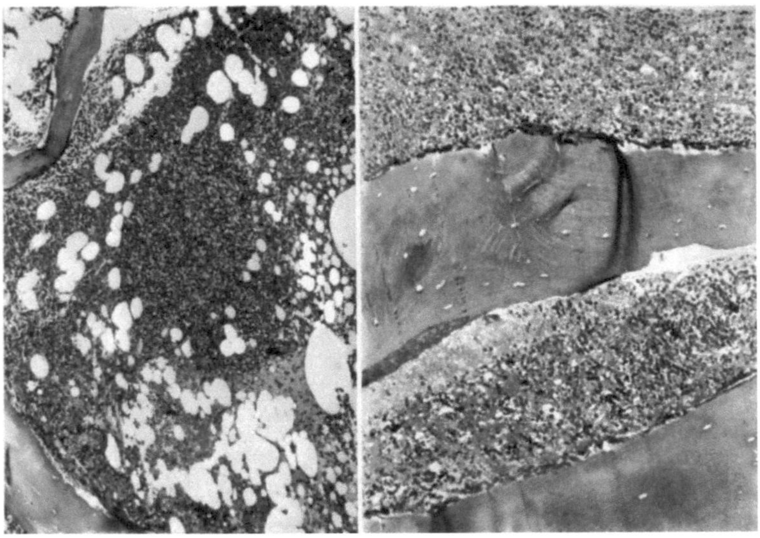

Fig. 1. Histologic aspects of bone marrow in stage IV (left) and in leukemic (or stage V) lymphosarcomas (right)

Table 1. *Differential diagnosis between stage IV lymphosarcoma and leukemic (stage V) lymphosarcoma*

	Smear myelogram after bone marrow punctures	*Histology of bone marrow biopsy*	*Blood cytology*	*Other fluids*
Stage IV	< 10% in *some sites* N[a] in other sites	*Circumscribed* nodules, *fat cells preserved*	No manifestation of bone marrow insufficiency	
Leukemic lymphosarcoma	> 10% in *all sites*	*Diffuse* infiltration *fat cells disappeared*	Manifestations of *bone marrow insufficiency*	
Intermediate stage (IV or V?)			Blood circulating neoplastic cells without leukemic myelogram or biopsy histology	Neoplastic cells in CFS fluid without apparent circulating neoplastic cells or/and without leukemic myelogram or biopsy histology

N[a]: normal.

1) plasmocytic LS and its possible conversion to plasmocytic leukemia, which has been the object of several studies [see 31], 2) the conversion of lymphoplasmocytic LS to systemic lymphoplasmocytic neoplasia called essential macroglobulinemia (Waldenström) (25), and 3) the conversion of so-called lymphocytic LS into chronic lymphoid leukemia, both having recently been reviewed by RAPPAPORT [25]. However, we feel it is necessary to make two remarks here: The frontier between localized circumscribed lymphoplasmocytic LS and systemic Waldenström's macroglobulinemia is different in LENNERT'S nomenclature [11, 12] and in others [5, 7, 14, 27] including the WHO classification [20]. LENNERT [11, 12]calls "immunocytoma" not only what the WHO classification calls a lymphoplasmocytic LS but also Waldenström's macroglobulinemia. The incidence of "true" nonleukemic lymphocytic LS, the differentiation of the stage of the cells being controlled by smear cytologic examination, and the leukemia sought by systematic bone marrow aspiration at the very beginning of the disease for cytologic study are very exceptional in our experience (less than 1/200), while RAPPAPORT'S group [25] reported 41 cases of lymphocytic LS, without absolute lymphocytosis or monoclonal serum immunoglobulin at the time of biopsy. The possible conversion of T-cell mycosis fungoïdes into the leukemic stage, called Sezary's syndrome, which has been reported recently will also not be discussed [6]. No remark will be made on leukemic conversion of Burkitt's LS. Hence, we will devote this paper to the *common types* of lymphosarcoma in the WHO categorization (Fig. 2): 1) the prolymphocytic, 2) the lymphoblastic, and 3) the immunoblastic types. Two studies were previously published by our group [18, 29] based on the nomenclature which we were using at the time of these publications [16]. We shall not discuss the difficulties that concern only the nomenclature of cases for which the necessary investigations mentioned above had not been made at all stages of the disease (difficulties which are frequent for so-called "lymphocytic" and "lymphoplasmocytic" LS as seen above). However, we shall consider the diagnostic and treatment difficulties brought up by conditions which appear transitional between some leukemic LS and chronic lymphoid leukemia (CLL).

Table 2. Types of leukemic conversion or LS secondarily in evolution or "d'emblée" (from the very beginning of the lymphosarcoma). Incidence of the different types

	Nonleukemic lymphosarcoma	Leukemic lymphosarcoma
Plasmocytic (B) LS	±	+
Lymphoplasmocytic (B) LS	±	(+)
Lymphocytic (B) LS	±	(+)
Prolymphocytic (B) Centrofoll nodular LS	+ +	±
Prolymphocytic (B) Centrofoll diffused LS	+ + +	$(\underline{++})$
(T) mycosis fungoides	+ +	± (Sezary's disease)
Lymphoblastic (null)	+ +	$(\underline{++})$
Lymphoblastic (T)	+ +	$(\underline{++})$
Burkitt's LS (B)	+	+
Immunoblastic (B)	+ +	(+)
Immunoblastic (T)	+ +	(±)

Common types of lymphosarcoma are in italic.
± to + + + indicate relative incidence of the disease presentations.

Patients and Methods

As seen in Table 3, the present study concerns 24 cases of *secondary* leukemic LS, i.e., which were converted to leukemia or stage V. Six were prolymphocytic (centrofollicular), one was

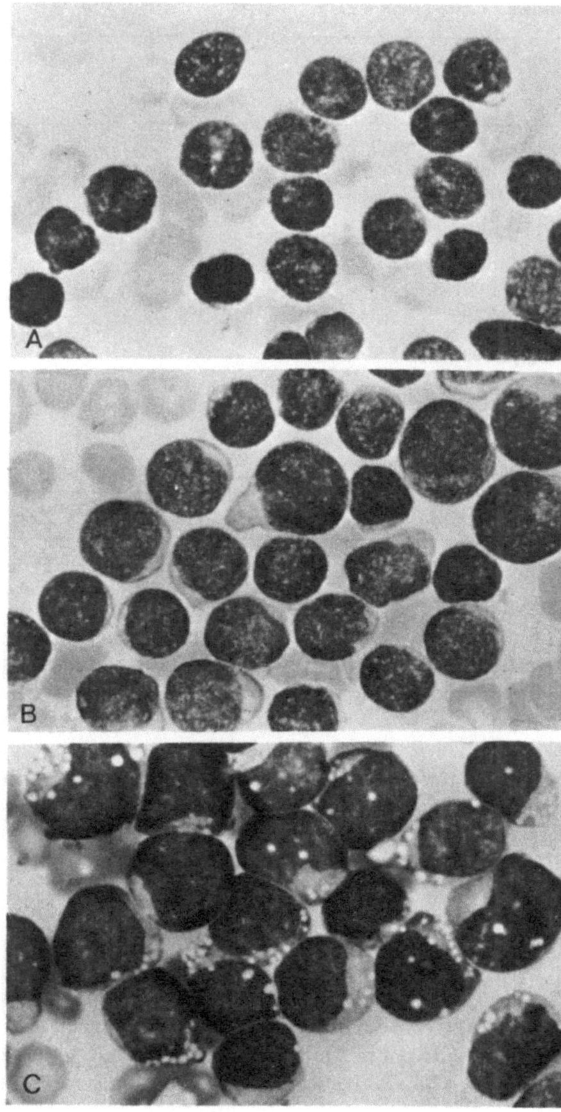

Fig. 2. Cytologic aspects of the three common types of leukemic LS.
(A) Prolymphocytic type;
(B) Lymphoblastic type;
(C) Immunoblastic type.

nodular, two were diffuse at the beginning of the disease; in three cases, the only pathologic material available at the time of leukemic conversion was taken at that time; six were lymphoblastic, three were immunoblastic; and nine were not classified because the only material available when we received these patients had been prepared outside our service. No further, more complete histocytologic study was subsequently undertaken by our service. This study also concerns 31 cases of "d'emblée" leukemic LS: six prolymphocytic, 14 lymphoblastic, three immunoblastic, and eight unclassified. Finally, we have followed ten cases (about which we are still hesitant) *between the diagnosis of leukemic lymphosarcoma and CLL.*

Age and sex of patients are given in Table 3. One sees that all types concern all ages, except the prolymphocytic LS and the neoplasia transitional between LS and CLL which do not appear in children. Males are more frequently affected than females by most of the types.

Table 3. Cases (1969–1977)

	LS observed	Leukemic LS	Age		Sex	
			Extremes	Median	M	F
Secondarily leukemic LS						
Prolymphocytic (centrofoll.) LS	36	6	18–55	35	3	3
Nodular	19	1				
Diffuse	14	2				
Dgc. at the leukemic phase	3	3				
Lymphoblastic LS	15	6	6–32	16	5	1
Immunoblastic LS	18	3	8–60	10	0	3
Unclassified LS	28	9	3–56	12	5	4
		24 (25%)				
D'emblée leukemic LS	31	31				
Prolymphocytic		6	12–45	21	5	1
Lymphoblastic		14	2–53	16	12	2
Immunoblastic		3	5–30	22	2	1
Unclassified		8	3–39	16	8	0
Transitional neoplasias between CLL	10(?)	10(?)	37–66	55	5	5
Reticulosarcoma	11	0	20–66	48	6	5

The patients were submitted to clinical, histocytologic, and when possible, immunologic investigations [2] for diagnosis, WHO typing [20], and staging [15].

Figure 3 shows the types of regimens which were followed before and after leukemic conversion. Before, we use a myelotoxic chemotherapy [24]. After, we apply the same regimen as is applied to primary acute leukemia patients [22], a regimen which is not myelotoxic because of the constant bone marrow insufficiency in the leukemic conditions.

Results and Discussion

Leukemic (Stage V)

The overall incidence of leukemic LS is 65 out of 138 disseminated LS (47%), if we include the ten patients whose disease is transitional between leukemic LS and CLL, and 55 out of 128 (43%), if we do not include these ten patients. Roughly, the leukemic conversion affects almost 50% of LS patients. Hence, this study of the leukemic stage is of primary importance—more important than it appears in the literature, where it is rarely studied [28].

Table 3 underlines the striking difference between LS and reticulosarcoma as far as their leukemic conversion is concerned. We saw no leukemic conversions among our 11 cases of reticulosarcoma (according to the WHO classification) [20].

Secondarily Leukemic LS

Overall Data and Considerations

The overall incidence of secondary leukemic conversion of all *common* types of LS is 25%, as seen in Table 3. This incidence is a little higher than that mentioned by Rosenberg et al. [28], who gave an incidence of between 5% and 10%. This may be due to the fact that in contrast to the Stanford group, our group receives more stages III and IV than stages I and II.

STAGE III AND IV LYMPHOSARCOMA

INDUCTION CHEMOTHERAPY									RADIOTHERAPY	COMPLEMENTARY CHEMOTHERAPY					IMMUNOTHERAPY
A	A	A	A	A	A	A	A	A	on "Icebergs" 3000 to 4000 rads	V	V	V	V	to be followed for one year	BCG + leukemic cells (beginning after about 20 months of chemotherapy)
VM	VM	VM	VM	VM	VM	VM	VM	VM		C	C	C	C		
C	C	C	C	C	C	C	C	C		P	P	P	P		
P	P	P	P	P	P	P	P	P							
0	1	2	3	4	5	6	7	8		0	1	2	3		

(time in months)

A	Adriamycin	50 mg/m2	D 1
VM	VM 26	60 mg/m2	D 2
C	Cyclophosphamide	300 mg/m2	D 3-4
P	Prednisone	40 mg/m2	D 3-7

V	Vincristine	1,5 mg/m2	D 1
C	Cyclophosphamide	300 mg/m2	D 2-5
P	Prednisone	40 mg/m2	D 2-6

LEUKAEMIC LYMPHOSARCOMA

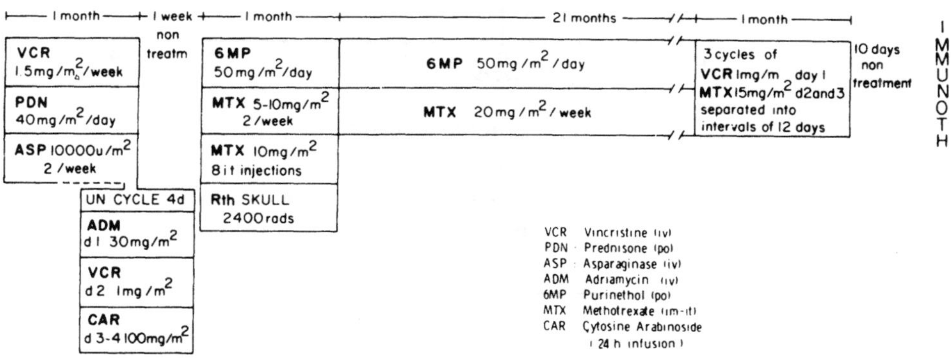

Fig. 3. Types of therapeutic regimens followed before (above) and after (below) leukemic conversion.

Data Considerations According to WHO LS Types (Fig. 4)

In WHO *prolymphocytic* (*centrofollicular*) *types*, the incidence of leukemic conversion was 17% (6 out of 36 cases). At the time of conversion, stage III was found in one patient and stage II in five patients. The duration of nonleukemic LS before conversion was 6 years for one patient and varied from 1 year to 4 months for the other five. The architecture before leukemic conversion was diffuse in two and still nodular in one out of the three cases in which it could be studied.

The presentation of the leukemic stage was variable. One case presented a mediastinal and pleural involvement, one case an abdominal mass, four cases large polyadenomegaly with hepatomegaly and pleural effusion in two, and nerve infiltrations in one. No central nervous system (CNS) involvement was observed. The bone marrow contained, at detection of leukemia, less than 50% LS cells in two cases, between 50% and 80% in two, and more that 80% in two. Such cells were found in the peripheral blood on routine hemogram in four patients.

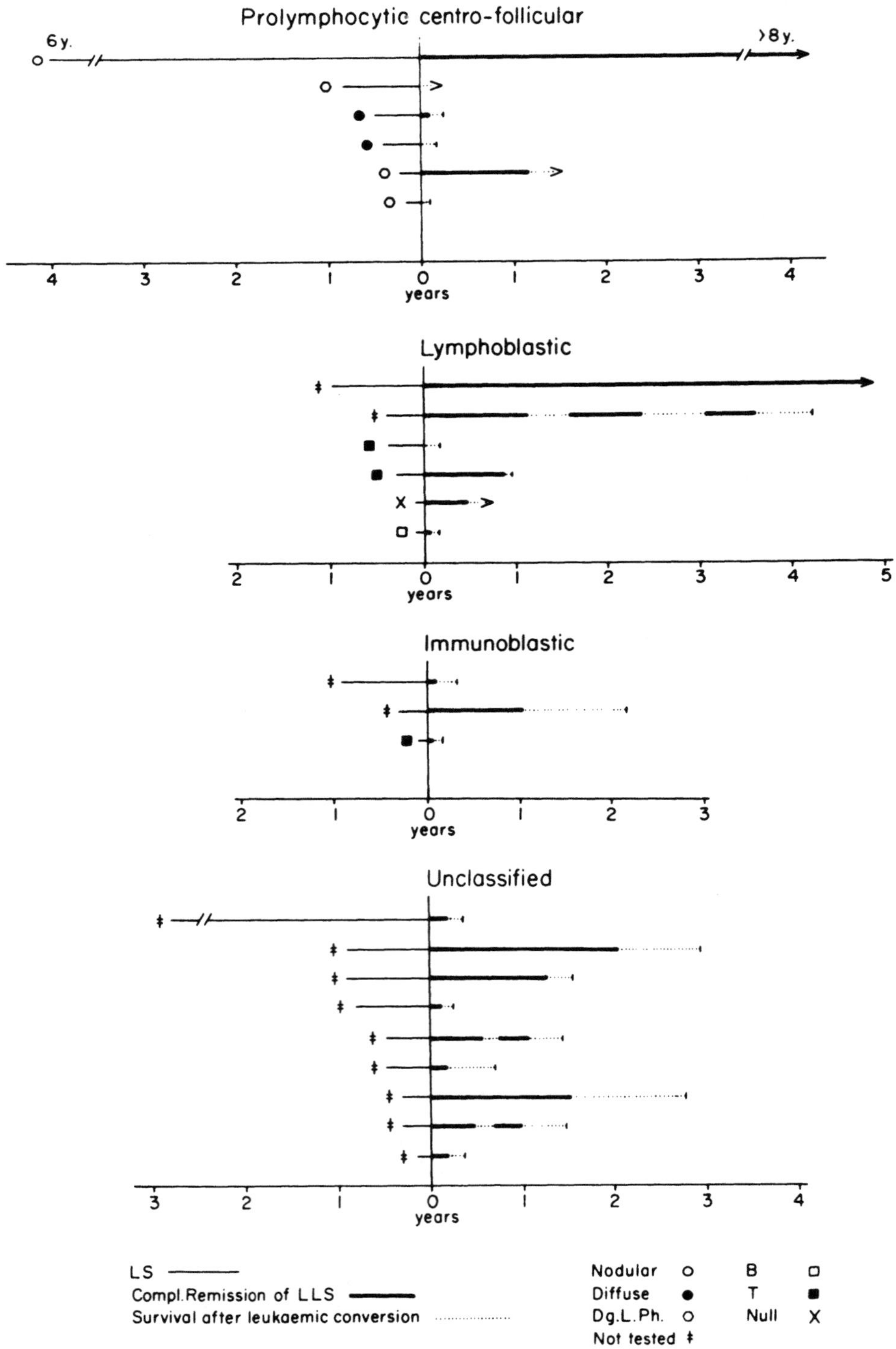

Fig. 4. Evolution before and after leukemic conversion of LS secondarily transformed into leukemia

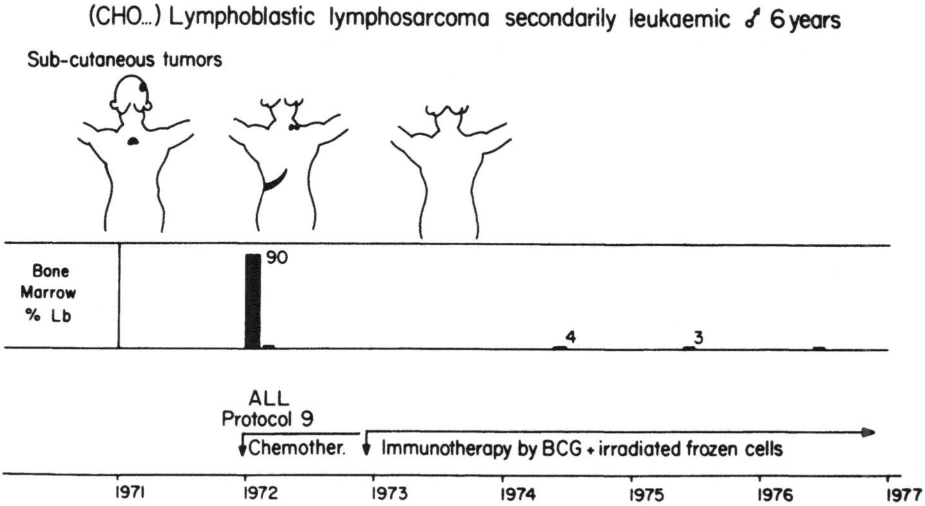

Fig. 5. The course of a patient treated in 1971 for a stage IV lymphoblastic LS (with mediastinal and skin involvements) converted into leukemia in 1972 and still in complete remission in 1977 after the application of our ALL protocol comprising systemic chemotherapy, CNS, chemoradiotherapy, and immunotherapy

Prognosis after leukemic conversion was poor except in two patients. One who was treated successively by chemoradiotherapy followed by active immunotherapy (the treatment applied by our group to acute lymphoid leukemia (ALL) patients) has been in complete remission for more than 8 years after leukemic conversion. It should be noted that this patient had the longest preleukemic phase (6 years) (Fig. 4). A second patient who had a short preleukemic phase (4 months) was in complete remission for more than 1½ years (Fig. 4).

In WHO *lymphoblastic types* the incidence of leukemic conversion was 40% (6 cases out of 15). The stages at the time of conversions were stage II for one patient (it was a case of mediastinal LS) and stage IV for five patients. The duration of nonleukemic LS before conversion varied from 1 year to 4 months as seen in Figure 4. The leukemic cells were T in two cases and null in one of the three cases in which they were studied for immune markers.

The presentation of the leukemic stage was different from that of the prolymphocytic type. Three cases presented a mediastinal involvement, four cases peripheral lymphoadenopathies, two cases pleural effusions, two cases hepatomegaly, one case skin lesions, one case an endonasal mass, and one case a CNS and meningeal involvement. The bone marrow contained, at detection of leukemia, less than 50% LS cells in two cases, between 50% and 80% in two cases, and more than 80% in two other cases. Such cells were found in the peripheral blood on routine hemogram in two cases.

Prognosis after leukemic conversion is variable and globally no different from that of the prolymphocytic type. One patient who successively received chemoradiochemotherapy and immunotherapy has been in perfect remission for more that 5 years (Figs. 4 and 5). Other patients relapsed and most of them died before 1 year (Fig. 4).

In WHO *immunoblastic types*, the incidence of leukemic conversion was only 17% (3 cases out of 18). This low incidence of conversion for this type of LS, the prognosis of which is the most severe [19], indicates that the severity of the type of LS is due rather to the large chemoresistant tumor masses than to the tendency for leukemic conversion.

Before conversion, two out of three patients were at stage II and one at stage IV. The duration of the nonleukemic LS before conversion was as short as in the lymphoblastic type cases; it also varied from 1 year to 4 months. The cells for only one patient were tested for the immune surface markers and they were T. The presentation of the leukemic stage was variable. One patient presented a mediastinal involvement; hence, such an involvement does not necessarily mean that the LS is lymphoblastic. One patient had an abdominal involvement, which is not rare in immunoblastic LS [19]. Three patients had peripheral lymphadenopathies. There was no case with CNS involvement.

The bone marrow contained, at detection of leukemia, less than 50% LS cells in one case and more than 80% in two. Such cells were not found in the circulating blood on routine hemogram in any of the three patients. Prognosis after leukemic conversion is poor. The three patients died 26, 4, and 2 months, respectively, after leukemic conversion. Only one had a long remission (of 1 year) (Fig. 4).

The duration of the *unclassified LS* before conversion and their prognosis after leukemic transformation are shown in Figure 4.

"D'emblée" Leukemic LS

This entity, characterized by the leukemic extension of the disease at its very beginning, includes, in our definition, the cases of lymphoid neoplasias with at least two parameters: 1) either large lymphoid or extralymphoid masses with bone marrow leukemic cell involvement inferior to 20% and 2) LS cell aspect of the leukemic cells. We have collected 31 cases (Tables 3 and 4); the extreme ages are 2—53 years, hence it is a disease of the first part of life. Twenty-seven males and four females. Thirteen patients had a mediastinal mass. Four cases presented only abdominal masses. Three patients had pleural effusions and one skeletal lesions. The lymphoid masses were very large in ten patients. LS cells were circulating in the peripheral blood of 23 patients.

As seen in Table 4, six patients had a WHO prolymphocytic type of LS, 14 a lymphoblastic, and three an immunoblastic type. Eight were not classified. Table 4 lists the main clinical presentations according to these histocytologic types and to the immune markers for the few patients who were studied for these markers. Most mediastinal forms were lymphoblastic type, and half of the abdominal forms were immunoblastic type. One case of prolymphocytic "d'emblée" leukemic LS was T, which is different from all secondarily converted prolymphocytic LS tested which were B. It brings to mind ALL, for which we described a prolymphocytic type which can be T or null [3, 17].

Table 4 also gives the incidence of complete remission obtained with the same regimen as that used in ALL (Fig. 3) [22]. This incidence is high, 87% (27 patients out of 31). It is especially high in the prolymphocytic (6/6) and lymphoblastic (13/14) types, but it is low (1/3) in the immunoblastic type.

The (direct) curves of cumulative remission and survival durations are shown in Figure 6. One sees that the curve of remission descends with a median at 5.5 months but is broken at the 18th month, after which it may form a plateau. Table 4 shows that the prognosis may be better for the lymphoblastic type than for the overall population, and Figure 7 shows the course of a patient still in remission 8 years after the beginning of the disease and 1.5 years after stopping immunotherapy.

There are now two questions to be discussed. Is "d'emblée" leukemic LS different from ALL? Tables 5 and 6 answer this question. Table 5 summarizes the differences. Concerning the immune markers, there are no T-convoluted lymphoblastic and no B-prolymphocytic subtypes in our ALL patients. The numbers of neoplastic cells in the bone marrow and in the peripheral blood are usually higher and the volumes of lymphoid and extralymphoid masses (tumors) usually larger in "d'emblée" leukemic LS than in ALL. Table 6 shows that the prognosis for ALL patients is better for all ages including children than for "d'emblée" leukemic LS. Hence, it seems useful to separate this entity from ALL.

Secondly, is "d'emblée" leukemic LS different from what Isaacs [10] and Schwartz [30] called

Table 4. "D'emblée" leukemic LS presentation and prognosis according to types

	Lymphoblastic: 14				Immunoblastic: 3		Prolymphocytic: 6				Unclassified: 8				Overall: 31
	Overall	T	Null	NT[a]	Overall	NT	Overall	T	Null	NT	Overall	B	Null	NT	
Clinical presentation															
Mediastinal masses	9				0		1				3				13
Abdominal masses	1				2		1				0				4
Skeletal masses	0				0		0				1				1
Others	4				1		4				5				13
Immune markers		2/14	4/14	8/14		3/3		1/6	2/6	3/6		1/8	1/8	6/8	
Prognosis															
Remission incidence	13/14	1/2	4/4	7/8	1/3		6/6	1/1	1/2	3/3	7/8	1/1	1/1	5/6	27/31 (87%)
Median	10 months														5.5 months
Plateau	50%?														27%?
Survival															
Median	14 months														13 months
Plateau	50%?														37%?

[a] NT = Not tested.

"lymphosarcoma cell leukemia"? The description is based on the aspect of the cells which are "atypical large lymphocytes with reticulated chromatin and a single nucleolus, with variable maturations;" the degree of bone marrow involvement is inferior to that of chronic lymphoid (lymphocytic) leukemia. In fact, SCHWARTZ [30] described two forms: an "acute" one, which corresponds to the above-described d'emblée leukemic LS (in photographs included in his paper, the author shows the different types of cells which we have described—prolymphocytic, lymphoblastic, and immunoblastic) and a "chronic" form, the cells of which are, according to the author, "lymphocytes." This last form corresponds to the third entity which we will now describe.

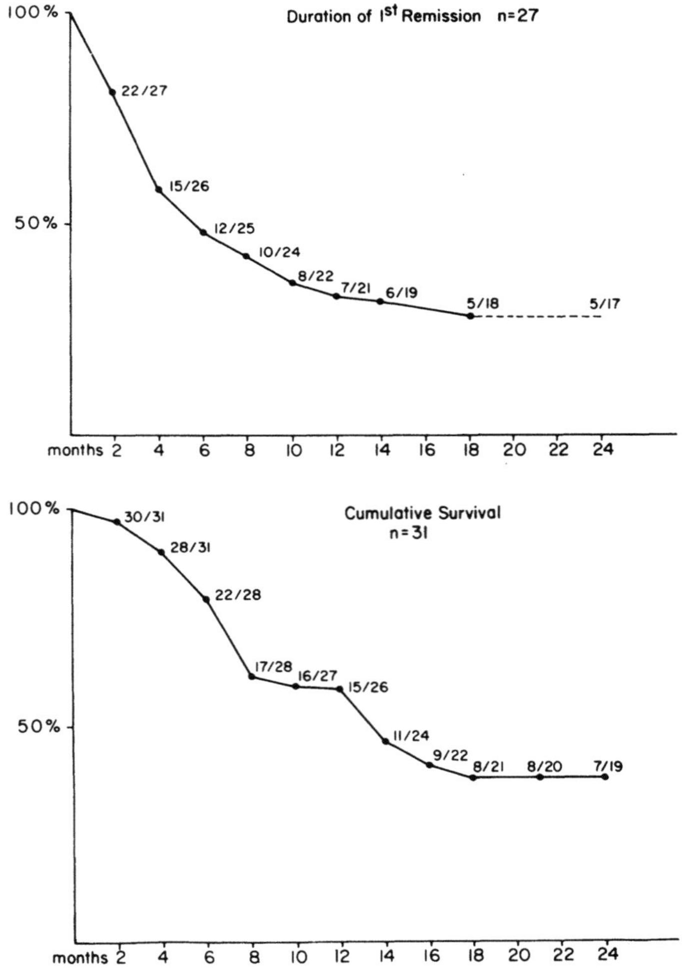

Fig. 6. Direct curves of cumulative duration of remission and survival of patients treated for "d'emblée" leukemic LS with chemo(radio)therapy followed by active immunotherapy

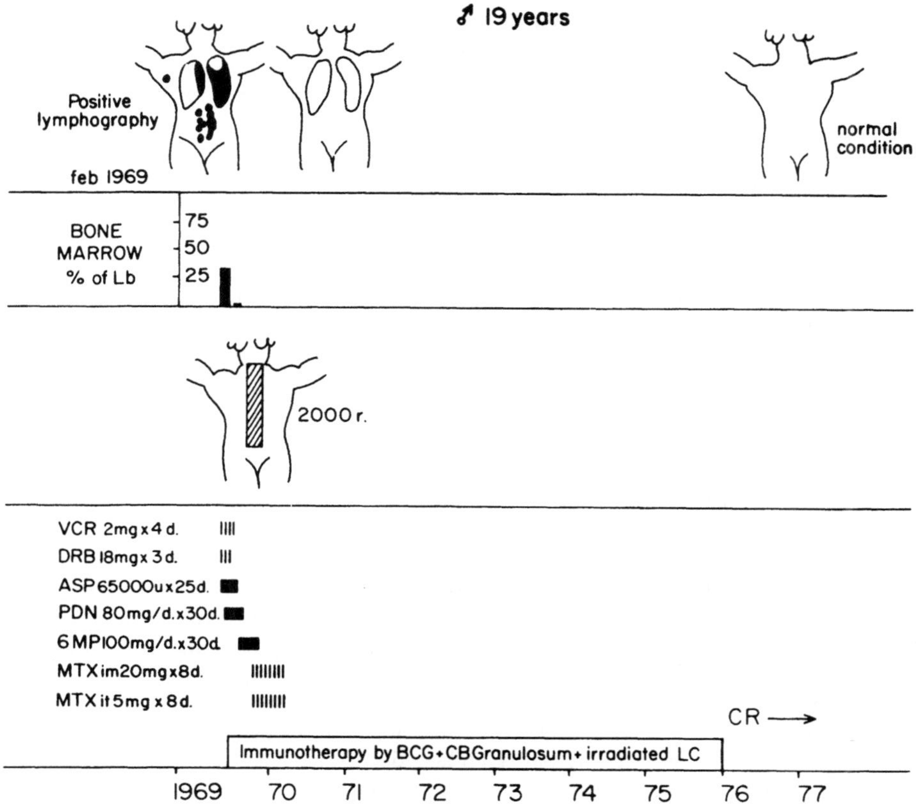

Fig. 7. The course of a patient treated in 1969 for a "d'emblée" leukemic LS by chemoradiotherapy followed by immunotherapy for 6½ years. He is still in complete remission. (LC: leukemic cells)

Table 5. Is d'emblée leukemic LS different from ALL?

Markers	Lymphoblastic			Immunoblastic			Prolymphocytic		
	T conv.[a]	T nonconv.	Null	T	B	Null	T	B	Null
Leukemic LS	+	+	+	+	+	+	+	+	+
ALL		+	+	+	+	+	+		+
Hematology									
Neoplastic cell number in bone marrow			ALL	>	LLS				
Neoplastic cell number in peripheral blood			ALL	>	LLS				
Clinical presentation									
Lymphoid masses			ALL	<	LLS				
Extralymphoid masses			ALL	<	LLS				

[a] T conv.: T-convoluted cells.

Table 6. Is d'emblée leukemic LS different from ALL?

		All ages	Children
Prognosis			
% of 1st remission	LLS[a]	87%	78%
	ALL[b]	89%	97
Median of 1st remission	LLS	5.5 months	5 months
	ALL	18 months	21months
Plateau of 1st remission	LLS	27% (?)	33% (?)
	ALL	37%	50%
Median of survival	LLS	13 months	7 months
	ALL	34 months	> 60 months
Plateau of survival	LLS	37% (?)	30% (?)
	ALL	45%	60%

[a] LLS: leukemic lymphosarcoma.
[b] Results of protocol ALL 9 (See 18).

Is there a lymphoid neoplasia transitional between leukemic LS and chronic lymphocytic leukemia?

Table 7 summarizes the data on the ten patients who posed this question. As seen in this Table, there was no sex predominance. The median age was 55 years, the extreme ages were 37 and 66 years; hence, this population is a little older than that of prolymphocytic LS and a little younger than that of chronic lymphocytic leukemia (CLL). All patients presented large adenopathies and one a pleural effusion. Three patients had circulating leukemic cells. The bone marrow of all patients contained more than 50% of mononuclear cells. They were called "prolymphocytic" in nine patients and "lymphocytic" in one. They were B cells in all patients, but their intensity of fluorescence in the immunofluorescence test was greater in these ten patients than it was in CLL, and as great as it is in prolymphocytic centrofollicular LS, an observation also made by Aisenberg et al. [1]. Thus, we were tempted to consider this disease as a leukemic prolymphocytic LS, but the leukemic LS regimen, i.e., the ALL regimen, failed to induce remission in six patients out of seven. In contrast, a therapeutic response of a type

Table 7. Can differential diagnosis between CLL and leukemic LS be difficult?

Transitional forms?		
Difficult cases: 10		
Sex: ♂ = 5; ♀ = 5		
Age: 37 – 66 years (median: 55)		
Clinical	Masses: adenopathies	10/10
	Mesothelial effusion	1/10
Cells	*prolymphocytic*	9
	lymphocytic	1
Number of patients with circulating leukemic cells 3/10		
Markers:[a] + = 0; +++ = 7/7		
Therapeutic response to CLL treatment: (prednimustine or chlorambucyl): 6/8		
Therapeutic response to LS treatment (Fig. 3): 1/3		
Therapeutic response to leukemic lymphosarcoma regimen (Fig. 3): 1/7		

[a] In typical CLL: +
In typical leukemic prolymphocytic LS: variable from + to +++. Same observation as those of Aisenberg (1976) and Clarkson (1977).

similar to that obtained in CLL was given by a CLL treatment (chlorambucil or prednimustine) [21] in six out of eight patients. The survival is as good as that of CLL (Fig. 8).

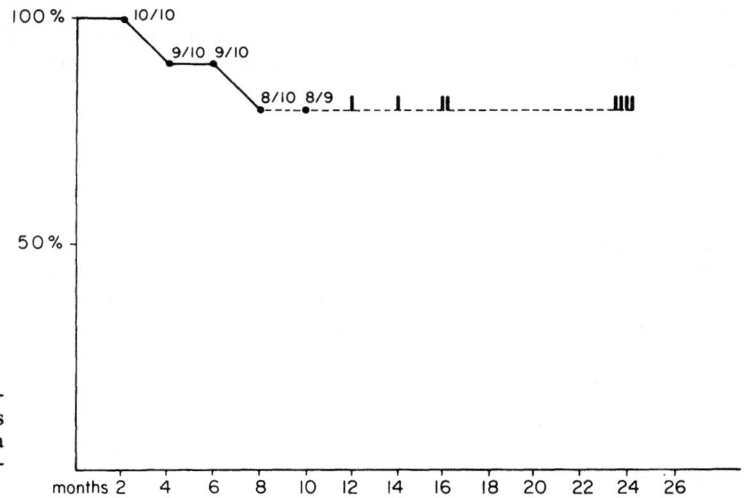

Fig. 8. Cumulative survival of ten patients presenting a neoplasia transitional between leukemic LS and CLL

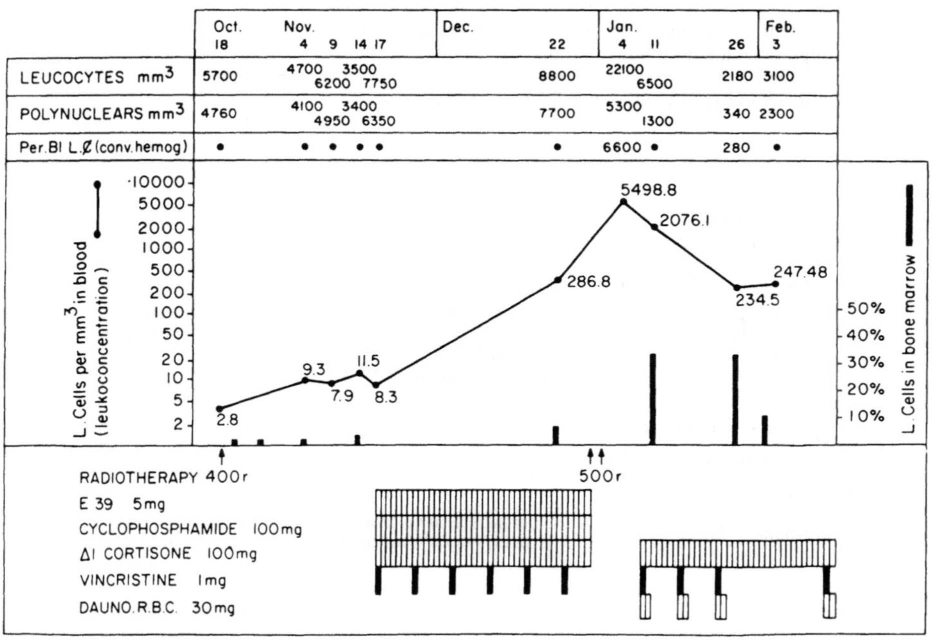

Fig. 9. Peripheral blood circulation of LS cells detected by blood leukoconcentrates before leukemic bone marrow invasion

Thus, those ten patients seem to carry a prolymphocytic leukemia having the cellular characteristics of prolymphocytic LS but the therapeutic sensitivity of CLL. This picture corresponds to the description of Galton's [8] prolymphocytic leukemia on the cell aspect but not on the leukemic cell content of the peripheral blood (which is high in Galton's leukemia) nor on the clinical presentation (which comprises a massive enlargement of the spleen and sometimes of the liver in Galton's leukemia), nor on the response to CLL treatment (which is poor in Galton's leukemia), nor on the survival (which is usually short in Galton's leukemia).

Frontiers Between Stages II, III, and IV and Leukemic (Stage V) LS: Immune Staging

We have discussed the frontiers between leukemic LS and leukemia, which are not clear-cut. The line of demarcation between leukemic LS and so-called nonleukemic LS remains equally ambiguous. As a matter of fact, this frontier depends on what tests are used. We have seen cases of LS with a few LS cells circulating in the peripheral blood without leukemic involvement of the marrow, as described in the introduction to this paper.

Table 8. Immune markers staging in the bone marrow and staging of lympho(sarco)ma

Detection by immune markers	B[a]	T (?)	Null (?)
Of blood circulation of neoplastic cells without leukemic microscopic involvement	5	0	1
Of bone marrow involvement without microscopically detectable involvement			
Bone marrow + blood	3		1
Bone marrow alone	4	2	3
Of blood circulation of neoplastic cells without leukemic microscopic involvement and without bone marrow involvement with cells carrying monoclonal immune markers	2		

[a] Proven monoclonality of lymphoid cells in all nine B-cell cases.

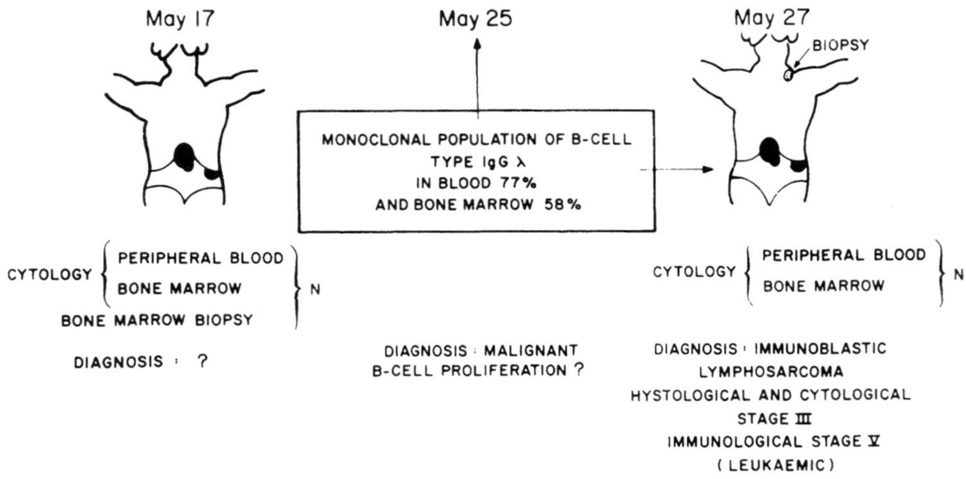

Fig. 10. Value of systematic immunologic membrane marker search in the peripheral blood and bone marrow for the diagnosis and staging of LS

Table 9. CNS Invasion in nonleukemic LS

Neoplastic cells in cerebrospinal fluid with normal blood and bone marrow	
No. of patients	8
First presentation	0
Relapse	8
CNS localization without blood detected lymphosarcoma cells	
Prolymphocytic (centrofollicular) type	0
Lymphoblastic type	5
Immunoblastic type	3

Using a method which concentrates mononuclear cells by blood centrifugation, we were able to detect cases in which the number of circulating LS cells was as high as $300/mm^3$, while there were no more than 2% of such cells on the bone marrow smears, which were considered normal. However, such a presence of LS cells in the blood announces leukemic invasion of the marrow after a short time (Fig. 9).

Moreover, we developed an original method [4] for detecting LS cells in the peripheral blood and in bone marrow. This consists of searching for B-mononuclear markers in cases of B-lymphosarcoma or looking for a high proportion of T-lymphocytes or of null lymphocytes in respective cases of T- or null cell LS. Table 8 shows our preliminary results, which we consider valid for B-lymphosarcoma and less valuable for T- and null cases. Figure 10 shows a case in which an IgG monoclonal population of B-secreting lymphocytes was found in the mononuclear cells of the blood (77% of cells) and bone marrow (58%) of a patient whose blood and marrow cytology was normal on routine examination and who was considered as being at a clinical stage III, while immune markers indicated that he really was at stage IV or leukemic. This evident frequent circulation of LS cells probably explains certain organ localizations such as CNS involvement (Table 9) during the so-called nonleukemic stages [9, 13, 26] and the frequent finding of organ infiltration of systematically made biopsies in patients clinically considered as being in the early stages [see 32].

Conclusion

There is a leukemic stage (stage V) of LS, but the frontier between this stage and other stages depends on the tests used, and we propose a very sensitive staging procedure based on searching for immune markers on the mononuclear cells. This procedure may be important because, although the distinction between the conventional stage IV (determined without immune markers) and the leukemic stage may be useful for indicating two different kinds of treatment which we determined a priori according to bone marrow function, and although there is a significant difference as far as cumulative duration of remission is concerned, there is no significant difference as far as survival curves are concerned (Fig. 11). It will be interesting to know if the new staging with immune markers will induce a difference.

Moreover, we have seen stage IV patients who were insensitive to our LS regimen and sensitive to our ALL regimen, as illustrated in Figure 12. Thus, detecting the leukemic stage with more sensitive markers may help in submitting the appropriate patients to the ALL regimen, which will include vindesine in the future. We have shown this drug to be active in cases of leukemic LS resistant to vincristine and to all other drugs (Fig. 13) [23].

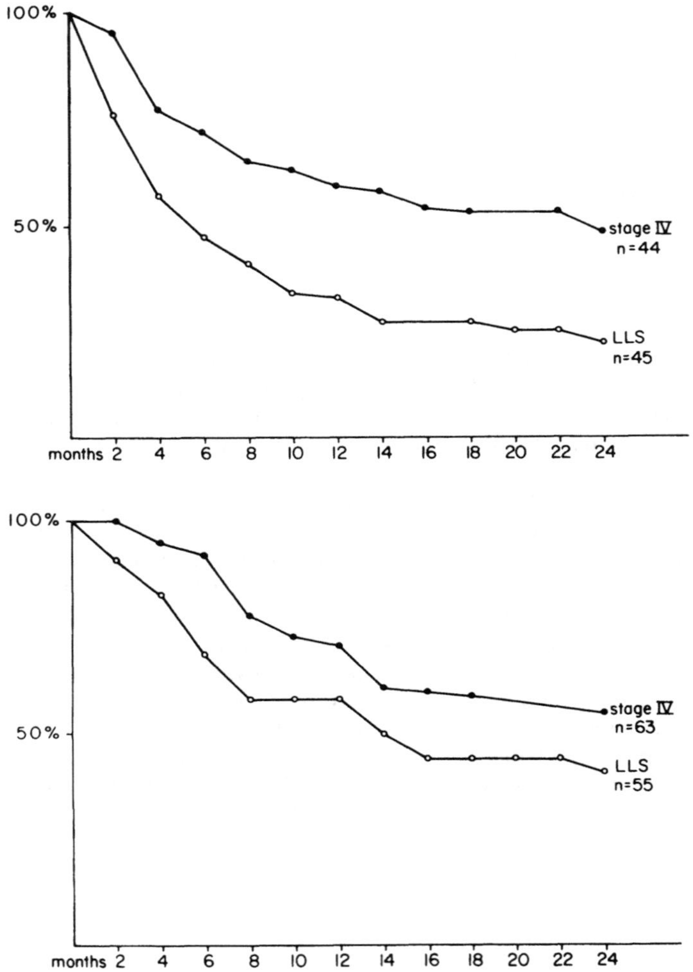

Fig. 11. Cumulative remission and survival duration curves of conventional stage IV and leukemic stages. (LLS: leukemic lymphosarcoma)

There is an acute "d' emblée" leukemic LS in which the frontier with ALL is not clear cut. This is not of great importance as the treatment of both of these entities is the same and gives the same result. The distinction is only important for prognosis prediction and for comparison of therapeutic trials conducted in different centers, as the prognosis of "d' emblée" Leukemic LS is not as good as that of ALL (Table 6).

There may be a chronic, mainly prolymphocytic leukemic LS. The frontier with CLL is also not clear-cut, as its sensitivity to CLL treatment is more frequent than its sensitivity to conventional LS and ALL treatments.

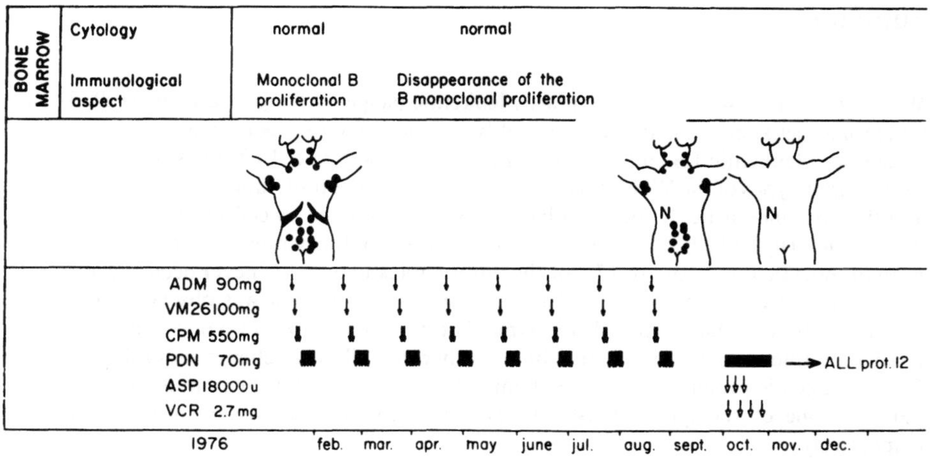

Fig. 12. Diffuse prolymphocytic conventional stage IV LS: failure of LS regimen; remission obtained with ALL regimen

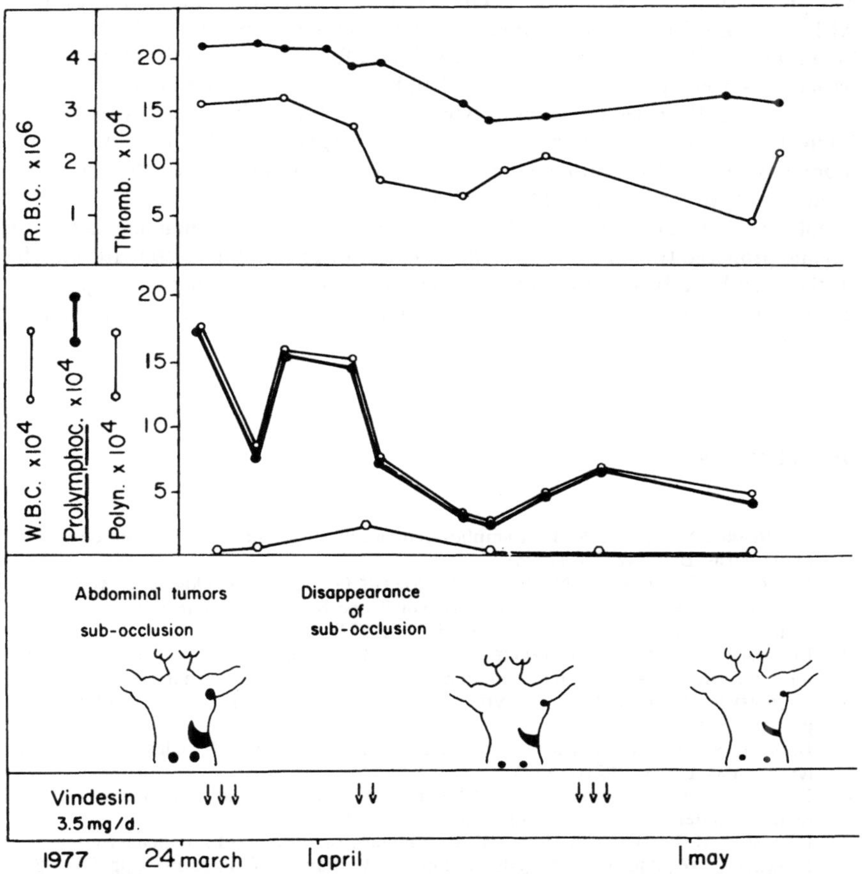

Fig. 13. Terminal case of prolymphocytic leukemic LS resistant to all available drugs including vincristine; sensitivity to vindesine

Summary

We have studied 24 cases of secondarily leukemic (stage V) lymphosarcoma (LS), 31 cases of "d'emblée" leukemic LS, and ten cases of lymphoid leukemic neoplasias transitional between "d'emblée" leukemic LS and chronic lymphocytic leukemia (CLL). These cases only concern the common types of the WHO classification of LS, i.e., the prolymphocytic, the lymphoblastic, and the immunoblastic. Some cases have also been classified by cell surface markers.

The secondarily leukemic conversion occurred in 40% of the lymphoblastic types, in 14% of the prolymphocytic types, and in 17% of the immunoblastic types. It never occurred at stage I but could occur after any other stage. The mediastinal involvement was observed in three types, but most often in the lymphoblastic type. The prognosis after an acute lymphoid leukemia (ALL) treatment comprising active immunotherapy following chemo(radio)therapy is better for the leukemic prolymphocytic and lymphoblastic LS than for the immunoblastic type. Two patients (one of the lymphoblastic type) are in complete remission after 8 and 5 years, respectively.

We have described ten cases of "d'emblée" leukemic LS with either large lymphoid or extra-lymphoid masses, bone marrow leukemic cell involvement, and LS aspects of neoplastic cells. Mediastinal, abdominal, or other tumor masses are frequent.

The prognosis for "d'emblée" leukemic LS following an ALL treatment is less favorable than ALL prognosis for patients of all ages including children. However, the first remission curve breaks at the 18th month and may form a plateau for about 30% of the patients of all ages. One patient has been in remission for more than 8 years after immunotherapy.

We have also described ten cases of lymphoid neoplasia, whose cells cytologically and by the intensity of Ig secretion resemble leukemic prolymphocytic LS cells. However, the disease is more sensitive to CLL treatment than to LS or ALL treatment. Hence, there may be transitional conditions between leukemic LS and CLL.

Finally, we have discussed the different possible frontiers between nonleukemic and leukemic LS and proposed two tests to detect the leukemic stage early: the systematic search for LS cells in the peripheral blood after concentration of nucleated cells by centrifugation and for cells carrying immune markers in the isolated mononuclear cell population of peripheral blood and the bone marrow.

References

1. Aisenberg, A. C., Wilkes, B.: Lymphosarcoma cell leukaemia: the contribution of cell surface study to diagnosis. Blood *48*, 707 (1976)
2. Belpomme, D., Lelarge, N., Joseph, R., Mathé G.: An immunological classification of leukemias and non-Hodgkin's hematosarcomas based on T and B-cell membrane markers with special reference to null "cell" disorders. Eur. J. Cancer *13*, 311 (1977)
3. Belpomme, D., Mathé, G., Davies, A. J. S.: Clinical significance and prognostic value of the T-B immunological classification of human primary acute lymphoid leukaemias. Lancet *1977/1*, 555
4. Belpomme, D., Mathé, G., Davies, A. J. S.: Immune marker staging of lymphosarcoma. (In preparation)
5. Bennet, M. H., Farrer-Brown, G., Henry, K., Jeliffe, A. M.: Classification of non-Hodgkin's lymphomas. Lancet *1974/1*, 1295
6. Brouet, J. C., Flandrin, G.: Clinical and hematological heterogeneity of T-cell derived lymphoproliferative diseases. Bull. Cancer *64*, 267 (1977)
7. Dorfman, R. F.: The non-Hodgkin's lymphomas. In: Reticulo-Endothelial System. Rebuck, J. W., Berard, C. W., Abell, M. R. (eds.) Baltimore: Williams & Wilkins 1975, pp. 262–283
8. Galton, D. A. G., Goldman, J. M., Wiltshaw, E., Catovski, D., Henry, K., Goldenberg, G. J.: Prolymphocytic leukaemia. Br. J. Haematol. *27*, 7 (1974)
9. Hayat, M., De Vassal, F., Gil, M. A., Mathe G.: Invasion of the central mervous system in

lymphosarcomas. In: "Lymphoid Neoplasias". MATHÉ, G., SELIGMAN, M., TUBIANA, M. (eds.) Heidelberg–New York: Springer-Verlag 1978 (in press)
10. ISAACS, R.: Lymphosarcoma cell leukemia. Ann. Intern. Med. *11*, 657 (1957)
11. LENNERT, K., MOHRI, N., STEIN, H., KAISERLING, E.: The histopathology of malignant lymphomas. Br. J. Haematol. *31*, Suppl. 193, 203 (1975)
12. LENNERT, K., STEIN, H.: Personal points of view on the Kiel classification. In: "Lymphoid Neoplasias II" (RRCR). MATHÉ, G., SELIGMAN, M., TUBIANA, M. (eds.), pp. 31–37. Heidelberg–New York: Springer-Verlag 1978
13. LONGPRE, B., LAMARCHE, J., ROCHON, M., LEPINE, M.: Involvement of the nervous system in non-Hodgkin's lymphomas. In: "Lymphoid Neoplasias II" (RRCR). MATHÉ, G., SELIGMAN, M., TUBIANA, M. (eds.), pp. 81–87. Berlin–Heidelberg–New York: Springer-Verlag 1978
14. LUKES, R. J., COLLINS, R. D.: A functional classification of malignant lymphomas. In: The Reticulo-Endothelial System. REBUCK, J. W., BERARD, C. W., ABELL, M. R. (eds.) Baltimore: Williams and Wilkins 1975, p. 213
15. MATHÉ, G.: Inventaire préthérapeutique des néoplasies, II. Les lympho et réticulosarcomes. Concours Médical *97*, 5012 (1975)
16. MATHÉ, G., SEMAN, G.: Aspects Histologiques et Cytologiques des Leucémies et Hematosarcomes. (Nomenclature, Classification, Diagnostic Atlas). Paris: Librairie Maloine 1963, Vol. I
17. MATHÉ, G., POUILLART, P., STERESCU, M., AMIEL, J. L., SCHWARZENBERG, L., SCHNEIDER, M., HAYAT, M., DE VASSAL, F., JASMIN, C., LAFLEUR, M.: Subdivision of classical varieties of acute leukemia. Correlation with prognosis and cure expectancy. Eur. J. Clin. Biol. Res. *16*, 554 (1971)
18. MATHÉ, G. POUILLART, P., SCHWARZENBERG, L., HAYAT, M., AMIEL, J. L., SCHLUMBERGER, J. R., DE VASSAL, F.: Transformation leucémique des hématosarcomes ("lymphomes") non-hodgkiniens. Efficacité de l'immunothérapie. Bull. Cancer (Paris) *16*, 69 (1974)
19. MATHÉ, G. BELPOMME, D., DANTCHEV, D., KHALIL, A., AFIFI, A. M., TALEB, M., POUILLART, P., SCHWARZENBERG, L., HAYAT, M., DE VASSAL, F., JASMIN, C., MISSET, J. L., MUSSET, M.: Immunoblastic lymphosarcoma. A cytological entity?. Biomed. *22*, 473 (1975)
20. MATHÉ, G., RAPPAPORT, H., O'CONOR, G. T., TORLONI, H.: Histological and Cytological Typing of Neoplastic Diseases of Heamatopoietic and Lymphoid Tissue. Geneva, W.H.O. Reference Center, Geneva, 1976
21. MATHÉ, G. BELPOMME, D., SCHWARZENBERG, L.: Prednimustine versus Chlorambucil in chronic lymphoid leukaemia. (In preparation) (1978)
22. MATHÉ, G., DE VASSAL, F., SCHWARZENBERG, L., DELGADO, M., WEINER, R., GIL, A. M., PENA-ANGULO, J., BELPOMME, D., POUILLART, P., MACHOVER, D., MISSET, J. L., PICO, J. L., JASMIN, CL., HAYAT, M., SCHNEIDER, M., CATTAN, A., AMIEL, J. L., MUSSET, M., ROSENFELD, C., RIBAUD, P.: Preliminary results of three protocols for the treatment of A.L.L. of children. Med. Pediatr. Oncol. *4*, 17 (1978)
23. MATHÉ, G., MISSET, J. L., DE VASSAL, F., GOUVEIA, J., HAYAT, M., MACHOVER, D., BELPOMME, D., SCHWARZENBERG, L., RIBAUD, P., MUSSET, M., JASMIN, CL.: Phase II clinical trial with vindesine for remission induction in acute leukaemia, blastic crisis of chronic myeloid leukaemia, lymphosarcoma and Hodgkin's disease. Absence of cross-resistance with vincristine. Cancer Treat. Report *62*, 805 (1978)
24. MISSET, J. L., MATHÉ, G., TUBIANA, M., CAILLOU, B., POUILLART, P., DE VASSAL, F., GIL, A. M., TENTAS, C., DELGADO, M: Preliminary results of chemo-radiotherapy followed or not by active immunotherapy of stage III and IV lymphosarcoma and reticulosarcoma. Correlation of the results with W.H.O. categorisation. Cancer Chemoth. Pharmacol., in press (1978)
25. PANGALIS, G. A., NATHWANI, B. H., RAPPAPORT, H.: Malignant lymphoma well differentiated lymphocytes. Its relationship with chronic lymphocytic leukaemia and macroglobulinemia of Waldenström. Cancer *39*, (1977)
26. POCHEDY, C.: Leukaemia and Lymphosarcoma in Nervous System. Springfield: C. C. Thomas 1977
27. RAPPAPORT, H.: Tumor of the hematopoietic system. In: Atlas of Tumor Pathology. Section 2, Fasc. 8. Washington D.C.: Armed Forces Institute Pathol. 1966
28. ROSENBERG, S. A., DIAMOND, H. D., JASLOWITZ, B., GRAVER, L. F.: Lymphosarcoma: a review of 129 cases. Medicine *40*, 31 (1961)
29. SCHLUMBERGER, J. R., MATHÉ, G., TEXIER, J. L., AMIEL, J. L., CATTAN, A., SCHWARZENBERG, L., SCHNEIDER, M., BERUMEN, L.: Plastic leukemia complicating reticulo-sarcoma and lympho-sarcoma. In: Advances in the Treatment of Acute (Blastic) Leukemias. MATHÉ, G. (ed.) Berlin–Heidelberg–New York: Springer-Verlag 1970, p. 162
30. SCHWARTZ, D. L., PIERRE, R. V., SCHEERRER, P. P., REED, E. C., LINMAN, J. W.: Lymphosarcoma cell leukaemia. Ann. J. Med. *38*, 778 (1965)
31. WALDENSTROM, J. G. D.: Diagnosis, and Treatment of Multiple Myeloma. New York: Grune & Stratton 1970
32. Workshop for classification of non-Hodgkin's lymphomas. Warrenton, Virginia, 4–5, Sept., 1975 Biomed. *22*, 466 (1975).

Comments on "Clinical Aspects: Staging and Therapeutic Implications"

S. Rosenberg and M. Tubiana

During this session, the results of pathologic staging in the non-Hodgkin's lymphomas from several large series were discussed for adults and children. The information obtained from routine multiple bone marrow biopsies and laparoscopy was reviewed. The staging experience of the past 10 years has clarified what new information will be gained from routine sequential bone marrow biopsy, laparoscopy, and laparotomy. The major questions were how to be selective in using the pathologic staging procedures and how the new information gained from the surgical procedures would influence therapeutic programs. It seemed clear that only after 10 years of experience with pathologic staging in Hodgkin's disease, its precise role and value was being realized. The less satisfactory and more controversial aspects of the classification, staging, and treatment of the non-Hodgkin's disease will make it more difficult to come to a consensus about the role of pathologic staging in the non-Hodgkin's lymphomas at this time. The situation seems different for the childhood age group. The reviews by Jaffe, Gout-Lemerle, confirmed by Murphy in the discussion period, conclude that staging laparotomy is rarely of value for children, although diagnostic laparotomy is performed for a significant proportion of the children. Even lymphography is of questionable value in the management of children, in contrast to adults. On the other hand, in multiple myeloma, clinical staging and kinetic data appear to begin to improve results of treatment. The possibility of assessing cell mass before and during treatment through M-component markers open new therapeutic approaches and helps to understand the reason for failures.

Part II

Treatment of Non-Hodgkin's Lymphomas

Radiotherapy of Extranodal Non-Hodgkin's Lymphoma

B. van der Werf-Messing

Introduction

Between 1950 and 1975, 1245 patients with non-Hodgkin's lymphoma were treated at the Rotterdam Radiotherapy Institute. Two hundred and thirty-two exhibited an apparently extranodal primary site. The purpose of this study is to assess for each site some characteristics of the malignancy, such as presenting signs and symptoms, pattern of spread, the simplest way to predict or discover relapses, and to assess the value of radiation therapy in each site as reflected by survival and relapse-free survival.

With increasing technical progress the patients have been submitted to an ever increasing number of investigations, some of which are both an inconvenience and a financial burden to the patient. An attempt has also been made to evaluate how much these investigations contributed to a better understanding and hence to a probably better treatment of the disease. Finally, an estimate has been made of the hypothetic benefit which could have been derived from elective "excellent" chemotherapy in those cases where failure could not be prevented by "good" radiation therapy, assuming that such chemotherapy might be developed in the future and disregarding the fact that the chemotherapy actually given—at that time considered to be good—has produced either only partial temporary remissions or no demonstrable beneficial influence at all.

Materials and Methods

Table 1 presents the various sites included in this study. The diagnosis was confirmed histologically in all instances. Unfortunately, the histology of all sites could not be reviewed due to shortage of pathologists. The influence of histology will be the subject of a later study.

All cases were classified either at the time of treatment or retrospectively according to the Ann Arbor classification. If no lymphography was done in sites where this examination could have increased the stage, clinical stage as determined by physical examination is indicated by stage $\geqslant$ I or $\geqslant$ II. Up to about 1965, routine treatment was limited to simple procedures but often included bone marrow examination; gradually after that period, more sophisticated investigations such as lymphangiography and liver-spleen scan were performed. Similarly, the routine procedures during follow-up became more complicated and numerous with the progression of time.

Patients without evidence of disseminated disease were treated by radiation therapy, up to 1965 by orthovoltage machines, and after that period usually by supervoltage facilities. In case of disseminated disease, either at first presentation or during the follow-up, chemotherapy was given. Since about 1970, adjuvant chemotherapy has been given electively after radiation therapy in some instances.

The average age for each site is reflected in Fig. 1. The presenting signs and symptoms for each site are listed in Table 2.

Table 1. Non-Hodgkin's lymphoma treated at Rotterdam Radiotherapy Institute (1950–1975)

Total No. of patients	1245	
Nodal	1013	
		(%)
Extranodal	232	100
Stomach	43	19
Bowel	40	17
(Para)nasal cavities	32	14
Testis	30	13
Skin	19	8
Parotis	14	6
CNS	12	5
Breast	11	5
Thyroid	10	4
Bladder	8	3.5
Bone	8	3.5
Orbital	5	2

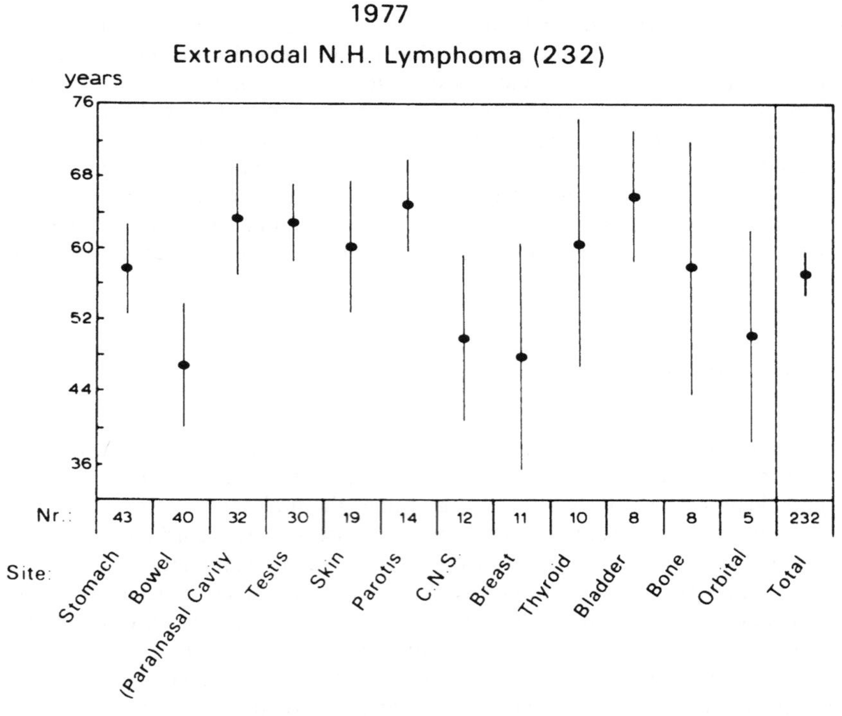

Fig. 1. Average age (with 95% confidence limits of average) by site. Patients with bowel, CNS, breast, and orbital lymphomas are younger than the average. Parotis and bladder patients are older

In 43 patients, the diagnosis of non-Hodgkin's lymphoma of the *stomach* was based on findings during surgery. No attempt was made to do routine radical surgery. The surgical findings also conveyed information about lymph node involvement. Before 1965, orthovoltage irradiation could only deliver a dose now considered insufficient. After that time, a dose of 2000 rad over

Table 2. Extranodal non-Hodgkin's lymphoma: presenting signs and symptoms

Site	No. treated	Signs and symptoms	
Stomach	43	Gastric pain/vomiting/bleeding	35
		Same with weight loss	8
Bowel	40		
Jejunum		Abd. pain, vomiting, diarrhoea	18
Ileum		Same with weight loss	4
Cecum		Same with abd. mass	6
		General malaise + back pain	2
		Acute abdomen	4
Colorectum		Abd. mass	1
		Back pain	1
		Constipation + diarrhoea	4
Nasal + paranasal cavities	32		
Nasal cavity		Bleeding/obstruction	6
Paranasal cavities		Ocular protrusion	2
		Swelling of cheek	7
		Nasal bleeding/ ± pain/ ± obstruction	17
Testis	30	Enlarged testis (with: pain in Testis 1, pain in groin 1, pain in loin 1)	30
Skin	19	Swelling (with pain 4)	19
Parotis	14	Swelling	14
CNS	12	Headache (with paresis 3)	7
		Disturbance of vision	4
		Aphasia	1
Breast	11	Lump in breast	11
Thyroid	10	Swelling of thyroid (with pain 1, with stridor 1)	8
		Myxoedema	2
Bladder	8	Hematuria	7
		Swelling of abdomen	1
Bone	8	Swelling	5
		Pain	1
		Fracture	1
		Paralysis	1
Orbital	5	Protusion of Eye	5

a period of about 3 weeks was given to the whole abdomen followed by a booster dose of ca. 2000 rad in 2 weeks to the gastric area.

Forty patients manifested a lymphoma of the *bowel*. Diagnosis was established by surgery. Subsequent radiation of the whole abdomen to ca. 2000 rad in 3 –4 weeks followed by a booster dose of ca. 2000 rad in 2 weeks to the involved area was considered "good" radiotherapy.

In 32 patients, a primary tumor was diagnosed in the *nasal or paranasal cavities*. Up to about 1970, irradiation was limited to large fields covering the involved areas at a dose equivalent to ca. 3000–4000 rad in 3–4 weeks; during the last 5 years, additional elective irradiation to the cervical lymph nodes has been given.

A non-Hodgkin's lymphoma of the *testis* was presented in 30 patients at the initial site. Since about 1962, routine investigation included a lymphangiography. After hemicastration, treatment consisted of irradiation of the lumbar and bilateral iliac lymph nodes. Since 1965, a dose of 3000–4000 rad in ca. 4 weeks could be delivered by a linear accelerator. Nineteen patients had a primary *skin* non-Hodgkin's lymphoma. Radiation therapy after 1965 consisted of electron beam irradiation covering the involved area and a wide margin of healthy tissue, delivered at a dose varying from 3000 to 4000 rad in 2–4 weeks.

In 14 patients, a lymphoma of the *parotis* was the presenting sign. Usually, irradiation was given to the involved parotis and a wide margin of healthy tissue; in cases of cervical lymph node involvement, this area was also included in the irradiation field. A dose of 3000–4000 rad in a period of 3–5 weeks was given. Incidentally, elective cervical irradiation was given in cases of parotis involvement only.

Neurosurgery yielded the diagnosis of primary tumor of the central nervous system (CNS) (brain) in 12 instances. Radiation therapy consisted of irradiation of the brain at a rate of 3000–4000 rad in 3–5 weeks. Since 1970, additional elective irradiation of the whole spinal cord has been administered, in some instances followed by adjuvant chemotherapy (CVP).

Non-Hodgkin's lymphoma of the *breast* was diagnosed by biopsy in 11 instances. Treatment consisted of irradiation of the breast, usually not including the regional lymph nodes. A dose of 3000–4000 rad was delivered in about 4 weeks. The *thyroid* was the primary site in ten instances. Irradiation was given to the thyroid region, including a wide margin of healthy tissue; regional lymph nodes were not routinely electively irradiated.

Eight patients exhibited a primary tumor of the *bladder*. Treatment before 1965 consisted of orthovoltage irradiation to the bladder region and a wide margin of healthy tissue. Since 1965, the whole pelvic region including the lymph nodes at the level of lumbar V have been included in the supervoltage irradiation field. A dose of 4000 rad in 4 weeks was given. A primary *bone* tumor was treated eight times. Irradiation, either by orthovoltage or by the supervoltage machine, was applied to the involved area and a wide margin of apparently healthy tissue. The dose was 3000–4000 rad in 3–4 weeks. In five *orbital* non-Hodgkin's lymphomas, irradiation of the involved area was given at a rate of 3000–4000 rad in 3–4 weeks.

Results of the Analysis

The uncorrected actuarial 5- and 10-year survival rate of all cases and in each site is presented in Fig. 2. Patients with the primary site in the stomach, skin, or parotis have a better prognosis than the average, whereas those with a primary site in the bowel, paranasal cavities, or bone fare worse.

The median survivals, the 5- and 10-year uncorrected actuarial survival rates, and the relapse-free survival rates for each site are listed in Table 3; where possible, subdivisions according to stage, type of treatment, histology, or other characteristics have been made.

In cases of stomach lymphoma, prognosis decreases with increasing stage. Prognosis becomes excellent after good radiation therapy. All good and bad histologic criteria were distributed equally in the group of good radiation therapy; hence, histologic characteristics apparently had no prognostic influence. Primary sites in the bowel have a significantly better prognosis if an adequate dose of irradiation is applied to a large field. Prognosis is extremely poor if the colorectal area is primarily involved. Patients with involvement of the nasal cavity have a considerably better prognosis than those with involvement of the paranasal cavities; adequate radiation dose and elective irradiation of cervical lymph nodes in clinical stage $\geq$I did not improve prognosis significantly. In cases of testis lymphoma, prognosis was excellent if no lymphographic evidence of lymph node involvement was demonstrable. If irradiation was given by supervoltage machines with an adequated dose of at least 3000–4000 rad in 3–4 weeks, prognosis improved in all cases without demonstrated dissemination (stages $<$IV). Histology had no demonstrable bearing on survival rates. Patients with lymphoma of the skin had a slightly better prognosis in cases with a solitary nodule than in cases with multiple nodules confined to one region.

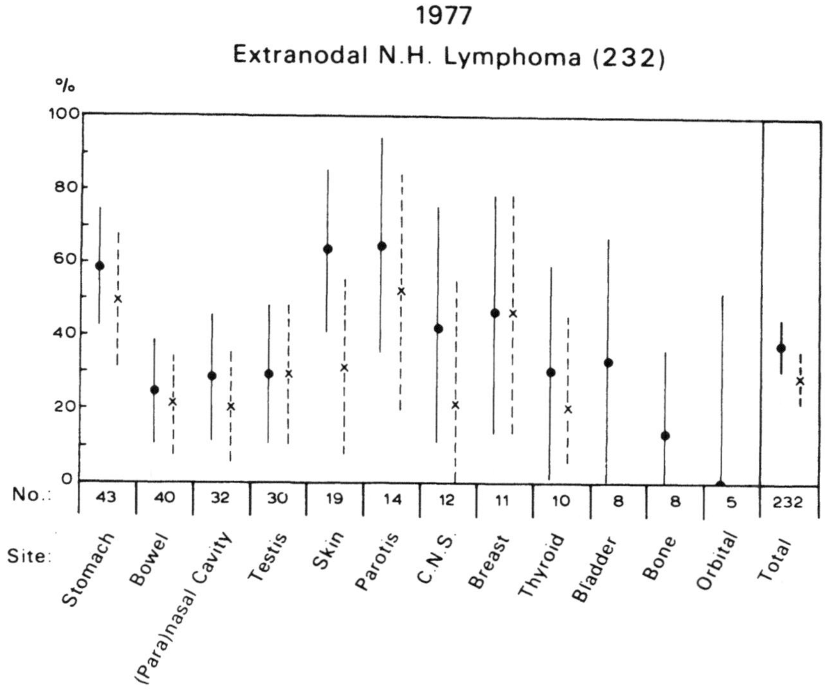

Fig. 2. Average uncorrected actuarial 5(•)- and 10(×)-year survival (with 95% conf. limits of average) by site. Patients with stomach, skin, and parotis lymphomas have a better prognosis. Prognosis is worse in case of bowel and bone lymphoma

Prognosis in cases of parotic involvement was excellent in stage ⩾I. Death was only due to intercurrent disease without evidence of malignancy. The prognosis in stage ⩾II was only slightly worse. The outlook for patients with involvement of the brain was poor: two patients treated with elective irradiation of the spinal cord fared no better than those without such extensive irradiation. One patient died within 3 months of brain and spinal cord irradiation followed by elective CVP chemotherapy. One stage IV patient was cured by radiation therapy of all clinical lesions and 1 year of elective Endoxan chemotherapy. A primary breast lesion implies a relatively good prognosis, the median survival being more than 120 months and the cure rate after 10 years being more than 50%. Both thyroid and bladder lymphoma patients have a gloomy prognosis; only 20%–30% are cured. However, the three cases of bladder lymphoma who received irradiation of the whole pelvis were cured. Prognosis in cases of bone involvement is extremely poor. Only one patient who displayed multiple bone lesions was cured by irradiation of all sites and additional Endoxan treatment during 1 year. Orbital lesions also had a poor prognosis; however, a bias is introduced due to two intercurrent deaths without clinical evidence of disease (one, however, had dubious postmortem findings).

In all sites, survival rates did not significantly differ from relapse-free survival rates. The uncorrected actuarial survival rate after the first relapse for each site is presented in Table 4. After relapse, 40% or more of the patients are alive in cases of primary skin and parotis involvements. In bladder, bone, and orbital lesions, a relapse implies death within 5 years. In all other sites, the chance of survival after 5 (and even 10) years is roughly 10%.

The pattern of spread for each site—where possible and relevant, subgroups were formed—is presented in Table 5. Most frequently no relapse was observed in low stages. In stage IV, all cases relapsed except two (one CNS, one bone). The pattern of spread varies from site to site, and no general rule can be derived from this Table. However, in the case of stomach and bowel

Table 3. Extranodal non-Hodgkin's lymphoma: 5- and 10-year uncorrected actuarial survival rates by sites and subgroups

Site	No. treated	Median survival (months)	Survival		Relapse-free survival	
			5 years (%)	10 years (%)	5 years (%)	10 years (%)
Stomach	43	72	60	50	55	45
Stage ⩾I	17	>120	93	72	87	70
Stage ⩾II	20	38	45	45	40	40
Stage IV	6	5	0	0	0	0
Well-irradiated stage ⩾I	16	>120	100	85	100	85
Well-irradiated stage ⩾II	10	>120	82	82	82	82
Bowel						
Total	40	12	25	23	23	20
Jejunum-ileum	20	12	35	35	26	26
Ileocecum	14	8	22	16	22	15
Colorectum	6	8	0	0	0	0
Stages <IV, well-irrad.	16	36	48	48	48	48
Stages <IV, poorly irrad.	18	6	10	6	10	6
Nasal Cavity	6	>120	80	53	80	53
Paranasal cavities	26	18	15	12	8	8
Stage ⩾I	14	24	24	24	20	20
Stage ⩾II	7	22	13	0	0	0
Stage IV	5	8	0	0	0	0
Stage ⩾I, Good ± elective node irradiation	10	34	35	35	35	35
Stage ⩾I, same with bone destruction	8	15	22	22	22	22
Testis	30	20	30	30	25	25
Stage I	4	> 60	100	—	100	—
Stage II	7	12	32	32	25	25
Stage ⩾I, <III	14	28	20	—	15	—
Stage IV	5	8	0	0	0	0
Stages <IV, well irradiated	13	>120	62	62	62	62
Poorly diff., diffuse lymphoblastic	18	12	38	38	33	33
Poorly diff., diffuse histiocytic	12	28	25	20	20	20
Poorly diff., diffuse lymphoblastic, without stage IV	13	12	49	49	46	46
Skin	19	75	65	30	32	21
Solitary	14	76	65	35	50	35
Multiple	5	66	60	20	20	20
Parotis	14	>120	65	52	45	30
Stage ⩾I (only intercurrent died)	6	>120	75	50	75	50
Stage ⩾II	7	>120	65	65	65	65
CNS	12	28	35	18	35	18
Stage IV	(2)	—	(1)	(1)	(1)	(1)
Breast	11	>120	53	53	53	53
Thyroid	10	6	30	20	30	20
Bladder	8	6	32	32	32	32
Bone (incl. two stage IV)	8	18	12	12	12	12
Orbital (two intercurrent died)	5	38	0	0	0	0

Table 4. Extranodal non-Hodgkin's lymphoma: uncorrected acturial survival rates after first relapse

Site	Relapse	Median survival in (months)	5-year survival (%)	10-year survival (%)
Stomach	18	15	12	12
Bowel	30	8	3	3
Nasal and paranasal cavities	20	18	13	9
Testis	23	10	18	18
Skin	12	60	50	20
Parotis	7	14	40	40
CNS	7	3	14	0
Breast	7[a]	35	17	–
Thyroid	7	5	15	0
Bladder	5	4	0	0
Bone	7	12	0	0
Orbital	3 (or 4)	38	0	0

[a] One relapse after surgery, cured after x-therapy.

lymphomas, good radiation therapy significantly reduced the incidence of relapses. In cases of testis lymphoma at stages above I, the high incidence of juxtaregional and regional recurrences is striking. After a local or (juxta) regional relapse, seven patients, five of whom had primary skin lesions, could still be cured. Table 6 shows which of the numerous investigations, done routinely during each follow-up, actually were the most reliable and sensitive indicators of an existing or threatening relapse. If pathologic physical examination results coincided with pathologic laboratory tests, only the simple physical examination has been recorded as a "relapse alarm"; in the same way, physical examination or simple laboratory tests had priority over pathologic results of more complicated investigations in defining the relapse alarm.

The first relapse alarm turned out to be just a good thorough physical examination in more than two-thirds of the cases. The sedimentation rate turned out to be the relapse alarm in one-third of the cases. In only five cases (4%) was a chest x-ray without other indicators the first relapse alarm. In only one instance were the results of bone marrow examination the only relapse alarm, without any other simpler indication of a relapse.

For each site, the intervals between the first treatment and the time it takes 50%, 90% and 100% of the relapse alarms to be noted, the relapse itself to be diagnosed, and dissemination to be confirmed are presented in Table 7. As quite often the relapse alarm was the result of physical examination, alarm and relapse coincided in a high percentage of cases. In a similar way, relapse could be identical with dissemination. However, more often dissemination was preceded by local or (juxta) regional recurrence. If cases presenting as stage IV are excluded from this analysis, the results do not change significantly.

Figure 3 shows the same intervals for all sites combined. Table 8 shows which simple criteria in each site established stage IV, disregarding results of more complicated investigations. In the majority of cases, a thorough physical examination or simple laboratory tests led to stage IV being diagnosed. Only twice did bone marrow examination and four times a chest x-ray establish a final staging.

The hypothetic or actual benefit of expensive routine investigations is listed for each primary site in Table 9. In cases of stomach and bowel lymphomas, it is doubtful whether after bad irradiation, which was followed by failure anyhow, additional investigations could have supplied information which would have resulted in superb chemotherapy that could have counterbalanced the bad radiation therapy; hence, data pertaining to the bad x-ray therapy group have been omitted. Although different conclusions are applicable for each site, they do not differ significantly from the overall conclusion that in about 11% of bone marrow lesions investigation might have contributed to better understanding of the disease and hence to a

Table 5. Extranodal non-Hodgkin's lymphoma: pattern of spread by site and subgroups

Site	No. treated	No. relapsed	Local recurrence	(Juxta) regional recurrence	Distant recurrence dissemination
Stomach	43				
Stage ⩾I	17	16	0	1[a]	0
Stage ⩾II	20	9	2[a]	2[a,b]	7[a]
Stage IV	6	0	0	0	6
Bowel	40				
Jejunum-ileum	20	7	2	3 (mediast. + supraclav. nodes)	8
Ileocecum					
Stages <IV	8	3	2	1 (mediast. + supraclav. nodes)	2
Stage IV	6	0	0	0	6
Colorectum	6	0	1	2 (mediast. + supraclav. nodes)	3
Stages <IV after good irradiation	16	9	0	3	4
Nasal + paranasal cavities	32				
Nasal cavity	6	4	1[c]	1	(1)[c]
Paranasal cavities	26				
Stage ⩾I	14	7	1	3[e]	3[d]
Stage ⩾II	7	1	1[g]	4[g]	1[f]
Stage IV	5	0	0	0	5
Testis	30				
Stage I	4	4	0	0	0
Stage II	7	1	0	5 (2 lumbar nodes 1 mediast. 2 groin	1 (pulm.)
Stages ⩾I, <III	14	2[h]	(1)[i]	6 (lumbar nodes)	6 (3 bone 2 skin 1 orbital)
Stage IV	5	0	0	0	5 (2 leukemia 2 brain mets 1 dissem.)

Skin	19				
Solitary	14	6	2[j]	3[k]	3
Multiple	5	1	3[l,m]	(1)[m]	1
Parotis	14				
Stages <IV	13	7	0	2	4 (2 lumber nodes with mediast. skip 1 pulm. m 1 leukemia)
CNS	12				
Stages <IV	10	4 (2 after local x 2 after local x + spinal cord x)	5 (4 after local x 1 after local x + chemoth.)	0	1 (after local x + elect. chemoth)
Stage IV	2	1 (after x-th. of all clin. lesions + 1 year Endoxan)	0	0	1 (pulm. m after local x + spinal cord x + elect. CVP)
Breast (No stage IV cases)	11	4	1[n]	1	5[o]
Thyroid	10				
Stages <IV	8	3	0	3 (cerv nodes)	2 (1 pulm. m 1 uterus m)
Stage IV	2	0	0	0	2
Bladder (No stage IV cases)	8	3	1	1 (scrotal)	3
Bone 8					
Stages <IV	6	0	1	1	4
Stage IV	2	1 (after x of all lesions, no chemotherapy)	0	0	1
Orbital (No. stage IV cases)	5	2 (1 interc. died with dubious P.M.)	1	0	2

[a] 11/12 After inadequate irradition; [b] 1 Cured after 2nd irradiation; [c] Same patient, leukemia, died 150 months intercurrent, no chemotherapy; [d] 3/3 No response to chemotherapy; [e] 1/3 Good response to chemotherapy; [f] After 56 months; [g] 3/5 No response to chemotherapy; [h] 1 2nd testis tumor after 14 years; [i] Combined with iliac recurrence; [j] 1/2 Cured after 2nd x-therapy; [k] 3/3 Cured after 2nd x-therapy (1 + natulan); [l] 1/3 Cured after 2nd x-therapy; [m] Same patient; [n] Cured after local x-ther.; [o] 1 blood picture "cured" after chemotherapy.

Table 6. Extranodal non-Hodgkin's lymphoma: relapse alarm by site (excluding stage IV)

Site	No. treated	Relapse	Physical exam.	Lab. tests	X-ray	Others
Stomach	37	12	6	4 (ESR)	2 (Chest)	
Bowel	34	24	12	12 (ESR: 8 APH: 3 Blood picture: 1)		
Nasal + paranasal cavities	27	15	11	4 (ESR: 2 APH: 2)		
Testis	25	18	13	2 (ESR)	3 (Chest)	
Skin	19	12	10	2 (ESR: 1 APH: 1)		
Parotis	13	6	3	2 (ESR)		1 (Bone marrow)
CNS	10	6	5	1 (ESR)		
Breast	11	7	6	1 (Blood picture)		
Thyroid	8	5	4	1 (ESR)		
Bladder	8	5	4	1 (ESR)		
Bone	6	6	5	1 (ESR)		
Orbital	5	4	2	2 (ESR)		
All sites	203	120	81 68%	33 27%	5 4%	1 1%

APH: alcaline phosphatase.

Table 7. Extranodal non-Hodgkin's lymphoma: cumulative distribution of intervals between 1st therapy and alarm, 1st relapse, and dissemination (in months)

Site of primary tumor	No. of relapses	50%	90%	100%	50%	90%	100%	50%	90%	100%
		of the alarms within:			of the relapses within:			of disseminations within:		
Stomach	18	6	26	33	6	26	33	8	26	33
Bowel	30	1	23	24	3	23	24	3	27	28
Nasal + paranasal	20	3	8	97	3	8	97	5	45	108
Testis	23	2	35	264	3	35	264	3	35	264
Skin	12	4	35	60	6	35	60	11	59	60
Parotis	7	3	35	60	5	35	60	6	35	85
CNS	7	4	50	74	4	50	74	4	50	74
Breast	7	10	23	36	10	23	36	10	26	36
Thyroid	7	3	16	72	4	16	72	5	27	72
Bladder	5	2	4	6	3	5	6	3	5	6
Bone	7	3	10	14	4	10	14	5	11	14
Orbital	3 (or 4)	6	31	36	7	31	36	14	32	36
All sites	144	3	25	264	3	25	264	5	37	264

better treatment. In 24% of all patients, a lymphangiography might have led to a better treatment; in cases of bowel and testicular lymphoma the benefit might even have been 40% and 30% respectively. A maximum of 6% improvement could have been the result of a reliable spleen-liver scan.

The hypothetic benefit from elective good chemotherapy for each site and all stages, excluding stage IV, is presented in Table 10. It is presumed that a local recurrence, a regional or juxtaregional recurrence, a distant recurrence, or dissemination, all occurring in spite of good radiation therapy, could have been prevented by excellent elective chemotherapy. If

Table 8. Extranodal non-Hodgkin's lymphoma: criteria for stage IV by site

Site	Stage IV/all treated cases	Criteria
Stomach	6/43	4 Findings during operation (2 pancreas, 2 liver + pancreas) combined with ESR >50, APH↗ 1 Chest x-ray (with ESR >50) 1 Liver scan with APH↗
Bowel	6/40 (All ileum-cecum)	1 Findings during operation 3 Physical examination (liver) 2 Blood picture + bone marrow
(Nasal +) paranasal cavities	5/32 (No nasal cavity stage IV)	3 Physical examination: 2 skin nod. 1 enlarged liver + thyroid + spleen 2 Chest x-ray
Testis	5/30	4 Physical examination: 1 other testis + liver 1 icteric + paralysis 1 paranasal cavity 1 diffuse tumor 1 Blood picture (with other testis +)
Skin	0/19	
Parotis	1/14	1 Bone marrow pos. (leukemia)
CNS	2/12	1 Clinical Examination (multiple bone lesions cured after local x + 1 year Endoxan) 1 Bone marrow (died 4 months after CVP)
Breast	0/11	
Thyroid	2/10	1 Physical examination (skin) 1 Chest x-ray
Bladder	0/8	
Bone	2/8	2 Physical examination: multiple bone lesions (1 with ly. nodes)
Orbital	0/5	
All sites	29/232	20 Physical examinations or findings at operation (bowel, stomach) 2 Blood picture (+ bone marrow) 4 Chest x-ray 1 APH↗/ + liver scan 2 Bone marrow

APH: alkaline phosphatase.

chemotherapy had been given electively or therapeutically with only partial response or no response at all, it is still assumed that a better chemotherapy could have prevented such relapses. Hence, Table 10 presents the *maximum* hypothetic benefit from such superb elective chemotherapy. This hypothetic benefit for all sites could be roughly 6% by preventing a local recurrence, 9% by preventing regional or juxtaregional recurrence, and 23% by preventing distant metastases or dissemination. This is the most audacious estimation, and for each site specific restrictions and doubts exist.

Discussion

Although depending on the site of the primary lesion, the average age of patients with non-Hodgkin's lymphomas differs, the disease mainly occurs in the older age groups. The resulting

Table 9. Extranodal non-Hodgkin's lymphoma: benefit from expensive routine investigations (excluding stage IV)

Site	Remarks	No. treated	Benefit from routine		
			Bone marrow	Lymphography	Spleen/liver scan
Stomach	After good x-therapy				
	Stage I and II	18	0/18	0/18	0/18
	Lymphography done (18 cured)				
	Stage ⩾I, <III	8	0/8	1/8	0/8
	No lymphography (1 mediast. rec.)			(for elect. med. x?)	
	After bad x-therapy (11/11 died)	11	?	?	?
	Total after "Good" x-Therapy	26	0/26	1/26	0/26
			0%	4%	0%
Bowel	After good x-therapy	16	3[a]/16	7[b]/16	0[c]/16
				(7 for elect. ch. th.?	
				3 for elect. med. x?)	
			19%	44%	0%
	[a] Bone marrow				
	Pos. 0				
	Dubious 2 — 1 Pulm. m. 1 month				
	Neg. 7 — 3 relapse				
	Not done 7 — 2 relapse: Pulm. m. 1 month; APH↗ 1 month				
	[b] Lymphography				
	Pos. 3 — 0 relapse				
	Neg. 1 — 0 relapse				
	Not done 12 — 7 relapse: 3 mediast.; 4 dissem. (alarm 1–6 months)				
	[c] No liver involv. without APH↗				
Nasal + paranasal cavities					
Nasal cavities		6	0/6	0/6	0/6
	1 Reg. relapse				
	1 Leukemia (L >8 years without ther.)				
Paranasal cavities		21	4/21?	4/21?	4/21?
			19%	19%	19%
	2 Skin mets, 1 Liver mets } not responding to Chemoth.				
	1 Bone mets after 56 months				

Testis				25	7[d]/25	18/25 (5[e] for elect. med. x 13[f] for elect. Ch. th.)	7[d]/25
					29%	32%	29%
	Lymphography						
	Neg.	4	4 cured				
	Pos.	7	1 cured				
			5[e] juxtareg. relapse				
			1[f] distant relapse				
	Not done	14	2 cured				
			6[f] locoreg. relapse (1 > 20 years P.M.)				
			6[f] Distant relapse				
	[d] After lymphography; if lymphography + : 7 distant mets						
Skin				19	3[g]/19	2[h]/19	0[i]/19
					16%	11%	0%
	[g]Bone marrow						
	Neg.	3	1 dissemination				
	Pos.	0					
	Not done	16	7 cured				
			3 interc.				
			3 loc. rec.				
			3 dissemination				
	[h]Lymphography						
	Pos.	1	1 cured				
	Not done	18	10 cured or interc. died				
			6 bone m. or loc. rec.				
			2 P.M. abd. ly. nodes				
	[i]Scan						
	Suspect	1	1 cured				
	Not done	18	1 liver m, APH↗ after 60 months				
Parotis	Stage ⩾I		6 cured	6	0/6	0/6	0/6
	Stage ⩾II		1 cured	7	2[j]/7?	2[k]/7	0/7
			1[j] pulm. mets				
			1[j] dissem. after elect. CVP				
			2[k] subdiaphragm. spread				
			2 cervic. relapse				
	Total stage ⩾I + ⩾II			13	2/13	2/13	0/13
					15%	15%	0%

Table 9 (continued)

Site	Remarks	No. treated	Benefit from routine		
			Bone marrow	Lymphography	Spleen/liver scan
CNS	Lymphography Neg. 6: 3 cured, 2 loc. rec., 1 dissem. after elective CVP Not done 4: 1 cured, 3 loc. rec.	10	0/10	0/10	0/10
Breast	4 Cured 7 Relapses ([l]bone marrow neg.): 5 distant organs involved [1 blood picture ("cured")] 2 locoreg. relapse (1 cured)	11	0[l]/11	0/11	0/11
Thyroid	2 Cured 6 Relapses: 1 distant involv. uterus 1 distant involv. lungs 4 reg. rec.	8	0/8	0/8	0/8
Bladder	3 Cured 5 Relapses: 1 loc. rec. 1 scrotal rec. 3 distant organs after poor? x-th. [m]Bone marrow was neg.: 8	8	0[m]/8	8/8? (to adapt x-th. fields?)	0/8
Bone	1 Loc. rec. 1 Reg. rec. 4 Distant organs preceded by alarm, no response to chemotherapy [n]Bone marrow was neg.: 6	6	0[n]/6	0/6	0/6

Orbital	1 Cured 1 Dubious P.M. after interc. died 1 Loc. rec. 2 Distant organs after alarm ° Bone marrow was neg.: 5	5	0°/5	0/5		0/5
All sites		174	19/174 11%	42/174 24%		? 11/174 6%

APH: alkaline phosphatase

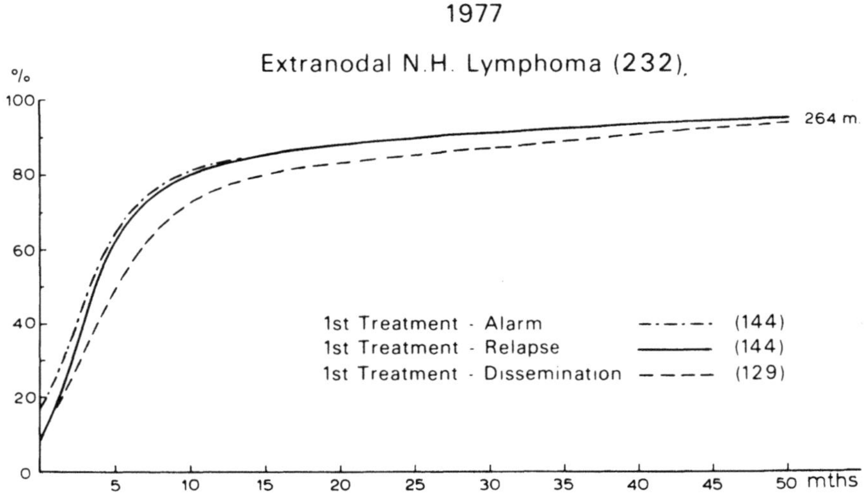

Fig. 3. Cumulative distribution of intervals. More than 90% of relapses occur within 50 months; 50% were diagnosed within 6 months. Usually, alarm precedes relapses and as a rule dissemination was not the first relapse

Table 10. Extranodal non-Hodgkin's lymphoma: hypothetic benefit from elective good chemotherapy by site (excluding stage IV)

Site	No. treated	Maximum hypothetic benefit to prevent (otherwise incurable?)		
		Loc. rec.	(Juxta) reg. rec.	Distant rec. dissem.
Stomach (after good x-therapy)	26	0	(1)[a]	0
Bowel (after good x-therapy)	16	0	3[b]	4
Nasal cavity	6	0	1[c]	0
Paranasal cavities	21	2[df]	7[d]	4[de]
Testis	25	0	(11)[g]	7
Skin	19	3	0[h]	4
Parotis	13	0[i]	(2)	4[i]
CNS	10	5	0	1[j]
Breast	11	0	1	5[k]
Thyroid	8	0	3	2
Bladder	8	(1)	(1)	3
Bone	6	(1)	1	4[l]
Orbital	5	1	0	2
All sites	174	11[n](+2) 6% (+1%)	16[n](+15) 9% (+9%)	40 23%

[a] Mediastinal nodes; [b] Mediastinal nodes; [c] Cervical nodes; [d] 1/11 Good response to therap. chemoth.; [e] 1 Distant mets after 56 months; [f] 1 No chemotherapy; [g] 8 Lumber rec. after orthovolt: 1 Mediast. rec: 2 Groin rec.; [h] 5 cured after 2nd x-th. (1 after x + Natulan); [i] 2 Subdiaphr. mets with mediast. skip.: 1 Dissem. after elect. CVP; [j] After local x + elective chemoth. (CVP); [k] 1 Pathol. blood picture, cured after chemoth.?; [l] 4 No response to therap. chemotherapy; [n] = could be prevented by adapted x-therapy

lower normal life expectancy will also be reflected in lower uncorrected survival rates after treatment. It will also have a bearing on the vigorousness with which primary treatment can be imposed on patients and will influence the feasibility of radical types of treatment with their inherent morbidity.

The chance of survival and of cure are to a large extent determined by the site of the primary tumor, by the stage of the disease at first treatment, by the effectiveness of radiation therapy, and perhaps—this is not yet fully explored—by the histologic type. After good radiation therapy, prognosis of stomach, bowel, testis, and bladder tumors is good, whereas for primary lesions in the bone or paranasal cavity prognosis is poor. The stage has a definite influence in cases of testicular tumors and paranasal cavity malignancies. No patients in stage IV, except for two, have been cured, in spite of therapeutic chemotherapy.

The pattern of spread, i.e., the first relapse, varies from site to site and is also dependent on the stage in which the disease is present. This pattern gives an indication of the possibilities of elective radiation therapy and perhaps of the possibilities of elective chemotherapy.

Although the treatment of patients before ca. 1965 was limited (usually excluding lymphography and liver-spleen scan but including bone marrow investigations), it could retrospectively be assessed from the course of the disease which investigations might have contributed additional knowledge so that therapy based on this information could have improved prognosis. In nearly all cases, stage IV could be based on simple physical examination or simple laboratory tests, and in the majority of cases the staging could be supported by more complicated investigations. In patients with stages less than IV, routine lymphography could have improved the diagnosis in 24% of the cases, and it might thus have contributed to a better treatment and hence a better survival. This applies mainly to testicular and bowel lymphomas. Bone marrow biopsy, usually performed, contributed only in 11% of the cases to a better understanding of the extent of the disease, whereas a conclusive and reliable bone-liver scan could have been beneficial in 6% of the cases.

During follow-up, the results of the physical examination and simple laboratory tests (sedimentation rate) supplied the most reliable relapse alarms, indicating an existing or threatening relapse; in the majority of instances, these findings could be supported by the results of more complicated isotope and x-ray examinations. In view of this finding, one should consider whether routine intensive and extensive investigations and both financially and psychologically expensive examinations are necessary or whether they could be postponed until a relapse alarm has been noticed, especially as non-Hodgkin's lymphomas usually occur in older patients. On the whole, survival after relapse is poor, although in some sites, such as skin and parotis, survival is good even after relapse. For each site, survival after relapse has to be considered against the background of the high age of these patients.

Elective chemotherapy could hypothetically benefit all those patients who relapsed either locally, regionally, or at a distance. However, from the data on this series it is evident that good radiation therapy to the involved area and, in certain sites, electivity to the regional lymph nodes is the sensible basis for good treatment. Moreover, with supervoltage machines, such radiation therapy is no great burden even on old patients.

In this series, no patient in stage IV was cured by chemotherapy only, two patients were cured after 1 year of Endoxan treatment preceded by vigorous irradiation of all involved areas. During follow-up, relapses treated by therapeutic chemotherapy responded either only temporarily or not at all. In spite of these discouraging results, it is assumed that future superb chemotherapy could prevent in some instances a local recurrence, a regional and juxtaregional relapse, and distant relapse or dissemination if previous adequate radiotherapy had dealt with the bulk of the malignancy. The hypothetic benefit of such elective chemotherapy has to be balanced against the age and general condition of the patient, the probable inherent morbidity of chemotherapy, and its psychologic and financial consequences; it has also to be balanced against the possibilities of cure and comfortable survival even with some remaining disease after treatment of the first relapse.

Summary

An analysis of 232 patients with extranodal non-Hodgkin's lymphomas has been presented. Prognosis of each site has been assessed. The influences of good radiation therapy and stage at the time of first treatment have been evaluated. Simple clinical examination and sedimentation rate appeared to be the first indicators of an existing or threatening relapse. This relapse alarm usually preceded distant relapse or dissemination. Retrospectively, the value of expensive (psychologically and financially to the patient) routine investigations has been evaluated with regard to the information they contributed to the understanding of the disease and hence to probably better treatment. In the same way, the hypothetic benefit from elective superb chemotherapy has been assessed, assuming that this might prevent relapses after good radiation therapy and disregarding the fact that the chemotherapy actually given resulted either in temporary partial response or no response at all.

Evaluation and Role of Single Chemotherapeutic Agents in Adult Non-Hodgkin's Lymphoma

H. L. DAVIS and D. D. VON HOFF

The non-Hodgkin's lymphomas are uniquely responsive to a broad range of chemotherapeutic agents of diverse chemical structure and mechanism of action. In the past decade, significant advances in histological diagnosis [86] and staging [20] have occurred documenting the importance of histology, nodal architecture, and stage upon intrinsic prognosis. Parallel to this, aggressive combination therapy has evolved and improved the prognosis in several subtypes, notably diffuse histiocytic and nodular mixed lymphocytic histiocytic lymphomas [15, 1]. In spite of these therapeutic advances, the majority of patients with non-Hodgkin's lymphoma relapse and ultimately die. The purpose of this review is to reexamine the role of old and new drugs. Combination programs will be mentioned in an illustrative fashion; however, the emphasis will be on single agent activity and its relevance for future investigations.

Survey of Standard Single Agents

Table 1 illustrates the major single agent activity in non-Hodgkin's lymphoma. This information is derived from data on file in the Investigational Drug Branch, Cancer Therapy Evaluation Program (CTEP), Division of Cancer Treatment (DCT), and from LIVINGSTON and CARTER [68] and BONADONNA and MONFARDINI [16], as well as specific references to be cited in the text. An agent is designated + + if there is major activity, + if there are hints of activity, − if inactive in at least 14 patients, and NE if activity is not evaluable.

Please note that the concept of response is *not* a uniform one; the modern concepts of comprehensive initial staging [22] and restaging of complete remission [54] have been applied mainly to recent studies involving combination chemotherapy. The majority of single agent studies reported before 1970 did not use the RAPPAPORT classification, and thus the terms "lymphosarcoma" reticulum cell sarcoma and simply "lymphoma" are used in most studies. It is further uncertain that all patients had non-Hodgkin's lymphoma; in some of the older studies, patients with Hodgkin's disease were included. Nevertheless, the number of active agents is impressive.

Ranking of Standard Agents

The overall activity of cyclophosphamide, adriamycin, vincristine, and corticosteroids is the highest of these many agents [15]. The activity of bleomycin, the nitrosoureas, and procarbazine has likewise resulted in their incorporation into combination programs. The antimetabolites, methotrexate, cytosine arabinoside, and 6-thioguanine have been incorporated into a few adult studies [28]. They are an integral part of the Memorial LSA_2L_2 study for childhood lymphoma [104].

Table 1. Single agent activity in non-Hodgkin's lymphoma

Agent	Activity[a]	Responses/total patients (%)		Total
		Lymphocytic (LSA)	Histiocytic (RCS)	
Alkylating agents				
Nitrogen mustard	++	75/154 (49%)	3/17 (18%)	85/197 (43%)
Cyclophosphamide	++	173/276 (65%)	122/219 (56%)	347/584 (59%)
Chlorambucil	++	61/90 (69%)	18/46 (39%)	95/159 (59%)
Melphalan	+	—	—	12/39 (31%)
Busulfan	+	—	—	6/24 (25%)
Antimetabolites				
Methotrexate	+	—	—	13/45 (29%)[b]
6-MP	+	—	—	13/35 (37%)[b]
5-FU	+	—	—	6/23 (26%)[b]
Hydroxyurea	NE	—	—	1/14[b]
Ara-C	+	—	—	15/23[bc]
Corticosteroids				
Prednisone	++	(60%–80%)	(20%–30%)	35/74
Vinca alkaloids	+	6/29	7/26	13/55 (24%)
Vinblastine		—	—	24/89 (27%)
Vincristine	++	51/118 (43%)	81/158 (51%)	132/276 (48%)
Antibiotics				
Actinomycin D	+	—	—	9/18
Mithramycin	NE	—	—	—
Chromomycin A_3	NE	—	—	—
Daunomycin	+	—	—	3/25
Adriamycin	++	12/35	19/34	31/69
Bleomycin	++	15/34	17/42	32/76
Mitomycin C	++	—	—	15/32
Porfiromycin	NE	—	—	—
Streptonigrin	++	—	—	43/98
Nitrosoureas				
BCNU	+	—	—	30/107
CCNU	+	—	—	13/52
MeCCNU	+	—	—	10/57
Streptozoticin	+	—	—	6/36
Miscellaneous				
Procarbazine	++	17/42 (40%)	12/33 (36%)	29/75 (39%)
Hexamethylmelamine	++	—	—	22/40
L-Asparaginase	+	—	—	7/11
DTIC	+	4/15	0/13	4/28
Methyl-GAG	+	—	—	5/11

[a] NE: nonevaluable; + : hint of activity; ++ : definite activity.
[b] Includes some with Hodgkin's disease.
[c] Very brief responses.

Alkylating Agents

The versatility of cyclophosphamide dosage and scheduling as well as its ease of administration has resulted in a deserved ranking of first among the active agents. The comparative study of Carbone and Spurr illustrated moderate superiority over vincristine as a single induction agent but emphasized the low percentage of complete remission (3%–6%) with either agent [21]. Direct comparisons with nitrogen mustard in two studies showed little overall preference for either agent in induction for lymphocytic lymphomas but more efficacy in reticulum cell sarcoma [49, 94]. Studies of maintenance therapy with single alkylating agents demonstrate prolongation of partial remission; the duration of the infrequent complete remissions is unaffected [21].

Antimetabolites

The early studies were simply activity seeking and noncomparative. In addition, Hodgkin's disease was frequently included (Table 1). Brief duration of moderate activity characterized these trials. Methotrexate has undergone a renaissance in combination programs for diffuse histiocytic lymphoma where it appears additive to cyclophosphamide and vincristine [62, 9].

Corticosteroids

Prednisone has become accepted as an integral part of the majority of combination programs. There is evidence that the addition of prednisone to cytoxan and vincristine results in an improved overall remission rate and duration, accounted for by an increased percentage of complete remissions [66]. Prednisone, however, was not additive to cytoxan in maintenance regimens [56].

Vinca Alkaloids

Although vinblastine is highly active in Hodgkin's disease, it has only moderate activity in non-Hodgkin's lymphoma [68] and is inferior to cyclophosphamide on direct comparison [62]. Vincristine is highly active in both lymphosarcoma and reticulum cell sarcoma [21], and its lack of myelosuppression made it a natural ingredient of combination programs.

Antitumor Antibiotics

Studies of actinomycin D are almost 2 decades old. Although they defy modern interpretation, they indicate a need to reexplore this agent in newer schedules, particularly in single intravenous doses given every 2–4 weeks, which has been successful in refractory melanoma [8].

Adriamycin represents a major advance, since high response rates were obtained initially in patients who had failed aggressive programs including alkylating agents and vinca alkaloids [81]. Adriamycin is active in a variety of schedules including single dosage q. 3 weeks and weekly maintenance regimens [81, 100]. A dose-response evaluation demonstrated significant response to single doses ranging from 25–75 mg/m^2 q. 3 weeks, allowing its effective use in patients who were heavily pretreated [80]. Thus, adriamycin is widely incorporated into induction combination programs, particularly for diffuse histiocytic lymphoma [15, 90]. Cardiotoxicity, however, limits its value to induction therapy.

Bleomycin is of special interest because it is essentially nonmyelosuppressive. Remissions are, however, generally brief, and thus its value as a single agent is limited both by duration of response and the hazard of pulmonary toxicity [14, 13]. However, both adriamycin and bleomycin remain among our most active induction agents in combination programs.

BCNU is the single *nitrosourea* utilized in major non-Hodgkin's lymphoma studies [7, 28]. The nitrosoureas are capable of producing responses after failure of alkylating agents (Table 1). Thus, they may offer promise in secondary therapy.

Miscellaneous Agents

Several classes of agents are active. Procarbazine has continued to be of major utility in Hodgkin's disease, but its use has waned in other lymphomas; it is rarely incorporated in the MOPP and COPP regimens [89, 95]. Similar conclusions hold for imidazole carboxamide. FREI found it totally inactive in histiocytic lymphoma, but there was activity in the lymphocytic histologies [34]. It might well be reconsidered; in Hodgkin's disease it is now part of a highly successful secondary combination [17].

Use of Standard Agents in Combination

Figure 1 details the incorporation of these standard agents into combination programs in diagrammatic form. The basis building blocks are cytoxan, vincristine, and prednisone to which have been added adriamycin, bleomycin, and less frequently, procarbazine and the antimetabolites, methotrexate and cytosine arabinoside. The detailed results of combination programs are presented elsewhere. Overall, there has been a major increase in the rate and duration of response. Some general conclusions are apparent.

1. The initial use of combination programs has increased the overall complete remission rate to 30%–70%, a feat not duplicated by any single agent [15].
2. Following induction therapy with active combinations, there is a substantial portion of patients with diffuse histiocytic and nodular mixed lymphocytic histiocytic lymphoma who enjoy long, probably permanent, unmaintained remission [15, 1, 28, 9, 90, 89].

Several problem areas remain.

1. A pattern of continuous late relapse is apparent for lymphocytic lymphomas [89, 52]. This may be reduced by combination therapy; results of current programs will take years to mature.
2. A varying portion of patients in all categories do not attain complete remission; this is characterized by eventual progression and lessened survival.
3. Single agent therapy given sequentially is apparently of similar benefit to cytoxan, vincristine, and prednisone in combination for nodular lymphomas [55, 85, 59]. Combination therapy including adriamycin and/or bleomycin may prove superior; ongoing studies are addressing this important issue.

Evaluation of Phase II Drugs in the United States

There are several obstacles to the evaluation of new agents in this group of disorders:

1. A reluctance of investigators to evaluate new agents until therapy with the present active combinations and radiation is exhausted.
2. The resultant frequent cumulative myelosuppression leading to impaired marrow reserve and intolerance to subsequent myelosuppressive therapy.
3. An advanced, often terminal, disease state may be present. Thus, it becomes difficult to decide at what point in the patient's course new agents can be introduced with reasonable chance of therapeutic benefit. It is a tribute to our current success that relatively few of our present armamentarium of investigational drugs have been adequately evaluated.
   This may, however, have ominous implications for the future.

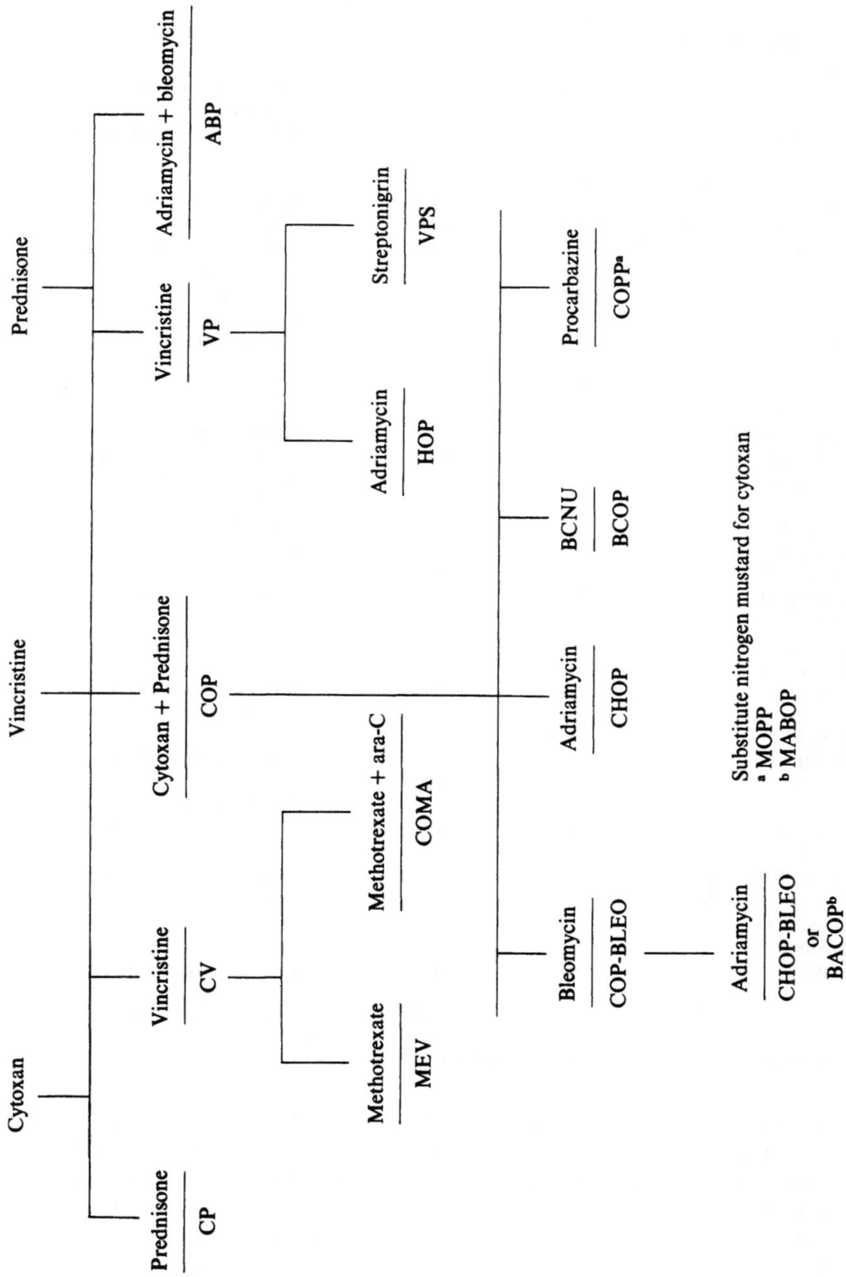

Fig. 1. Use of standard agents in combination

Table 2. Activity of investigational drugs in non-Hodgkin's lymphoma

Agent (NSC No.)	Activity[a]	No. responses/ No. evaluable	Comments
High-dose methotrexate (740)	++	23/40	Duration response 1.5–2 months
Azaserine (742)	NE	—	—
Cycloleucine (1026)	NE	—	Adequately tested only in soft tissue sarcomas
Hexamethylmelamine (13875)	+	22/40	Activity promising; includes Hodgkin's disease
Dichloromethotrexate (29630)	NE	—	—
Methyl-GAG (32946)	+	5/11	Prohibitively toxic
Trimethylcolchicinic acid (36354)	+	6/29	4/9 in DH
Streptonigrin (45383)	++	43/98	Activity being investigated by CALGB
Tubercidin (56408)	NE	—	—
Porfiromycin (56410)	NE	—	—
Chromomycin A_3 (58514)	NE	—	IND recently discontinued
β-TGDR (71261)	NE	—	—
F_3 TdR (75520)	NE	—	—
Daunomycin (82151)	+	3/25 (Adults)	—
Streptozotocin (85998)	+	6/36	Nonmyelosuppressive
MeCCNU (95441)	+	10/57	No advantage over other analogues
Camptothecin (100880)	NE	—	Being reinvestigated on weekly schedule
Yoshi 864 (102627)	+	3/5	One CR
5-Azacytidine (102816)	+	2/12	Brief PR in COG study
Dibromodulcitol (104800)	+	5/7	Duration 5–36 months
Cytembena (104801)	NE	—	Not tested—nonmyelosuppresive
L-Asparaginase (109229)	+	7/11	—
Isophosphamide (108724)	+	7/15	—
Diglycoaldehyde (118994)	NE	—	—
Cis-platinum (119875)	NE	9/35	Includes Hodgkin's disease and minor responses
VM 26 (122819)	++	28/77	—
VP 16 (141540)	+	17/80	Now in combination programs
ICRF 159 (129843)	+	8/27	Candidate for combination
Dianhydrogalactitol (132213)	NE	2/4	Highly myelosuppressive
Piperazindione (135758)	NE	3/16	highly myelosuppressive
Baker's antifol (139105)	NE	—	—
Pyrazofurin (143095)	NE	0/10	Eight minor responses—little myelosuppression
Cyclocytidine (145668)	NE	—	—
Ftorafur (148985)	NE	—	—
Azapicyl (68626)	NE	1/4	Little myelosuppression; similar to procarbazine with CNS toxicity
Prednimustine (LEO 1031)	++	26/40	Chlorambucil ester of prednisolone

[a] NE: non-evaluable; +: hint of activity; ++: definite activity.

Table 2 represents a selected list of investigational drugs being tested. Activity is documented as in Table 1. Numerous discontinued drugs have been inadequately tested in non-Hodgkin's lymphoma; for details, the reader is referred to a recent review [99]. Of the 36 drugs displayed, 17 have demonstrated activity; the rest are nonevaluable for a variety of reasons. In recommending agents for further testing, some basic observations can be made:

1. The alkylating agents would seem to offer little advantage over cyclophosphamide. Yoshi 864, dibromodulcitol, piperazinedione, and dianhydrogalactital are all quite myelosuppressive [3, 5, 53, 39]. Isophosphamide, though active and less myelosuppresive, is less attractive because of the high incidence of hemorrhagic cystitis [25]. Streptonigrin is being actively tested in combination with vincristine and prednisone as an induction regimen [12].

2. The chlorambucil ester of prednisolone (prednimustine LEO 1031) is active with only moderate myelosuppression [77, 56]. It may offer a therapeutic advantage to single alkylating agent therapy.

3. High-dose methotrexate is highly active in adults and children with diffuse lymphomas [27, 84] and has been effective in the COMA regimen (Fig. 1) for diffuse histiocytic lymphoma where it is combined with vincristine, cytoxan, and cytosine arabinoside [9]. Note that the MEV regimen (Fig. 1) uses the conventional dose of 20 mg/m^2 on day 2, following vincristine and cytoxan on day 1 [62]. It too is very active in lymphocytic, and especially histiocytic, lymphoma (56% vs. 93% complete remissions; overall, 73% complete remissions). This raises the question of relative efficacy of the more inconvenient high-dose schedule, which has never been directly tested in a comparative schedule in this disease.

4. VM 26, highly active in reticulum cell sarcoma in European studies [70, 71, 69, 30], has received a preliminary trial in combination with adriamycin, cytoxan, and prednisone. It replaces vincristine as the "synchronizing agent" and initial results are highly encouraging. However, this combination is not demonstrably superior to the combinations including vincristine. [75, 73]. VP 16 has received its first combination trial combined with adriamycin and prednisone. It is well-tolerated; however, responses may not be greater than those seen with adriamycin as a single agent (5/15 partial remission in heavily pretreated patients) [79]. The remainder of the drugs displayed in Table 2 are more tentative, and of those tested, results are inconclusive.

Table 3 lists those drugs which the authors feel should be studied in future trials. Nonmyelosuppressive agents worthy of careful evaluation include:

Table 3. Phase II drugs recommended for further testing

Drug	Phase II activity[a]	Basis for recommendation	References
Methotrexate	++	Forms basis for effective combinations in diffuse histiocytic lymphoma (DHL)	*10, 27, 59, 81*
Hexamethylmelamime	+	May find place in noncross-resistant combinations; new soluble analogues under development	*60*
Trimethylcolchicinic acid	+	Active in DHL (4/9) in phase II study	*94*
Diglycoaldehyde	NE	Relatively nonmyelosuppressive	*55*
Streptonigrin	++	Under active investigation in combination with vincristine and prednisone	*13*
Streptozotocin	+	Nonmyelosuppressive	*89*
Camptothecin	NE	Weekly schedule well-tolerated; highly active in animal screen	*35, 75*
Cytembena	NE	Nonmyelosuppressive; never tested in non-Hodgkin's lymphoma	*7, 32*
L-Asparaginase	+	Nonmyelosuppressive; could be integrated into induction therapy	*103*
Cis platinum	NE	Not adequately tested in NHL; new analogues under development	43, 86
VM 26	++	Both agents introduced into combination program	*30, 66, 68, 72, 76*
VP 16	+		
ICRF 159	+	Oral form has established activity; new parenteral (IV) enantiomer under development	*33*
LEO 1031	++	Highly active with only moderate toxicity	*54, 74*
AAFC	NE	Analogue of 5-fluorocystine; active in gastric carcinoma on weekly schedule	*2, 6*
Actinomycin D	+	Single dose schedule q. 3 weeks may be optimum	*9*

[a] NE: nonevaluable; +: hint of activity; ++: definite activity.

1. Cisplatinum diamminedichloride (DDP): thus far, activity has been meager in heavily pretreated patients [43]. In view of high levels of activity in a variety of solid tumors [88], it would seem appropriate to conduct a careful phase II trial.

2. Streptozotocin: dose-limiting renal toxicity has been troublesome; however, lack of myelosuppression suggests a need for reevaluation [91].

3. Cytembena: trials in breast and ovarian cancer and sarcoma have proved negative in the United States [6, 32]. It has never been tested in non-Hodgkin's lymphoma.

4. L-asparaginase: the LSA_2L_2 program for childhood lymphoma incorporates L-asparaginase as part of the consolidation program [104]. Sequential administration of methotrexate and L-asparaginase given on days 1 and 2 at 10–14 day intervals seems to allow an enhanced therapeutic effect and lesser toxicity in acute lymphocytic leukemia [19]. Such a trial would seem appropriate in lymphocytic lymphoma.

Antimetabolites of Interest

1. Anhydro-arabinosyl fluorocytidine (AAFC): a relatively slow metabolic disposition allows for a weekly schedule which has been effective in gastric cancer and acute myelogenous leukemia [2, 45].
2. Diglycoaldehyde: The dose-limiting toxicities are renal and metabolic (hypocalcemia) [58]. Myelosuppression is minimal.

Miscellaneous Agents

1. Hexamethylmelamine (HMM): the more soluble analogue, pentamethylmelamine, is under formulation in the DCT drug development program [105]. The oral preparation of HMM has had wide usage in lung cancer [61], less so in lymphomas [63]. Nausea, vomiting, and the necessity for continuous administration thus far have limited its utility.

2. ICRF 159: The oral racemic mixture has adequate activity in phase II testing in non-Hodgkin's lymphoma [33]. There is the possibility of therapeutic synergism with adriamycin and cis platinum [82]. A parenteral enantiomer (D +) is under development and should enter clinical trial soon.

3. Actinomycin D showed activity in older trials, and the single intermittent dose schedule is worthy of testing in non-Hodgkin's lymphoma [68, 8]. A note of caution is provided in a recent report testing this schedule in refractory childhood acute leukemia where prohibitive myelosuppression was frequent [36]

4. Trimethylocolchinic acid (TMCA) may be chiefly of historical interest, although activity in diffuse histiocytic lymphoma is impressive [96]. There would seem to be adequate numbers of antimitotic agents under study at this time.

5. Campothecin: this plant alkaloid has had essentially negative results in trials on colon cancer and melanoma [76, 35]. Myelosuppression and cystitis are drawbacks to a q. 3-week schedule but are more easily arranged on a weekly schedule [78]. Because of excellent experimental activity, a trial has been planned for non-Hodgkin's lymphoma.

6. Azapicyl (1-acetyl-2-picolinoyhydrazine) shows promising activity in embryonal rhabdomyosarcoma [98]. Severe, though reversible, neurotoxicity was dose limiting in reported trials and myelosuppression was absent [61].

Agents Recently Completing Phase I Trials

Rubidazone (NSC 164011) demonstrates less cardiotoxicity in the rat model as compared to its analogues daunomycin and adriamycin [107]. Extensive French experience has demonstrated definite activity in acute myelocytic leukemia and hints of activity in non-Hodgkin's lymphoma [50, 11, 51]. If this compound proves less cardiotoxic and equally active, it may be a substitute for adriamycin in lymphoma therapy.

Anguidine (NSC 141537) is a cytotoxic alkaloid derived from a parasitic plant fungus [26, 41]. In addition to moderate activity in P388, L1210, and AKR leukemia, it possesses a high degree of activity in a transplantable mouse colon tumor [24]. This drug has proved difficult to handle in phase I trials with considerable gastrointestinal and central nervous system toxicity [38].

Chlorozotocin (NSC 178248) is the 2-chloroethyl analogue of streptozotocin possessing less carbamylating and greater alkylating activity than BCNU and its analogues. It was selected for clinical trials because it was less myelosuppressive in animal systems [92]. Preliminary clinical studies using a single intravenous dose q. 6 weeks showed little myelosuppression [44].

Maytansine (NSC 153–858) is an ansa macrolide chemically related to the ansamycin antibiotics but differs from them in being a mitotic inhibitor similar to the vinca alkaloids and epidophyllotoxins [87, 106, 42]. It is experimentally effective in extremely low dosage but is cross-resistant with vincristine. Phase I studies have used single dose q. 3 weeks and three daily doses q. 3 weeks, both intravenously [23, 18]. Dose-limiting toxicity has been gastrointestinal with little myelosuppression. Diarrhea has been severe above the maximum tolerated doses.

Neocarzinostatin (NSC 157356) is a high molecular weight (11,000) polypeptide developed in Japan in 1965 and studied extensively in acute leukemia [64] where it showed moderate activity. In phase I trials, the agent was given intravenously by rapid injection on a schedule of five daily doses with the dose-limiting toxicity, myelosuppression; in addition, vomiting, chills and fever were regularly observed [37].

Gallium nitrate (NSC 15200) was developed for clinical trial following demonstration of uptake of radiolabeled gallium citrate in a variety of human tumors including lymphomas [103]. Gallium nitrate is active mainly in the Walker 256 tumor and is inactive in L1210, P388, B16, and sarcoma 180 [1]. In phase I studies, there is no true dose-limiting toxicity, although proteinuria becomes progressively more frequent with repeated courses at higher dose levels [72]. It is anticipated that limited phase II trials in lung, melanoma, and possibly lymphomas will follow. The absence of a firm maximum tolerated dose and absolute lack of antitumor activity in phase I trials remain disturbing.

Vindesdine (NSC 245467) (desacetylvinblastine amide, DVA) is a vinca alkaloid under study sponsored by the Eli Lilly Company. Clinical experience was recently summarized [46]; the most widely used schedules were single doses q. 1–2 weeks. At the lower doses, the limiting toxicity was moderate myelosuppression and mild neuropathy; at higher dosage, constipation and ileus became more prominent. Scattered responses have been noted in a variety of neoplasms, including acute lymphocytic leukemia. It is unclear at present whether this analogue offers a therapeutic advantage in tumors presently treated with standard vinca alkaloids.

New Agents and Approaches With Potential for Clinical Trial

Anthracycline Analogues

Because of the potential for cardiotoxicity of adriamycin [65], there is considerable interest in analogue development with the hope of obviating this dose-limiting property. Carminomycin, closely related to daunomycin, has been extensively evaluated in Russia (N. I. Perivochdikova, personal communication) [83]. This agent is active in experimental systems at considerably lower dosage that daunomycin. Human studies have demonstrated activity in non-Hodgkin's lymphoma. The potential for cardiotoxicity has not been fully evaluated by the Russian investigators; they have imposed a maximum allowable cumulative dose and have not observed cardiomyopathy. N-Trifluoroacetyladriamycin-14-valerate (AD32) was synthesized by the Sidney Farber Cancer Institute and found to have superior activity in P388 and L1210 leukemia [48]. Rapid intracellular penetration has been demonstrated [60] as well as remarkably different hepatic metabolism and biliary secretion [101], possibly supporting the hypothesis of a different mechanism of action from adriamycin.

A new approach to prevention of adriamycin cardiotoxicity was presented by Meyers and associates [74]. They have demonstrated peroxidation of cardiac lipids in mice by adriamycin and prevention of cardiac toxicity by simultaneous treatment with tocopherol as a free radical scavenger. These preliminary results, if confirmed, may allow more intensive use of current anthracycline antibiotics and human tumors and obviate the difficult search for noncardiotoxic analogues.

Platinum Analogues

As previously mentioned, cis platinum is highly effective in a variety of human tumors. Nephrotoxicity remains a threat even though it is minimized by hydration and diuresis [40]. A number of analogues are under investigation. PHM (Malanato-1, 2-diamine-cyclohexane platinum) has received clinical trial at the Wadley Institute [43]. Results indicated less nephrotoxicity at relatively high doses. Activity-seeking trials have been carried out in a few patients with acute leukemia where responses have been noted.

Bruceantin (NSC 165563)

This compound is a plant product which inhibits protein synthesis thus varying from the more common mechanisms of action of antineoplastic agents [67, 93]. Major activity is seen in the P388 system at single dose and chronic daily adminstration. Large animal toxicology is complete and indicates reversible features; thus, clinical trials should be forthcoming soon.

Pyrazoloimidazole (NSC 51143)

This compound may be unique as a long-acting nucleotide reductase inhibitor which does not exhibit schedule dependency in the L1210 system, in contrast to other nucleotide reductase inhibitors [29, 7, 47]. It is also rapidly reversible. It offers the possibility of inhibition of DNA synthesis, with a more intermittent dosage than is possible with hydroxyurea.

Discussion

The content of this review supports the conclusion that non-Hodgkin's lymphoma should be a prime signal tumor; in fact, it can be regarded as a "human screen" for drug activity. It follows that an agent truly inactive in this disorder would be unlikely to have a major impact on the common solid tumors.

As previously described, there are obstacles to the testing of many new agents in this disease, and it would follow that routine testing of all agents might be medically and ethically unwise. Our current success with combination programs is a testimony to the past achievements of drug development. At this time, the investigator can be more particular and select compounds of special interest for development.

The application of the clinically relevant histologic classification of RAPPAPORT allows prognostic classification into favorable and unfavorable subtypes [52, 31]. A priority schema for the major subtypes should define the point at which new agents could be logically and ethically introduced. In the diffuse unfavorable group, it would be appropriate to insist that initial therapy should consist of an active combination, a noncross-resistant combination for attempt at reinduction upon first relapse, selecting agents of proven efficacy in both instances. Following this, trial with promising single agents is indicated with a view toward improving initial or secondary combination therapy. This approach has been successful in Hodgkin's disease [17].

Since the role of combination therapy is less secure in favorable presentations, the first relapse might be an appropriate time to introduce selected new agents. Highly active agents might even be introduced as first line therapy in comparison with combination programs.

The potential for cross-resistance would seem to be of less clinical importance, as illustrated by successful sequential trials of alkylating agents in myeloma [10], and the realization (Table 2) that the majority of patients responding to investigational alkylating agents had failed previous trials of cytoxan.

In selecting directions for new agent development, several factors could be considered:

1. The value of nonmyelosuppresive agents. Agents of high activity should easily be integrated into combination programs.
2. Unusual mechanisms of action could lead to agents active in consolidation programs, e.g., protein synthesis inhibition with L-asparaginase or bruceantin.
3. Analogues with a more favorable therapeutic index.

In summary, non-Hodgkin's lymphoma forms a unique human tumor for testing new agents and hypotheses of effective drug treatment. It is hoped that this review will stimulate interest in the many agents available and further enhance the therapeutic progress in this disease.

References

1. ADAMSON, R. H., CANELLOS, G. P., SIEBER, S. M.: Studies on the antitumor activity of gallium nitrate (NSC 15200) and other Group III-a metal salts. Cancer Chemother. Rep. *59*, 599–610 (1975)
2. ALBERTO, P., GANGJI, D., KENIS, Y., BRUGAROLAS, A., CLARYSSE, A., SYLVESTER, R., (EORTC Early Clinical Trials Group): Phase II Study of anhydro-ara-5 fluorocytidine (AAFC). Proc. AACR and ASCO *18*, 231 (AACR abs. 923) (1977)
3. ALTMAN, S. J., FLETCHER, W. S., ANDREWS, N. C., WILSON, W. L., PISCHER, T.: Yoshi 864, a new Phase I study. Cancer *35*, 1145–1147 (1975)
4. ANDERSON, T., DE VITA, V., BENDER, R., MANN, R., CHABNER, B., YOUNG, R.: Nodular lymphomas (NL): an important correlation of survival with complete remission induction. Proc. AACR and ASCO *18*, 326 (ASCO abstr. C 238) (1977)
5. ANDREWS, N. C., WEISS, A. J., WILSON, W., NEALON, T.: Phase II study of dibromodulcitol (NSC 104800). Cancer Chemother. Rep. *58*, 653–660 (1974)
6. BAKER, L. J., SAMSON, M. K., IZBICKI, R. M.: Phase I and II evaluation of cytembena in disseminated epithelial ovarian cancers and sarcomas. Cancer Treat. Rep. *60*, (9), 1389–1391 (Sept. 1976)
7. BEER, C. T., KAJIWARA, K., MUELLER, G. C.: Synchronization of HeLa cells with 2,3-dihydro-1H-imidazo (1,2-b)-pyrazole. Biochem. Pharmacol, *23*, 1112–1115 (1974)
8. BENJAMIN, R. S., HALL, S. W., BURGESS, M. A., WHEELER, W. L., MURPHY, W. K., BLUMENSCHEIN, G. R., GOTTLIEB, J. A.: A pharmacokinetically based Phase I-II study of single dose actinomycin D (NSC 3053). Cancer Treat. Rep. *60*, 289–291 (1976)
9. BERD, D., CORNOG, J., DI CONTI, R., LEVITT, M., BERTINO, J. R.,: Long term remission in diffuse histiocytic lymphoma treated with combination sequential chemotherapy. Cancer *35*, 1050–1054 (1975)

10. Bergsagel, D. E., Cowan, D. H., Hasselback, R.: Plasma cell myeloma: response of melphalan-resistant patients to high dose intermittent cyclophosphamide. Can. Med. Assoc. J. *107*, 851–855 (1972)
11. Bernard, J., Jacquillat, Cl., Boiron, M., Weil, M., German, M. F., Izrael, V., Schaison, G., Delobel, J.: Cinquante-Sept. observations de leucemies aiques. Essai de traitmente par un derive semi-synthetique de la daunorubicine: le 22050 R.P. Nouv. Presse Med. *1*, 2149–2152 (1972)
12. Blom, J. and Cancer and Leukemia Group B: Treatment of stage II & IV diffuse lymphocytic and histiocytic lymphoma with vincristine/prednisone/bleomycin/streptonigrin induction, cyclophosphamide/vincristine/prednisone maintenance with and without consolidation with vinblastine/CCNU/prednisone. Proc. AACR and ASCO *18*, 332 (ASCO abstr. C-261) (1977)
13. Blum, R. H., Carter, S. K., Agre, K.; A clinical review of bleomycin: a new antineoplastic agent. Cancer *31*, 903–913 (1973).
14. Bonadonna, G., De Lena, M., Monfardini, S., Bartoli, C., Bajetta, E., Baretta, G., Fossati-Bellani, F.: Clinical trials with bleomycin in lymphomas and solid tumors. Eur. J. Cancer *8*, 205–215 (1972)
15. Bonadonna, G., Lattuada, A., Banfi, A.: Recent trends in the treatment of non-Hodgkin's lymphomas. Eur. J. Cancer *12*, 661–673 (1975)
16. Bonadonna, G., Monfardini, S.: Chemotherapy of non-Hodgkin's lymphomas. Cancer Treat. Rev. *1*, 167–181 (1974)
17. Bonadonna, G., Zucalli, R., Monfardini, S., De Lena, M., Vslenghi, C.: Combination chemotherapy of Hodgkin's disease with adriamycin, bleomycin, vinblastine and imidazole carboxamide versus MOPP. Cancer *36*, 252–259 (1975)
18. Cabanillas, F., Rodriguez, V., Bodey, G. P., Benjamin, R. S.: Phase I-II study of maytansine (NSC 153,858). Proc. AACR and ASCO *18*, 206 (AACR abstr. 823) (1977)
19. Capizzi, R. L.: Improvement in the therapeutic index of methotrexate (NSC 740) by L-asparaginase (NSC 109229). Cancer Chemother. Rep. *6* (3), 37–41 (1975)
20. Carbone, P. P., Kaplan, H. S., Musshof, K., Smithers, D. W., Tubiana, M.: Report of the committee on Hodgkin's disease staging classification. Cancer Res. *31*, 1860–1861 (1971)
21. Carbone, P. P., Spurr, C.: Management of patients with malignant lymphoma. A comparative study of cyclophosphamide and vinca alkaloids. Cancer Res. *28*, 811-822 (1968)
22. Chabner, B. A., Johnson, R. E., Young, R. C., Canellos, G. P., Hubbard, S. P., De Vita, V. T., Jr.: Sequential nonsurgical and surgical staging in non-Hodgkin's lymphoma. Ann. Intern. Med. *85*, 149–154 (1976)
23. Chabner, B., Levine, A., Adamson, R., Johnson, B., Whangpeng, J., Young, R.: Initial clinical and pharmacological studies of maytansine. Proc. AACR and ASCO *18*, 129 (AACR abstr. 515) (1977)
24. Corbett, T. H., Griswold, D. P.: Treatment of colon adencarcinomas in mice with anguidine (NSC-141537) and anguidine + 5-FU (NSC-19893). Proc. AACR and ASCO *18*, 115 (AACR abstr. 457) (1977)
25. Creaven, P. J., Allen, L. M., Cohen, M. H., Nelson, R. L.; Studies on the clinical pharmacology and toxicology of isophosphamide (NSC 109724). Cancer Treat. Rep. *60*, 445–449 (1976)
26. Dawkins, A. W., Grove, J. F., Tidd, B. K.: Diacetoxyscirpenol and some related compounds. Chem. Community *2*, 27 (1965)
27. Djerassi, I,. Kim, J. S.: Methotrexate and citrovorum factor rescue in the management of childhood lymphosarcoma and reticulum cell sarcoma (non-Hodgkin's lymphomas) prolonged unmaintained remission. Cancer *38*, 1043–1051
28. Durant, J. R., Gams, R. A., Bartolucci, A. A., Dorfman, R. F.: BCNU with and without COP and cycle active therapy in non-Hodgkin's lymphoma. Cancer Treat. Rep. (in press, 1977)
29. Ennis, H. L., Moller, L., Wang, J. J., Selawry, O. S.: 2,3-dihydro-1H-imidazo (1,2-b)-pyrazole. A new inhibitor of deoxyribonucleic acid synthesis. Biochem. Pharmacol *20*, 2639–2646 (1971)
30. European Organization for Research on the Treatment of Cancer, Co-operative Group for Leukaemias and Haematosarcomas: Clinical Screening of epipodophyllotoxin VM 26 in malignant lymphomas and solid tumours. Br. Med. J. *2*, 744–748 (1972)
31. Edzinli, E., Pocock, S., Berard, C. W., Aungst, C. W., Silverstein, M., Horton, J., Bennett, J., Bakemeier, R., Stolbach, L., Perlia, C., Brunk, S. F., Lenhard, R. E., Klaasen, D. J., Richter, O., Carbone. P.: Comparison of intensive versus moderate chemotherapy of lymphocytic lymphomas. Cancer *38*, 1060–1068 (Sept. 1976)
32. Falkson, H. C., Falkson, G.: Phase II trial of cytembena in patients with advanced ovarian and breast cancer. Cancer Treat. Rep. *60* (11), 1655–1658 (1976)
33. Flannery, E. P., Corder, M. P., Sheehan, W. W., Bateman, J. R.: Phase II evaluation of ICRF-159 (NSC-129943) in non-Hodgkin's lymphomas. Proc. AACR and ASCO *17*, 289 (ASCO abstr. C-209) (1976)

34. Frei, E., III, Luce, J. K., Talley, R. W., Vaitkevicius, V. K., Wilson, H. E. 5 (3,3 dimethyl-triazeno) imidazole-4-carboxamide (NSC-45388) in the treatment of lymphoma. Cancer Chemother. Rep. *56*, 667–670 (1972)
35. Gottlieb, J. A., Luce, J. K. Treatment of malignant melanoma with campothecin (NSC 100880). Cancer Chemother. Rep. *56*, 103 (1972)
36. Green, D., Sallan, S., Krishan, A.: Single dose actinomycin D in relapsed childhood leukemia. Proc. AACR and ASCO *18*, 302 1977 (ASCO abstr. C-144)
37. Griffin, R. L., Comis, R. L., Lokich, J., Canellos, G.: Neocarzinostatin: phase I study. Proc. AACR and ASCO *18*, 302 (ASCO abstr. C-142) (1977)
38. Haas, C., Goodwin, W., Leite, C., Stephens, R., Hoogstraten, B.: Phase I study of anguidine diacetoxyscirpenol (NSC 141537). Proc. AACR and ASCO *18*, 296 (ASCO abstr. C-120) (1977)
39. Haas, C. D., Stephens, R. L., Hollister, M., Hoogstraten, B.: Phase I evaluation of dianhydrogalactitol (NSC 132313). Cancer Treat. Rep. *60*, 611–614 (1976)
40. Hayes, D., Cvitkovic, E., Golbey, R., Scheiner, E., Krakoff, I. H.: Amelioration of renal toxicity of high dose cis platinum diammine dichloride (CPPD) by mannitol induced diuresis. Proc. AACE and ASCO *17*, 169 (1976)
41. Helman, L., Henney, J., Slavik, M.: Clinical brochure—anguidine (NSC 141537). Investigational Drug Branch Cancer Therapy Evaluation Program, Division of Cancer Treatment, National Cancer Institute, Bethesda, Md.
42. Helman, L., Henney, J., Slavik, M. Clinical brochure—Maytansine (NSC 153858). Investigational Drug Branch, Cancer Therapy Evaluation Program, Division of Cancer Treatment, National Cancer Institute, Bethesda, Md.
43. Hill, J. M., Loeb, E., Pardue, A. S., Khan, A., Hill, N. O., King, J. J., Hill, R. W.: Platinum coordination compounds in the treatment of acute leukemia and other malignant diseases with particular reference to malanato 1,2-di-aminocyclohexane platinum (II). J. Clin. Haematol Oncology *7*, 681–700 (1977)
44. Hoth, D., Schein, P., McDonald, J., Buscaglia, D., Haller, D.: Phase I trial and clinical pharmacology of chlorozotocin (CL 2). Proc. AACR and ASCO *18*, 309 (1977)
45. Investigational Drug Branch, Cancer Therapy Evaluation Program, Division of Cancer Treatment, National Cancer Institute, Bethesda, Md.: Ara-C-analogues. In: Minutes of New Drug Liaison Meeting 186–242 (Feb. 17–18, 1977)
46. Investigational Drug Branch, Cancer Therapy Evaluation Program, Division of Cancer Treatment, National Cancer Institute, Bethesda, Md.: Vindesine. In: Minutes of New Drug Liaison Meeting (Feb. 17–18, 1977)
47. Investigational Drug Branch, Cancer Therapy Evaluation Program, Division of Cancer Treatment, National Cancer Institute, Bethesda, Md.: Pyrazolo imidazole. In: Minutes of the Phase I Working Group Meeting (Oct. 7, 1976)
48. Israel, M., Modest, E. J., Frei, E., III: N-trifluoroacetyl adriamycin-14-valerate—an analogue with greater experimental antitumor activity and less toxicity than adriamycin. Cancer Res. *35*, 1365–1368 (1975)
49. Jacobs, E. M., Peters, F. C., Luce, J. K., et al: Mechlorethiamine (HCL) and cyclophosphamide in the treatment of Hodgkin's disease and the lymphomas. JAMA *203*, 392–398 (1969)
50. Jacquillat, Cl., Weill, M., Geman-Auclerc, M. F., Izrael, V., Bussed, A., Boiron, M., Bernard, T.: Clinical study of rubidazone (22050 R. P.), a new daunorubicin-derived compound, in 170 patients with leukemias and other malignancies. Cancer *37*, 653–659 (1976)
51. Jacquillat, Cl., Weil, M., Geman, M. F., Izrael, V., Schaison, G., Boiron, M., Bernard, J.: Treatment of acute myeloblastic leukemia with R.P. 22050. Br. Med. J. *4*, 468–469 (1972)
52. Jones, S. E., Fuks, Z., Bull, M., Kadin, M., Dorfam, R., Kaplan, H. S., Rosenberg, S. A.: Non-Hodgkin's lymphomas IV—clinicopathologic correlation in 405 cases. Cancer 31, 806–823 (1973)
53. Jones, S. E., Salmon, S., Members of the Southwest Oncology Group: Phase II trial of piperazinedione (Crystal-line antibiotic) in lymphoma and multiple myeloma. Proc. AACR and ASCO *17*, 45 (AACR abstr. 179) (1976)
54. Jones, S. E., Salmon, S. E., Moon, T. E., Butler, J. J., Members of the Southwest Oncology Group (Swog): Chemo-immunotherapy of non-Hodgkin's lymphoma (NHL). Proc. AACR and ASCO *18*, 291 (ASCO abstr. C-100) (1977)
55. Jones, S. E., Rosenberg, S. A., Kaplan, H. S., Kadin, M. E., Dorfman, R. F.: Non-Hodgkin's lymphomas II. Single agent chemotherapy. Cancer *30*, 31–38 (1972)
56. Kaufman, J. H., Ezdinli, E., Aungst, C. W., Stutzman, L.: Lymphosarcoma—a comparison of extended to conservative chemotherapy. Cancer *37*, 1283–1292 (1976)
57. Kaufman, J. H., Hanjina, G. L., Mittleman, A., Aungst, C. W., Murphy, G. P.: Study of LEO 1031 (NSC 134087) in lymphocytic lymphoma and chronic lymphocytic leukemia. Cancer Treat. Rep. *60*, 277–279 (1976)

58. Kaufman, J. H., Mittleman, A.: Clinical phase I trial of imosine dialdehyde (NSC 118954). Cancer Chemother. Rep. *59*, 1007–1014 (1975)
59. Kennedy, B. J., Hill, J., Bloomfield, C. D., Kiang, D., Fortuny, I., Theologides, A.: Combination (COP) versus successive single agent chemotherapy (C-O-P) in lymphocytic lymphoma. Proc. AACR and ASCO *16*, 142 (AACR abstr. 568) (1975)
60. Krishan, A., Frei, E., III, Paika, K,: Studies on the biological action of adriamycin analog, N-trifluoro-acetyl-adriamycin (AD 32). Proc. AACR and ASCO *18*, 188 (AACR abstr. 751) (1977)
61. Laszlo. J., Durant, J., Loeb, V.: Clinical pharmacological study of 1-acetyl-2-picolinoylhydrazine (NSC 68626). Cancer Chemother. Rep. *53*, 131–134 (1969)
62. Lauria, F., Baccarani, M., Fiacchini, M.: Methotrexate cyclophosphamide and vincristine (MEV regimen) for non-Hodgkin's lymphoma. Eur. J. Cancer *11*, 343–349 (1975)
63. Legha, S. S., Slavik, M., Carter, S. K.: Hexamethylmelamine. An evaluation of its role in the therapy of cancer. Cancer *38*, 27–35 (1976)
64. Legha, S. S., Von Hoff, D. D., Slavik, M., Muggia, F. M.: Neocarzinostatin (NSC 157365)—a new cancerostatic compound. Oncology *33*, 265–270 (1976)
65. Lenaz, L., Page, J. A.: Cardiotoxicity of adriamycin and related anthracyclines. Cancer Treat. Rev. *3*, 111–120 (1976)
66. Lenhard, R. E., Jr., Prentice, R. L., Owens, A. H., Jr., Bakmeier, R., Horton, J. H., Shnider, B. I., Stolbach, L., Berard, C. W., Carbone, P.: Combination chemotherapy of the malignant lymphomas—a controlled clinical trial. Cancer *38*, 1052–1059 (1976)
67. Lias, L. L., Kupchan, S. M., Horwitz, S. B.: Mode of action of the antitumor compound bruceantin, an inhibitor of protein synthesis. Mol. Pharmacol. *12*, 167–176 (1976)
68. Livingston, R. B., Carter, S. K.: Single agents in cancer chemotherapy. New York–Washington–London: IFI/Plenum, 1970, p. 405
69. Mathé, G., Schwarzenberg, P., Pouillart, R., Oldham, R., Weiner, R., Jasmin, C., Rosenfeld, C., Hayat, M., Misset, J. L., Musset, M., Schneider, M., Amiel, J. L., De Vassal, F.: Two épipodophyllotoxin deratives, VN 26 and VP 16213, in the treatment of leukemias, hématosarcomas, and lymphomas. Cancer *34* (4), 985–992 (1974)
70. Mathé, G., Schwartzenberg, P., Pouillart, P., Weiner, R., Oldham, R., Jasmin, C., Rosenfeld, C., Hayat, M., Schneider, M., Amiel, J. L., Céoara, B., Steresco-Musset, M., De Vassal, F.: Essai de traitment de divers hématosarcomes par le 4-déméthyl-épipodophyllotoxine β D. thénylidème glucoside (VM 26 ou EPT). Nouve. Presse Med. *23*, 447–451 (1974)
71. Mathé, G., Schwartzenbergerg, P., Pouillart, P., Weiner, R., Oldham, R., Jasmin, C., Rosenfeld, C., Hayat, M., Schneider, M., Amiel, J. L., Céoara, B., Steresco-Musset, M., De Vassal, F.: Leucémies aiguës et hématosarcomes divers. Essai de traitement par un second dérivé de la podophyllotoxine (le 4-demethyl-epipodophyllotoxine beta.D. ethylidene glucoside VP 16213 ou EPE). Nouv. Presse Med. *2*, 521–524 (1974)
72. McKelvey, E. M.: Gallium nitrate in minutes of the phase I working group meeting, April 26–27, 1977. Investigational Drug Branch, Cancer Therapy Evaluation Program, Division of Cancer Treatment, National Cancer Institute, Bethesda, Md.
73. McKelvey, E. M., Gottlieb, J. A., Wilson, H. E., Haut, A., Talley, R. W., Stephens, R., Lane, M., Gamble, J. F., Jones, S. E., Grozea, P. N., Gutterman, J., Coltman, C., Jr., Moon, T.: Hydroxyldaunomycin (adriamycin combination chemotherapy in malignant lymphoma. Cancer *38* (4), 1484–1493, (1976)
74. Meyers, G. E., McGuire, W., Young, R. C.: Adriamycin: amelioration of toxicity by α-tocopheral. Cancer Treat. Rep. *60*, 961–962 (1976)
75. Misset, J. L., Pouillart, P., Belpomme, L., Schwarzenberg, L., Delgado, M., Gil, M., Jasmin, C., Hayat, M., Mathé, G.: Combination chemotherapy with adriamycine, VM 26, cyclophosphamide and prednisone in lymphosarcoma and reticulosarcoma stage III and IV. Eur. J. Cancer *13*, 411–414 (1977)
76. Moertel, C. G., Schutt, et al.: Phase II study of campothecin (NSC 100880) in the treatment of advanced gastrointestinal cancer. Cancer Chemother. Rep. *56*, 95 (1972)
77 Möller, T. R., Brandt, L., Könynes, I., Lindberg, L. G.: Therapeutic effects of Leo 1031, an alkylating corticosteroid ester in lymphoproliferative disorders—II lymphocytic lymphoma. Acta Med. Scand. *197*, 323–327 (1975)
78. Muggia, F. M., Creaven, P. J., Hansen, H. H., Et Al; Phase I clinical trial of weekly and daily treatment with campothecin (NSC 100880): correlation with preclinical studies. Cancer Chemother. Rep. *56*, 515–521 (1972)
79. O'Connell, M. J., Silverstein, M. J., Silverstein, M. N., Kiely, J. M., White, W. L.: Pilot study of two adriamycin-based regimens in patients with advanced malignant lymphomas. Cancer Treat. Rep. *61*, (1), 65–68 (1977)
80. O'Bryan, R. M., Baker, L. H., Gottlieb, J. A., Rivkin, S. E., Balcerak, S. P., Grumet, G. N., Salmon, S. E., Moon, T. E., Hoogstraten, B.: Dose response evaluation of adriamycin in human neoplasia. Cancer *39*, 1940–1948 (1977)

81. O'Bryan, R. M., Luce, J. K., Talley, R. W., Gottlieb, J. A., Baker, L. J., Bonadonna, G.: Phase II evaluation of adriamycin in human neoplasia. Cancer *32*, 1–8 (1973)
82. Page, R. H., Talley, R. W., Bukagiar, J.: The enhanced anti-tumor activity of cis-diammedichloroplatinum (II) against murine tumors when combined with other agents. J. Clin. Haematol. Oncology 7, 96–104 (1977)
83. Perevodchikova, N. I., Gorbunova, V. A., Lichinitser, M. P., Borisov, V. I., Alekseev, N. A., Vygodskaya, L.: Phase I clinical trial of carminomycin in a new anthracycline antibiotic. Proc. AACR and ASCO (AACR abstr 437) *17*, 110 (1976)
84. Pittman, S., Frei, E., III: Weekly methotrexate citrovorum (MTX-CF) with alkalinization: tumor response in a phase II study. Proc. AACR and ASCO *18*, 124 (AACR abstr. 494) (1977)
85. Portlock, C. S., Rosenberg, S. A., Glatstein, E., Kaplan, H. S.: Treatment of advanced non-Hodgkin's lymphomas with favorable histologies: Preliminary results of a prospective trial. Blood *47*, 747–756 (1976)
86. Rappaport, H.: Tumors of the hematopoetic system. In: Atlas of Tumor Pathology, Sec. 3, Fasc. 8. Washington, D.C.: Armed Forces Institute of Pathology, 1966
87. Remillard, S., et al: Antimitotic activity of the potent tumor inhibitor maytansine. Science *189*, 1002–1005 (1975)
88. Rozencweig, M., Von Hoff, D. D., Slavik, M., Muggia, F. M.: Cis-diamminedichloroplatinum II: a new anticancer drug with significant clinical activity. Ann. Intern. Med. *86*, 803–812 (1977)
89. Schein, P. S., Chabner, B. A., Canellos, G. P., Young, R. C., Berard, C. W., De Vita, V. T., Jr.: Potential for prolonged disease-free survival following combination chemotherapy of non-Hodgkin's lymphomas. Blood *43*, 181–190 (1974)
90. Schein, P. S., De Vita, V. T., Jr., Hubbard, S., Chabner, B. A., Canellos, G. P., Berard, C., Young, R. C.: Bleomycin, adriamycin, cyclophosphamide, vincristine and prednisone (BACOP) in the treatment of advanced diffuse histiocytic lymphoma. Ann. Intern. Med. *85*, 417–422 (1976)
91. Schein, P. S., O'Connell, M. J., Blom, J., Hubbard, S., Magrath, I. T., Bergevin, P., Wiernik, P. H., Ziegler, J. L., De Vita, V. T.: Clinical antitumor activity and toxicity of streptozotocin (NSC-85998) Cancer *34*, 993–1000 (1974)
92. Schein, P. S., Panasci, L., Woolley, P. V., Anderson, T.: Pharmacology of chlorozotocin (NSC-178248), a new nitrosourea antitumor agent. Cancer Treat. Rep. *60*, 801–805 (1976)
93. Sieber, S. M., Mead, J. A. R., Adamson, R. H.: Pharmacology of antitumor agents from higher plants. Cancer Treat. Rep. *60*, 1127–1139 (1976)
94. Spear, P. W., Patno, M. E.: A comparative study of the effectiveness of HN_2 and cyclophosphamide in bronchogenic carcinoma, Hodgkin's disease and lymphosarcoma. Cancer Chemother. Rep. *16*, 413–415 (1962)
95. Stein, T. S., Moran, E. M., Desser, R. K., Miller, J. B., Golomb, H. M., Ultman, J. E.: Combination chemotherapy of lymphomas other than Hodgkin's disease. Ann. Intern. Med. *81*, 601 (1974)
96. Stolinsky, D. C., Jacobs, E. M., Irwin, L. E., Bateman, J. R.: Study of trimethylcolchicinic acid methyl ether d-tartrate (TMCA; NSC.-36354) in Hodgkin's and non-Hodgkin's lymphoma. Proc. AACR and ASCO *17*, 237 (ASCO abstr. C-1) (1976)
97. Stitzman, L., Ezdinli, E. Z., Stutzman, M. A.: Vinblastine sulfate vs. cyclophosphamide in the therapy of lymphoma. JAMA *195*, 173–178 (1966)
98. Sutow, W. W., Komp. D., Vietti, T. J., Pinkerton, D.: Clinical trials with 1-acetyl-2-picolinoylhydrazine (NSC-68626) in children. Cancer Chemother. Rep. 59, 341–344 (1975)
99. Von Hoff, D. D., Rozencweig, M., Soper, W. T., Helman, L. J., Davis, H. L., Penta, J. S., Muggia, F. M.: Whatever happened to NSC——? Cancer Treat. Rep. *61*, 759–768 (1977)
100. Weiss, A. J., Metter, G. E., Fletcher, W. S., Wilson, W. L., Grage, R. B., Ramirez, G.; Studies on adriamycin using a weekly regimen demonstrating its clinical effectiveness and lack of cardiac toxicity. Cancer Treat. Rep. *60*, 813–822 (1976)
101. Wilkinson, P. M., Israel, M., Pegg, W. J., Frei, E., III: Comparative hepatobiliary metabolism and excretion of adriamycin (ADR) and N-tri-flouroacetyladriamycin-14-valerate (AD-32). Proc. AACR and ASCO *18*, 188 (AACR abstr. 752) (1977)
102. Wilson, W. L., Weiss, A. J., Frelich, R. W.: A phase III study in lung cancer comparing hexamethylmelamine with dibromodulcital. Oncology *31*, 289–305 (1975)
103. Winchell, H. S., Sanchez, P. D., Watanabe, C. K., Hollander, L., Auger, H. O., McCrae, I.: Visualization of tumors in humans using ^{67}Ga-citrate and the Auger whole-body scanner, scintillation camera and tomographic scanner. J. Nucl. Med. *11*, 459–466 (1970)
104. Wollner, N., Burchenal, J. H., Lieberman, P. H., Exelby, P., D'Angio, G. J., Murphy, M. L.: Non Hodgkin's lymphoma in children. A comparative study of two modalities of therapy. Cancer *37*, 123–134 (1976)
105. Worzolla, J. F., Kaiman, B. D., Johnson, B. M., Ramirez, G., Bryan, G. T.: Metabolism of hexamethylmelamine-ring C in rats and man. Cancer Res. *34*, 2669–2674 (1974)

106. Yang, S. S.: Rifamycin antibiotics: Inhibitors of Rauscher murine leukemia virus reverse transcriptase and of purified DNA polymerases from human normal and leukemic lymphoblasts. J. Natl. Cancer Inst. *49*, 7–25 (1972
107. Zbinden, G., Brandle, E.: Toxicologic screening of daunorubicin (NSC 82151), adriamycin (NSC 123127) and their derivatives in rats. Cancer Chemother. Rep. *59*, 707–715 (1975)

General Strategy of Staging and Therapy of Non-Hodgkin's Lymphomas

CH. E. MYERS and B. A. CHABNEV

The classification of lymphomas proposed by RAPPAPORT et al. [1] in 1966 brought order to the chaos surrounding the non-Hodgkin's lymphomas. This classification, based on the presence or absence of a nodular pattern of nodal involvement and on the degree of differentiation of the malignant cells, stimulated much of the work presented at this symposium. It served a useful purpose in identifying the nodular pattern as carrying a favorable prognostic import when compared to the diffuse pattern. In addition, it called attention to the differing natural histories and patterns of disease progression associated with the major RAPPAPORT classifications. It was in this context that, in 1971, the National Cancer Insititute (NCI) initiated a study of the patterns of organ involvement and response to therapy of each of the lymphoma subclasses (2). An important aspect of this study was the ordered, sequential nature of the staging procedures used (Table 1). The staging approach used involved an initial battery of procedures including lymphangiogram, bone marrow, and percutaneous liver biopsy which served to identify a significant proportion of those with stage IV disease. Those patients with negative percutaneous liver biopsies were subject to peritoneoscopy with multiple liver biopsies and if still negative with respect to liver disease, then laparotomy. Table 2 illustrates the upstaging which resulted from the procedures used. It also emphasizes that a majority of the patients were staged

Table 1. Staging of non-Hodgkin's lymphoma

1. Routine Diagnostic Procedures (after physical exam)
   A. Clinical Chemistries, Hemogram
   B. Chest and Bone Films
   C. Gallium and Bone Scans
   D. Lymphangiogram
   E. Bone Marrow Biopsy
   F. Percutaneous Liver Biopsy
2. Peritoneoscopy with Multiple Liver Biopsies—in stage I-III patients.
3. Staging Laparotomy—in all stage I-III patients after above tests.
   A. Splenectomy
   B. Splenic, Portal, Mesenteric and Para-aortic Nodes
   C. Wedge Liver Biopsy

Table 2. 170 Patients with non-Hodgkin's lymphoma: change in stage during work-up

	Percentage of patients in each stage			
	I	II	III	IV
Clinical stage on referral	12	21	42	24
After lymphangiogram	8	15	54	24
After bone marrow	7	13	33	48
After closed liver biopsies	6	11	25	58
After laparotomy	6	8	21	65

adequately without laparotomy. Thus, this staging approach gave all of the advantages of aggressive clinical staging while limiting laparotomy to the minority of patients where it is of value. This NCI study and the work of others have served to clarify the natural history of the non-Hodgkin's lymphomas (Table 3). What has been particularly disconcerting is the similarities in patterns of disease extension between the various RAPPAPORT classifications (Table 4). For example, nodular poorly differentiated lymphoma (PDL), nodular mixed, and diffuse PDL were all found to have a high frequency of liver and marrow involvement. The diffuse PDL, in fact, differed from the nodular types only in its increased incidence of extranodal primaries, with the increase being confined to the gastrointestinal tract, bone, and skin (Table 5). In addition, the justification for making a distinction between the two main types of nodular lymphomas, PDL and mixed cellularity, would depend on there being a difference in response to therapy not demonstrable at this time.

The RAPPAPORT classification does distinguish at least one unique group, diffuse histiocytic lymphoma (DHL), from the other histologies. Yet, there is growing evidence that DHL is a heterogenous group on several counts. In terms of presentation, the gastrointestinal primary DHLs clearly represent a distinct group with a propensity for extensive local spread and poorer prognosis. In terms of immunologic markers, DHL is heterogeneous with approximately 10% of T-cell origin and the rest classified as null cells. Finally, in our hands there are two clearly defined groups with regard to therapeutic response: 40%–50% attain complete remission with

Table 3. Natural history of non-Hodgkin's lymphomas

1. Not often localized
2. Often spreads in an unpredictable fashion
3. Tendency to disseminate and spread unpredictably related to histologic subtype and nodularity
4. Extranodal sites of origin are common
5. Bone marrow and liver often involved early without signs of organ dysfunction
6. Absence of symptoms does not favorably influence prognosis

Table 4. Yield of non-surgical procedures in non-Hodgkin's lymphoma

	Lymph gram	Bone marrow Bx	Liver biopsy	
			Perc.	Perit.
Nodular	62/69 (90%)	31/79 (39%)	18/72 (25%)	16/51 (32%)
Diffuse				
Hist. and mixed	27/44 (61%)	8/45 (18%)	3/37 (8%)	5/31 (16%)
Other[a]	13/19 (68%)	19/35 (54%)	5/18 (28%)	5/8 (63%)

[a] Includes stem cell and poorly-differentiated lymphocytic lymphoma.

Table 5. Diffuse histiocytic lymphoma. Staging of patients with extranodal primary presentation and comparison with nodal primary patients

Site	No. pts.	L gram	Bone marrow Bx	Liver biopsy	Final stage IV
Bone	7	4/6	2/7	0/5	6/7
Gastro-intestinal tract	17	11/15	2/17	2/17	14/17
Skin	3	2/3	0/3	1/3	2/3
Total	27	17/25 (68%)	4/27 (15%)	3/25 (12%)	22/27 (81%)
Nodal histiocytics	26	15/26 (58%)	5/26 (19%)	4/24 (17%)	7/26[a] (27%)

[a] $p < 0.05$.

relative ease, and this group contains a relatively high percentage of long-term remitters. The remainder achieve no response or a partial response and have a median survival of less than 1 year. Do we design our regimens in order to achieve durable remissions in the responsive group with as little morbidity as possible, or do we risk potentially lethal toxicity to more effectively treat the drug-resistant patients? The best answer would be to have a system of lymphoma classification which would do a better job of segregating patients according to natural history and therapeutic responsiveness than does the present pathologic classification.

Rather than discard pathology because of these inadequacies, it seems to us that it should be expanded by the use of the growing list of biochemical and immunologic parameters by which one lymphomatous malignancy has been shown to differ from another. Perhaps it would be more constructive to view pathology as only one of the windows through which we examine the non-Hodgkin's lymphomas.

The division of lymphomas according to B- or T-cell markers is particularly attractive and is being actively pursued at several institutions including NCI. For acute lymphocytic leukemia (ALCL) such a division has provided information of major prognostic importance (3). While a similar clear-cut prognostic value for B- and T-cell classification has yet to be demonstrated for non-Hodgkin's lymphomas, studies to date have shed some light on the nature of the disease process (4). This immunologic typing may have as yet unexplored therapeutic implications; for example, type-specific antilymphocyte serum may allow serotherapy of selected lymphomas. Finally, the recent discovery of the helper and inhibitor T-cell subtypes are of particular interest and may help one understand the nature of the various T-cell malignancies (5).

In addition to these immunologic markers, we have a growing list of biochemical markers which serve to separate lymphomas into distinct groups. M. Lippman and co-workers have shown a clear relationship between the presence of the glucocorticoid receptor and the response to prednisone in ALCL [6]. The favorable prognosis associated with the presence of this hormone appears to be independent of the T- or B-cell classification of the leukemia. In the same vein, it would be of value to determine the prognostic value of the gluecocorticoid receptor in the non-Hodgkin's lymphomas and further to study how receptor presence correlates with the current pathologic classification.

Adenosine deaminase, the enzyme which converts adenosine to inosine, is elevated to T-cell ALCL and Sezary's syndrome but decreased in chronic lymphocytic leukemia (CLCL), a B-cell malignancy [7]. In addition to its potential use as a marker for the subclassification of lymphomas, presence or absence of this enzyme may have therapeutic implications. Lymphomas with a high content of this enzyme may be sensitive to inhibitors of this enzyme, such as deoxycoformicin, whereas tumors with low levels of the enzyme would be unable to clear the drug Ara A and might thus be responsive to this drug.

The enzyme, terminal transferase, has been shown to be characteristic of immature lymphocytes of thymus origin, ALCL cells, and certain lymphoblastic chronic mylogenous leukemia lines [8]. The role which this enzyme plays in vivo is not clear; however, its ability to generate genetic material without a template suggest it may act as a mechanism to generate genetic diversity. The distribution of this enzyme might not only provide more information upon which to classify lymphomas but might also shed light on how these tumors evolve drug resistance or shift their histologic pattern.

This obviously partial listing is meant only to illustrate the range of windows through which the lymphomas may be viewed. Certainly, a lymphoma classification which includes pathologic, immunologic, and biochemical parameters would provide a more comprehensive view of the disease process involved. It seems likely that such a classification would be better at predicting the natural history and therapeutic responsiveness of the lymphomas than the current one. Finally, as an added benefit, the immunologic and biochemical information might allow the prediction of the success of specific forms of therapy such as response to glucocorticoid or Ara A.

References

1. Broder, S., Humphrey, R., Durm, M., Blackman, M., Meade, B., Goldman, C., Strober, W., Waldmann. T.: Impaired Synthesis of Polyclonal Immunoglobulins by circulating lymphocytes from Patients with Multiple Myeloma. N. Engl. J. Med. *293*, 887 (1975)
2. Chabner, B. A., Johnson, R. E., Young, R. C., Canellos, G. P., Hubbard, S. P., Johnson, S. K., DeVita, V. T.: Sequential Non-Surgical and Surgical Staging of non-Hodgkin's Lymphoma. Ann. Inter. Med. *85*, 149 (1976)
3. Dow, L. W., George, S. L., Mauer, A. M.: Predictive Models for Lymphoblastic leukemia. Proc. Am. Assoc. Cancer Res. *18*, 63 (1977)
4. Jaffe, E. S., Shevach, E. M., Frank, M. M., Bernard, C. W., Green, I.: Nodular lymphoma-Evidence for Origin from Follicular B Lymphocytes. N. Engl. J. Med. *290*, 813 (1974)
5. Konior, G. S., Lippman, M. E., Johnson, G. E., Leventhal, B. G.: Correlation of Glucocorticoid Receptor Levels and Complete Remission Duration in Poor Prognosis Acute lymphocytic leukemia. Proc. Am. Soc. Clin. Oncology *18*, C346 (1977)
6. McCaffrey, R., Harrison, T. A., Parkman, R., Baltimore, D.: Terminal Deoxynucleotidyl Transferase Activity in Human Leukemic Cells and in Normal Human Thymocytes. N. Engl. J. Med. *292*: 775 (1975)
7. Rappaport, H., Winter, W. J., Hicks, E. B.: A Re-evaluation of its Position in the Scheme of malignant lymphoma, Based on Survey of 253 cases. Cancer *9*, 792 (1956)
8. Smythe, J., Poplack, D. G., Holiman, B. J., Leventhal, B. J., Magrath, I. T.: Correlation of Adenosine Deaminase Activity and Cell Surface Markers in Leukemic Lymphoblasts. Proc. Am. Assoc. Cancer Res. *18*, 856 (1977)

Chemotherapy in Non-Hodgkin's Malignant Lymphomas According to Potential Evolutive Groups

J. J. Sotto, M. Michallet, M. F. Sotto, B. Lachet, H. Martin, R. Schaerer, C. Vrousos, and D. Hollard

Histology and cytology show us the strong heterogeneity of non-Hodgkin's malignant lymphomas (NHML). Numerous classifications have been proposed. They contain 6–12 classes [18, 25] which more or less match [5, 9, 10, 12, 17, 18, 20, 25]. If, with luck, a nonsophisticated and reproducible classification could predict the evolution, we would have to take it into account and suit the treatment to it. Nevertheless, none of the present classification systems are able to solve the problem for all the patients with NHML. The aim of a practical classification is to clearly distinguish the morphologic groups with the same predictable evolution possibly to cancel those in which the prognosis is still confused. Such well-defined groups have already been described, e.g., African Burkitt's lymphoma [1], immunoblastic sarcoma [19], convoluted cell lymphosarcoma [18, 30], nodular well-differentiated lymphomas [4, 16], and histiocytosarcoma [22]. Nevertheless, it is still difficult to compare the potential evolution of the morphologic groups from one center to another. There are several causes: the reproducibility is not easy, the treatments are different, and even the frontiers of the disease are badly separated from the chronic lymphocytic leukemia or the acute leukemia.

Our aim in this study was: 1) to define evolutive groups in a retrospective study with patients having an homogeneous treatment and 2) to recognize these groups by a cytologic classification described elsewhere [28, 29] in order to suggest in a prospective study different treatments in relation to their potential evolution. The retrospective study was performed on 147 patients treated from 1967–1975. There were 91 male patients (61%) and 60 female patients (39%). The median age was 55 years. The staging method particularly consisted in performing x-ray examination of the mediastinum, lymphography, laparoscopy, liver biopsy, and bone marrow examination. Thus, the clinical stage according to the Rye classification [26] separated 62 localized forms of stages I and II (41%) from 89 disseminated forms of stages III and IV (59%). All of the patients were examined histologically according to the Kiel classification [12]. The histologic distribution is shown in Table 1. We noticed the usual predominance of centrofollicular lymphomas (51%), but there were few nodular forms in our experience, i.e., 15 cases (10%). The treatment was decided on only in relation to the clinical stage. We applied

Table 1. Histologic distribution according to Kiel classification

Histologic type	No. of patients	Percentage
Lymphocytic	5	3
Centrocytic	29	20
Mixed	20	14
Centroblastic	25	17
Lymphoblastic	31	21
Immunoblastic	25	17
Reticulosarcoma	7	5
Nonclassified	4	3
Total	146	

regional radiotherapy in stages I and II, and in disseminated forms, we gave various slightly modified chemotherapies. The main variations in treatment were in relation to the age, but all the treatments contained vincristine, cyclophosphamide, and prednisone. In patients under 50 years of age, we performed a meningeal prophylaxis.

Definition of the Evolutive Groups

Considering that this treatment schedule was applied for the entire patient population, we have been able to describe four evolutive groups using four parameters:

1. The patient's survival
2. The behavior of the disease in relation to remission status
3. The spreading patterns of the disease
4. The initial clinical stage

The survival data are shown in Fig. 1. Each patient is recorded at the time of death or at the time of survey while still alive. Patients who died from other causes are indicated. We noticed that the development for the whole population is divided into four periods. During the first two periods (0–7 and 9–15 months), deaths were frequent. The last two periods from 18 months onward contain mainly patients who are still alive.

The second parameter takes the remission status into account (Fig. 2). Here again, we can divide the whole population into four groups:

1. Patients not in complete remission (CR): 49 patients.
2. Patients in short CR < 5 months.
3. Patients in CR for longer than 7 months: 28 patients. We noticed that these patients later often had several relapses.
4. Patients who are still in first CR: 30 patients.

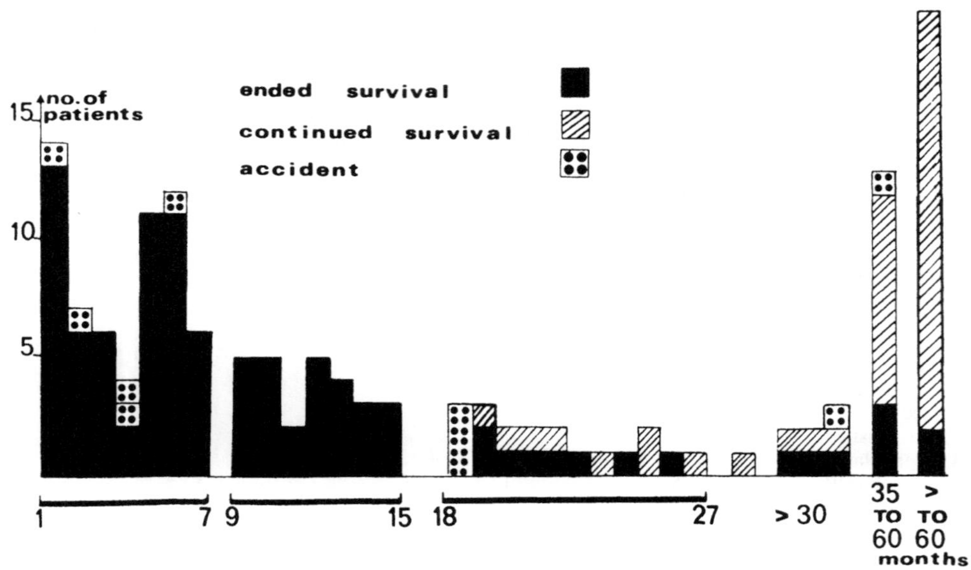

Fig. 1. Survival duration of the total patient population (147 patients)

Figure 3 shows the survival periods in terms of the remission status. With these two parameters, the distribution of the patients falls into two well-defined groups:

1. A bad prognosis group (81 patients). They had no CR or a short CR (< 5 months) in relation to the survival time (15 months). Only 4 out of 15 patients who relapsed between 7 and 12 months (Fig. 2) died before 15 months.
2. A good prognosis group (61 patients) in which survival was longer than 18 months. We can divide this group into two subgroups: one in which 30 patients are still in first CR (25 alive plus 5 patients who are allocated to this group because they died in first CR due to another cause) and another subgroup in which the patients had relapsed; in this case, the first relapse most often occurred after 7 months (24 patients); it was seldom before or absent (7 patients). The third parameter takes the spreading pattern of the disease into account. It enables one to separate an acute leukemic type from a metastatic type. Our criteria for the group with an acute leukemic evolution are:

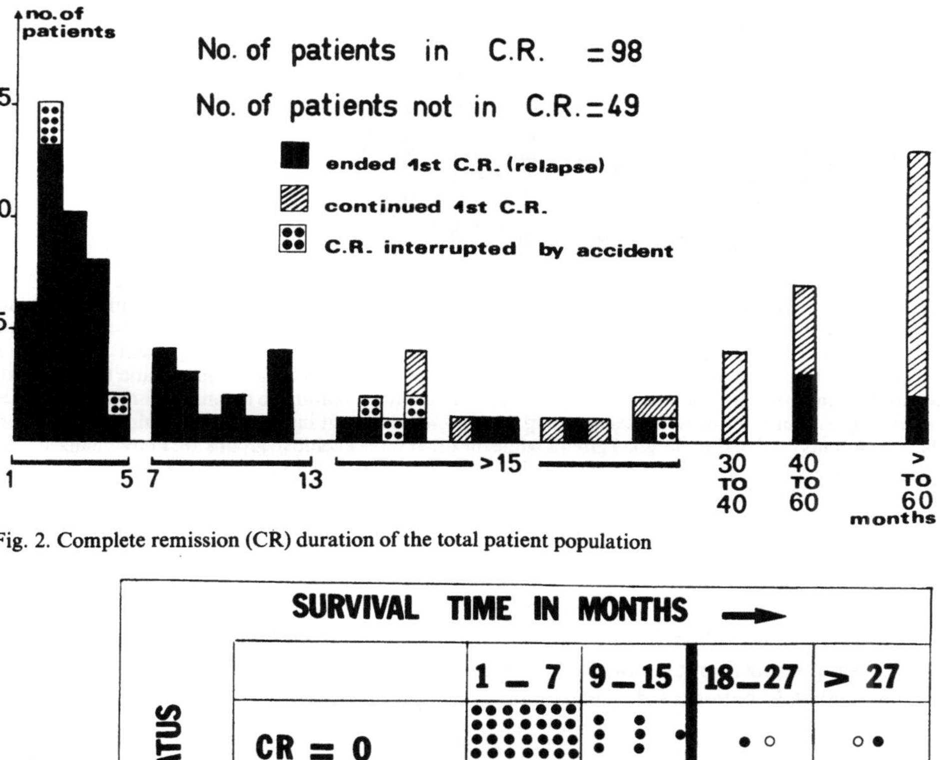

Fig. 2. Complete remission (CR) duration of the total patient population

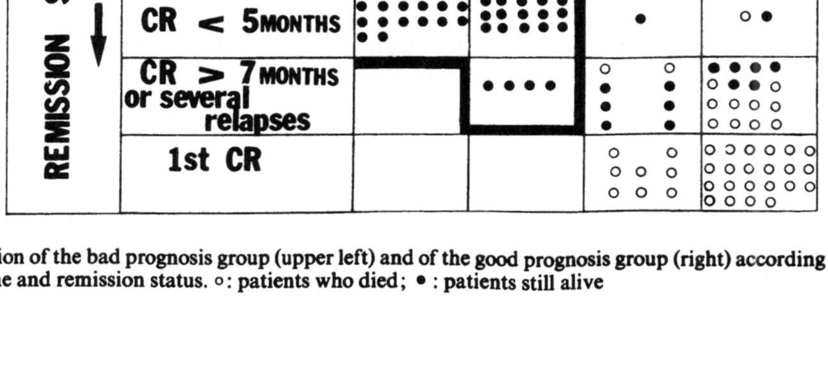

Fig. 3. Definition of the bad prognosis group (upper left) and of the good prognosis group (right) according to survival time and remission status. o: patients who died; •: patients still alive

1. At presentation, patients must have no or only partial involvement of the bone marrow and < 5% circulating blasts in order to separate NHML from acute leukemia.
2. During the progresssion of the disease, patients must not only have a diffused bone marrow involvement but also a depression of normal hematopoiesis and a rapid progression either of the tumor or of the bone marrow involvement.

All the other patients with progression of the disease are classified as having metastastic evolution. The fourth parameter is the initial clinical status, which indicated either a localized or diffused disease. The four parameters for defining the four evolutive groups are assembled in Figure 4. Five patients who died quickly due to other causes are excluded; 142 evaluable patients remain.

INITIAL CLINICAL FEATURES	EVOLUTION				
	BAD		GOOD		
	leuk.	metast.	leuk.	chronic metast.	free of disease
stage III+IV	24	33	4	15	7
stage I+II	8	16	1	11	23

Fig. 4. The four parameters assembled to define the four evolutive groups in 142 evaluable patients. The first two parameters (patient's survival and remission status) allows us to set up two major columns corresponding to the bad evolution and to the good evolution. The second parameter is used only in the good cases in order to specify whether the patients are free of disease or if they present a progressive disease. The third parameter separates the acute leukemic type (leuk.) from the metastatic type (metast.) in both bad and good groups. The two rows classify the patients according to the initial clinical stages. The evolutive groups are: the acute leukemic group (leuk.)—which is split into two parts within the bad groups (24 + 8 patients) and within the good groups while the other three evolutive groups are individualized—the bad and metastatic group (33 + 16 patients), the good chronic and diffused groups (15 + 11 + 7 patients), and the good and localized groups (23 patients)

Leukemic Evolutive Group

This group represents 26% of the patients. Thirty-two were in the bad prognosis group and five in the good prognosis group, only by reason of the efficiency of the chemotherapy. Within this group, 9 out of 37 patients (24%) had an initially localized stage.

Bad and Metastatic Evolutive Group

Patients in this group behave as do those with solid tumors. They represent 35% of the patients; 16 out of 49 (34%) had an initially localized stage.

Good Chronic and Diffused Evolutive Group

This group contains patients with long survival who had one or several relapses. We added patients still free of disease who had initially a diffused clinical stage. It represents 23% of the patients.

Good and Localized Evolutive Group

This group contains patients with a long survival who were free of disease after only a regional treatment. This truly localized disease represents 16% of the patients. On the whole, the notion of an evolutive group seems practical to us. It involves almost all the factors which occur in the therapeutic indications.

Usefulness of a Cytologic Classification in Predicting the Evolutive Group

We need a method that enables us to recognize the evolutive group of each patient at the onset of his disease. To this end, we developed a cytologic classification [28, 29] comprising nine classes, assembled in three groups of classes. The nomenclature which abstracts the physiologic terms consists in the association of a number and a letter (1a, 1b, 1c, 2a, 2b, 2c, 3a, 3b, 3c). Several statistical techniques were performed on a basic data table constituted by 51 columns, each corresponding to a well-defined cytologic elementary characteristic and 144 rows each corresponding to an individual patient. The results led us to substitute a quantitative description for a qualitative one. The most representative of the cytologic traits selected by this statistical analysis are: the size of the cells, the aspects of the chromatin, the basophilia, and the homogeneity of the cytoplasm. These properties are reproducible and generally applicable to clinical practice and lend strong support to this system.

Among the 147 patients in the retrospective study, 120 had a good cytologic study. We did not have cytologic material for 13 patients with localized disease, and nine smears were rejected because of the bad quality of the smears.

Table 2 gives the distribution of the nine cytologic classes in each evolutive groups. In the leukemic group, 90% of the patients are in cytologic class 2. In the bad and metastic group, 76% belong to cytologic class 3. In this group, the 21% of patients with cytologic class 1 had in most cases a bad evolution due to overtreatment and advanced age. In the good chronic and diffused group, 81% of the patients belong to cytologic class 1, and in the good and localized group, 80% are in cytologic class 1. If we examine the distribution of evolution groups in each cytologic class (Table 3), the correlation between evolutive group and cytologic class is very strong.

1. 84% of the patients in class 1a were in the good prognosis groups.
2. 94% of the patients in class 2 were in the leukemic group.
3. 89% of the patients in class 3b and 3c are in the bad and metastatic group.

For the classes 1b and 1c, the correlation is less strong: 63% are in the good prognosis groups;

Table 2. Distribution of cytologic classes in four evolutive groups

Evolutive groups	Leukemic	Bad and metastatic	Good chronic and diffused	Good and localized
No. of cytologic studies/ Total No. of patients in the group	37/37	42/49	31/33	10/23
Patients from cytologic classes (%) 1a + 1b + 1c	5	21	81	80
Patients from cytologic classes (%) 2a + 2b + 2c	90	3	3	0
Patients from cytologic classes (%) 3a + 3b + 3c	5	76	16	20

it is also less strong for class 3a whose distribution, with a rather bad prognosis, remains dispersed. On the whole, most cytologic classes (75% of the patients studied cytologically) showed a strong correlation with the evolutive groups.

Table 3. Distribution of evolutive groups in nine cytologic classes

	No. of valid cytologic studies	Leukemic group (%)	Bad and metastic group (%)	Good chronic and diffused group (%)	Good and localized group (%)
1a	25	4	12	72	12
1b	9	5	32	37	26
1c	10				
2a	14				
2b	12	94	3	3	0
2c	9				
3a	13	15	54	23	8
3b	16	0	89	7	4
3c	12				

Chemotherapy Adapted to the Evolutive Groups

Starting in January 1976 the cytologic classification was used in defining the evolution groups. Thus, we have suggested three modalities of treatment according to the three potential situations. Fourty-one patients took part in the new regimen. Here we will only describe the chemotherapy part of the treatment.

For the cytologic classes 2a, 2b, and 2c, we perform as for acute leukemia. Such a group has already been described by Mathé [21], also with three cytologic classes. For these patients, the surgical staging is useless because irrespective of the clinical stage we apply an intensive chemotherapy with meningeal prophylaxis. Figure 5 illustrates the induction treatment for the patients less than 50 years of age according to regimen 71-L.S.-01 (Bernard, Jacquillat; Paris, St Louis): once a week an association of vincristine, cyclophosphamide, and daunorubicin is given intravenously. We add methyl prednisolone i.m. or i.v. 2 mg/kg/day for 6 weeks. The hematologic toxicity is high, and we are often obliged to withold the therapy. After this period,

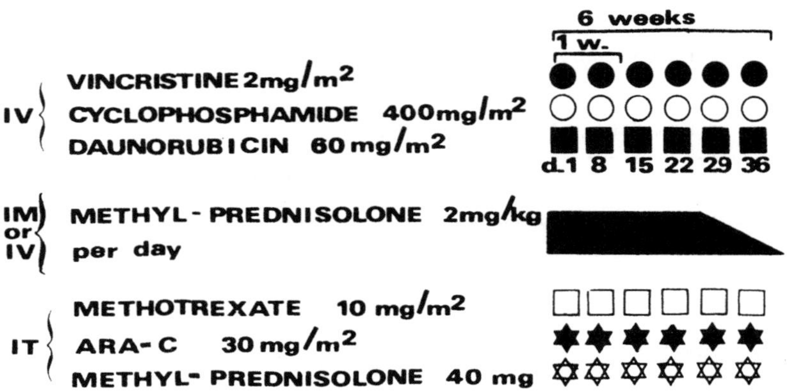

Fig. 5. Induction treatment for non-Hodgkin's malignant lymphoma (NHML) with a potentially leukemic evolution for patients less than 50 years of age. IT: intrathecal

we begin the therapeutic reinforcement (Fig. 6): for 1 month we give 6-mercaptopurine (6-MP) and methotrexate while simultaneously applying a central nervous system irradiation [15]. This is followed by three identical monthly courses of the association of adriamycin and Ara C followed by L-asparaginase. These drugs are known to be active in NHML and acute lymphocytic leukemia [3, 8, 11, 23], and we used this association, called "3A", because during the previous regimen we had applied it in some relapses or resistant lymphomas and observed a very good rate of secondary CR, i.e., 18 out of 29 patients (62%). Here again, the hematologic toxicity is very high, and patients often need intensive suppportive care. Lastly, Figure 7 illustrates the maintenance treatment in which we alternate vincristine and cyclophosphamide, then 6-MP and methotrexate, and then adriamycin and Ara C for 3 years.

For patients with cytologic class 1a and the majority of other patients over 50 years of age, the

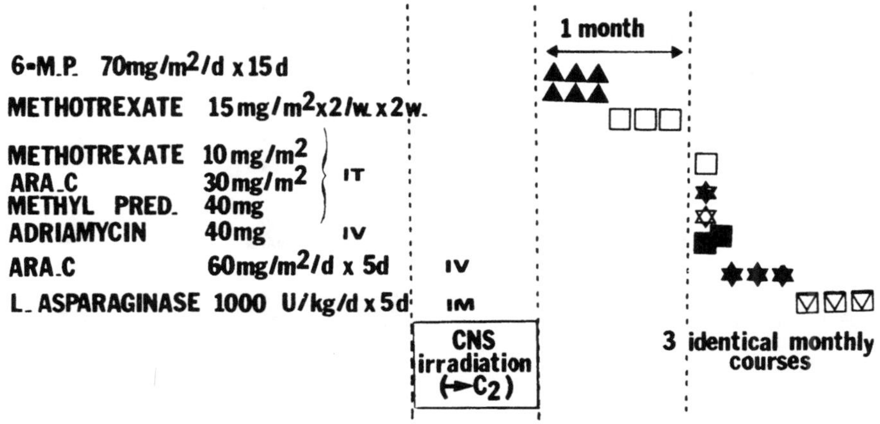

Fig. 6. Therapeutic reinforcement for non-Hodgkin's malignant lymphoma with a potentially leukemic evolution. 6-MP: 6-mercaptopurin

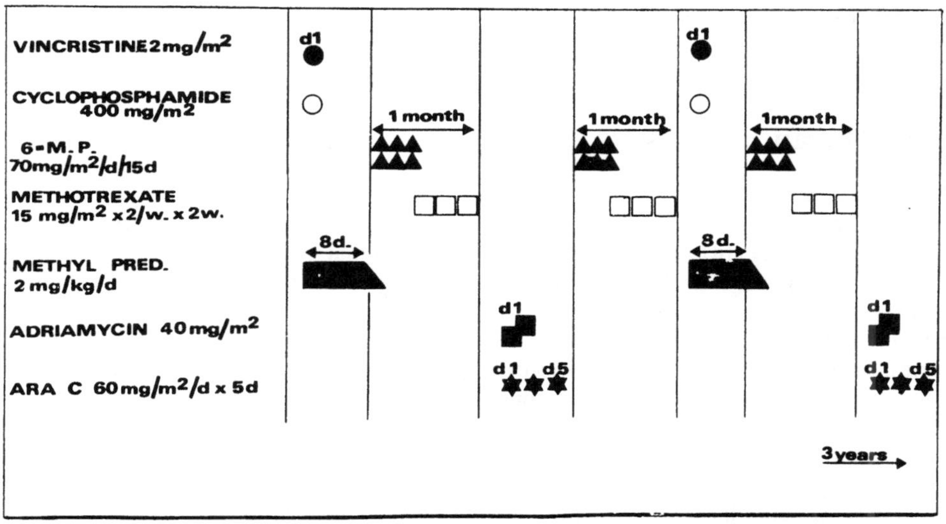

Fig. 7. Maintenance treatment for non-Hodgkin's malignant lymphoma with potentially leukemic evolution. Methyl pred.: methyl prednisolone

staging remains useful in order to apply only a regional radiotherapy for the localized stages, but the surgical staging which is often dangerous in NHML [13] must be avoided. In those patients the prognosis is most often favorable even if the disease is not eradicated by a locoregional treatment. In diffused clinical stages, we use a moderate chemotherapy (Fig. 8). After two consecutive courses of the association of vincristine, cyclophosphamide, daunorubicin, and methotrexate, we give one course monthly for 6 months and then once every 3 months. From time to time, we also use iceberg irradiation in the 6th month [2, 24], according to the initial or persistent volume of the lymph nodes.

As for the patients with a potentially bad metastatic evolution, i.e., cytologic classes 3a, 3b, and 3c and for patients younger than 50 years of age belonging to class 1b and 1c, the management is as follows. The surgical staging remains useful [7, 31] in apparent localized clinical stages. If it is confirmed, we apply regional radiotherapy followed by a prophylactic chemotherapy for 6 months. It is the same as the one given to elderly patients as curative chemotherapy (Fig. 8). In diffused clinical stages, we used an intensive chemotherapy. The association is the same as for the leukemic group but without meningeal prophylaxis, which in this case is useless and sometimes dangerous [14].

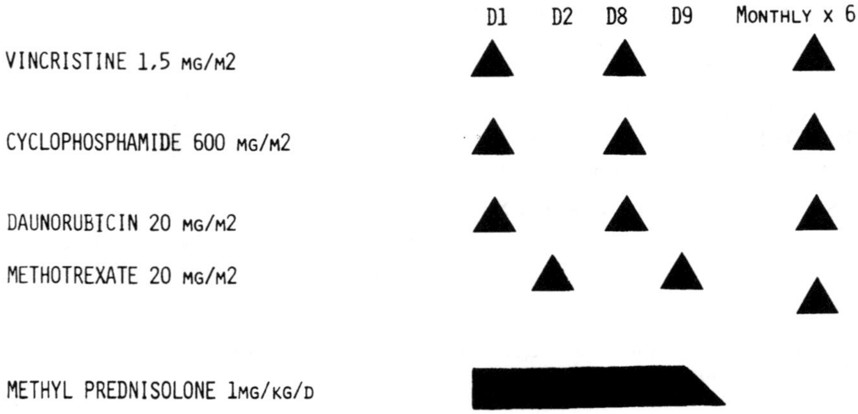

Fig. 8. Chemotherapy for non-Hodgkin's malignant lymphoma in patients older than 50 years of age

First Therapeutic Results

In order to draw our first conclusions, we compared the survival of the patients from the retrospective study (147 patients from 1967–1975) with that of the patients from the current regimen (41 patients since January, 1976) (Fig. 9). There are some difficulties in the statistical analysis because the two follow-up examinations in these studies are different. In order to avoid penalizing the most recent series by taking into account the long-term survivals of the first series, we proceeded as if all the patients from the first series had a 20 month maximum survey. This was indeed the follow-up of the second series.

We observed an improvement in the survival with a median survival of 13 months in the first series as compared with 18 months in the second series. The statistical analysis using the exponential fitting of survival $S = e^{-\lambda t}$ and the comparison of the fitted curves by the χ^2 test [6] as well as the actuarial survival by the method of unique information at fixed date [26] show, for the moment, a nonsignificant difference: $\chi^2 = 1.532 < \chi^2_{0.05(1)} = 3.841$. Thus, if we consider the elderly patients, our impression is that the results are not improved by the proposed

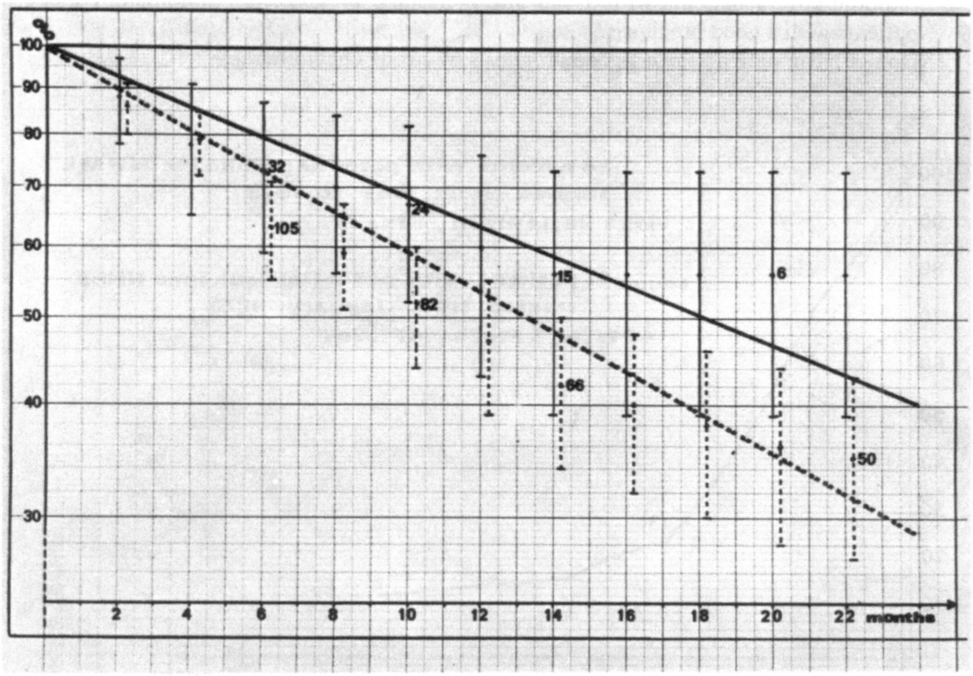

Fig. 9. Actuarial survival and exponential fitting from the retrospective study and those from the current regimen. Current regimen (solid lines): 41 patients; previous regimen (dashed lines) : 147 patients. For the moment, these two groups are not found significantly different ($\chi^2 = 1.532 < \chi^2_{0.05\,(1)} = 3.841$)

chemotherapy if they belong to the bad prognosis group. The chemotherapy is not strong enough. In most cases we cannot obtain or maintain CR. If their cytologic prognosis is good, the chemotherapy proposed is sufficient for maintaining a CR. Moreover, we believe that no patient ever died from a therapeutic complication as was the case in the first regimen.

As for the youngest patients, our first impression is very good, expecially with the potential leukemic group. In Figure 10, the survival curve of patients with potential leukemic evolution (cytology classes 2a, 2b, and 2c are compared) is shown. The survival of the first series was very bad with a median survival of 6 months. Considering the insufficient survey and the small number of patients, the difference in survival is not significant, but the analysis of these curves seems interesting to us. The two curves overlap up to 6 months, which means that the improvement in the hematologic reanimation had not changed the immediate prognosis. But, up to now, we have observed relapses and deaths after 6 months in the second regimen. Six out of 11 patients are still in first CR after 9 months. If this fact is confirmed, the curve would demonstrate the efficiency of the therapeutic reinforcement by the 3A association. The fact that the curves (Fig. 10) overlap up to 6 months demonstrates that progress in the supportive care is not involved. The improvement beyond 6 months is correlated with chemotherapy.

In summary, at present it seems to us very important to separate patients with the same potential evolution in order to perform treatments adapted to the evolution of these diseases. The main directives in the treatment of NHML are for us the following:

1. Reinforce the chemotherapy in the two bad prognosis groups.
2. Individualize the leukemic groups in order to perform meningeal prophylaxis.
3. Make a distinction between the localized forms in order to perform either a leukemic-like treatment in patients with such a potential evolution or a prophylactic chemotherapy after

radiotherapy in patients with a bad and metastatic prognosis or radiotherapy alone in patients with a good prognosis.

4. Do not harm patients with a good prognosis by strong chemotherapy.

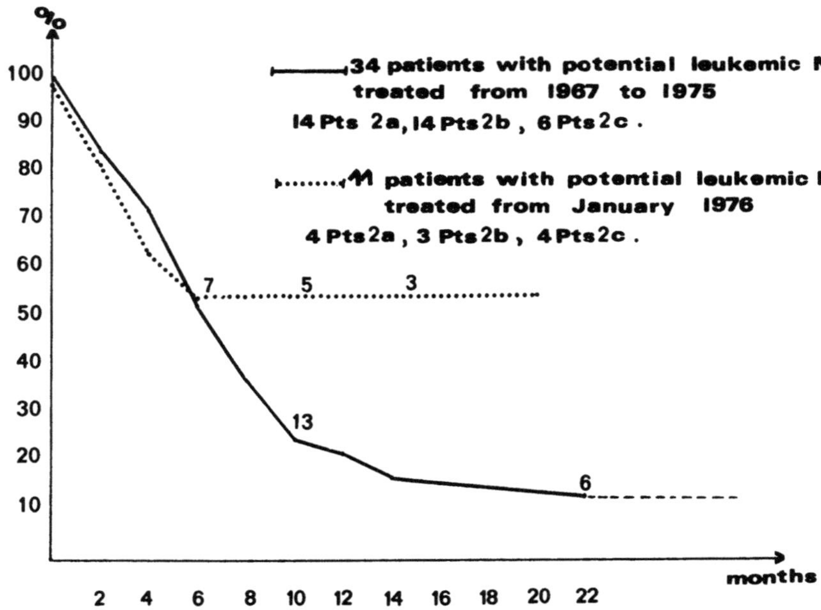

Fig. 10. Actuarial survival curve of non-Hodgkin's malignant lymphoma patients with potential leukemic evolution

References

1. Berard, C., O'Conor, G. T., Thomas, L. B., Torloni, H.: Histopathological definition of Burkitt's tumour. Bull. W.H.O., *40*, 601 (1969)
2. Bonnadonna, G., De Lena, M., Lattuada, A., Milani, F., Monfardini, S., Beretta, G.: Combination chemotherapy and radiotherapy in non-Hodgkin's lymphomata. Brit. J. Cancer, 31 Suppl. *2*, 481–488 (1975)
3. Bonnadonna, G., Monfardini. S., De Lena, M., Fossati-Bellani, F., Beretta, G.: Clinical trials with adriamycin. In: International Symposium on Adriamycin, Berlin. Heidelberg. New York: Springer, 1972
4. Brown, T. C., Peters, M. V., Bergsagel, D. E., Reid, J.: A retrospective analysis of the clinical results in relation to the Rappaport histological classification. Br. J. Cancer, 31 Suppl. II, 174–186 (1975)
5. Bryon, P. A., Gentilhomme, O., Fiere, D.: Classification histocytologique des lymphomes malins non hodgkiniens. Nouv. Presse med., *5*, 514–515 (1976)
6. Byar, D. P.: Analysis of survival data in heterogeneous populations. In: Recent Developments in Statistics, Amsterdam: North Holland, 1977, 51–68
7. Carbone, P. P., Kaplan, H. S., Musshoff, K., Smither, D. W., Tubiana, M.: Report of the committee on Hodgkin's disease staging classification. Cancer Res. *31*, 1860–1861 (1971)
8. Cimo, P., Rudders, R. A., Hensleigh, D.: A clinical trial of adriamycin in the malignant lymphomas. Cancer, *34*, 1571–1575 (1974)
9. Diebold, J.: Proposition pour classer les hématosarcomes lymphoïdes non hodgkiniens. Ann. Anat. Pathol., *20*, 35–42 (1975)
10. Dorfmann, R. F.: Classification of non-Hodgkin's lymphomas. Lancet, *1*, 1295–1296 (1974)

11. EKERT, H., COLEBATCH, J. H., MATTHEWS, R. N.: Short courses of cytosine arabinoside and L-asparaginase in children with acute leukemia. Cancer, *30*, 643–647 (1972)
12. GERARD-MARCHANT, R. I., HAMLIN, I., LENNERT, K., RILKE, F., STANSFELD, A. G., VAN UHNIK, J. A. M.: Classification of non-Hodgkin's lymphomas. Lancet, *2*, 406–408 (1974)
13. GOFFINET, D. R., CASTELLINO, R. A., KIM, H., DORFMAN, R. F., FUKS, Z., ROSENBERG, S. A., NELSEN, T., KAPLAN, H. S.: Staging laparotomies in unselected previously untreated patients with non-Hodgkin's lymphomas. Cancer, *32*, 672–681 (1973)
14. HENDIN, B., DEVIVO, D. C., TORACK, R., LELL, M. E., ABDELSALAM, H. R., VIETTI, T. J.: Parenchymatous degeneration of the central nervous system in childhood leukemia. Cancer, *34*, 468–482 (1974)
15. HUSTU, H. O., AUR, R. J. A., VERZOSA, M. S., SIMONE, J. V., PINKEL, D.: Prevention of central nervous system leukemia by irradiation. Cancer, *32*, 585–597 (1973)
16. JONES, S. E., FUKS, Z., BULL, M., KADIN, M. E., DORFMAN, R. F., KAPLAN, H. S., ROSENBERG, S. A., KIM, H.: Non-Hodgkin's lymphomas. IV. Clinico pathologic correlation in 405 cases. Cancer, *31*, 806–823 (1973)
17. LENNERT, K., MOHRI, N., STEIN, H., KAISERLING, E.: The histopathology of malignant lymphoma. Br. J. Haematol., *31* Suppl., 72, 193–203 (1975)
18. LUKES, R. J., COLLINS, R. D.: New approaches to the classification of the lymphomata. Br. J. Cancer, 31, Suppl. II, 1–28 (1975)
19. MATHE, G., BELPOMME, D., DANTCHEV, D., KHALIL, A., AFIFI, A. M., TALEB, N., POUILLART, P., SCHWARSENBERG, L., HAYAT, M., DE VASSAL, F., JASMIN, C., MISSET, J. L., MUSSET, M.: Immunoblastic lymphosarcomata, a cytological and clinical entity? Biomedicine, *22*, 473–488 (1975)
20. MATHE, G., BELPOMME, D., DANTCHEV, D., POUILLART, P.: Progress in the classification of lymphoid and/or monocytoid leukemias and of lympho and reticulo sarcomas (Non-Hodgkin's lymphomas). Biomedicine, *22*, 177–185 (1975)
21. MATHE, G., BELPOMME, D., DANTCHEV, D., POUILLART, P., SCHLUMBERGER, J. R., LAFLEUR, M.: Leukaemic lymphosarcomas: respective prognosis of the three types: prolymphocytic, lymphoblastic (or lymphoblastoid) and immunoblastic. Blood Cells, *1*, 25–36 (1975)
22. MATHE, G., GERARD-MARCHANT, R., TEXIER, J. L., SCHLUMBERGER, J. R., BERUMEN, L., PAINTRAND, M.: The two varieties of lymphoid tissue "reticulosarcomas" histiocytic and histioblastic types. Br. J. Cancer, *24*, 687–695 (1970)
23. MCELWAIN, T. J., HARDISTY, R. M.: Remission induction with cytosine arabinoside and L-asparaginase in acute lymphoblastic leukaemia. Br. Med. J., *4*, 596–598 (1969)
24. POUILLART, P., AMEIL, J. L., MATHE, G., TUBIANA, M.: Le traitement des lymphoréticulosarcomes de l'adulte (à l'exclusion des formes du carrefour aérodigestif supérieur). Nouv. Presse med., *4*, 247–252 (1975)
25. RAPPAPORT, H.: Tumors of the haematopoietic system. In: Atlas of Tumor Pathology, Section 3, Fascicle 8, Ed.: Washington D.C.. Armed Forces Institute of Pathology, 1966
26. ROSENGERG, S. A.: Report of the committee on the staging of Hodgkin's disease. Cancer Res., *26*, 1310 (1966)
27. SCHWARTZ, D., FLAMANT, R., LELLOUCH, J.: L'essai thérapeutique chez l'homme, Paris: Flammarion, 1970
28. SOTTO, J. J., CAILLOT, P., SOTTO, M. F., LACHET, B., MARTIN, H., BENSA, J. C., HOLLARD, D.: A cytological classification of non-Hodgkin's malignant lymphomas based on a statistical analysis. (Submitted for publication in Br. J. Cancer)
29. SOTTO, J. J., SOTTO, M. F., BRAMBILLA, E., MARTIN, H., MICHALLET, M., BENSA, J. C., VROUSOS, C., HOLLARD, D.: Non-Hodgkin's lymphoma (NHL): Multifactorial analysis of prognostic factors; special value of the cytology. 16th Intern. Congr. Hematol., Kyoto, 1976
30. STEIN, H., PETERSON, N., GAEDICKE, G., LENNERT, K., LANDBECK, G.: Lymphoblastic lymphoma of convoluted or acid phosphatase type—a tumor of T precursor cells. Intern. J. Cancer, *17*, 292–295 (1976)
31. TUBIANA M., LE BOURGEOIS, J. P.: La classification et le bilan des hématosarcomes. Bull. Cancer, *61*, 39–50 (1974)

BCG in the Immunotherapy of Non-Hodgkin's Malignant Lymphomas: Preliminary Results of a Controlled Trial

B. HŒRNI, M. DURAND, A. DE MASCAREL, P. RICHAUD, G. HŒRNI-SIMON, J. CHAUVERGNE, and C. LAGARDE

In a previous paper, we presented our current results of a randomized trial of the efficacy of BCG to maintain complete remission in patients with malignant lymphoma in whom complete remission had previously been induced by an association of chemo- and radiotherapy [3]. There was a significant difference in the duration of complete remission in favor of patients treated with BCG scarifications as compared with the control group; this difference was about the same for patients with Hodgkin's disease (who constituted two-thirds of the patients) and for the other patients suffering from non-Hodgkin's lymphoma. We have concluded that BCG may be useful in maintaining complete remission and that a 3-year treatment seems sufficient. After obtaining these results, we continued this trial for non-Hodgkin's lymphomas, and we present here the current results of this study.

Materials and Methods

From January, 1973–January, 1977, 33 patients were included in this trial. According to the design of the trial, all of them were less than 65 years old and had one or more criteria of poor prognosis. These criteria were: 1) a high grade malignancy histologically, 2) clinical stage III or IV, and 3) a case history of first or later relapse. For all patients a clinical staging was performed according to the Rye classification for Hodgkin's disease [7], with chest x-rays and abdominal lymphography and without systematic biopsies of bone marrow or liver or laparotomy. According to previous personal data, the expected survival of these patients could be evaluated at ca. 40%–50%.

Five patients were excluded from this analysis. Four of them were excluded after histologic review according to the Kiel classification (4): out of three patients classified as anaplastic carcinoma, two are dead and one is alive 7 months after randomization and one patient with testicular dysembryoma is alive and in complete remission 26 months after randomization. Unfortunately, these four patients were all in the treated group. Lastly, one patient was randomized for treatment but refused BCG and is still in complete remission after 11 months. The main prognostic criteria of the two groups of patients are shown in Table 1. There is no significant difference between the two groups on these criteria nor on other ancillary criteria not shown here.

Treatment

All patients were first put into complete remission with an association of chemo- and radiotherapy. Chemotherapy was an association of cyclophosphamide, vincristine, and

Table 1. Distribution of main prognostic criteria among evaluable patients

	All patients[a]	BCG	Control
Total	28 (10)	11 (2)	17 (8)
Age:			
<50	15 (5)	7 (1)	8 (4)
⩾ 50	13 (5)	4 (1)	9 (4)
Histology:			
low grade	16 (4)	6 (1)	10 (3)
high grade	12 (6)	5 (1)	7 (5)
Visible phase:			
No. 1	19 (9)	7 (2)	12 (7)
No. 2 +	9 (1)	4 (0)	5 (1)
Clinical stage:			
I	12 (3)	7 (0)	5 (3)
II	6 (3)	1 (1)	5 (2)
III	7 (4)	2 (1)	5 (3)
IV	3 (0)	1 (0)	2 (0)

[a] The number in brackets represents the number of patients in relapse.

prednisone (CVP) according to a published schedule [2] or an association of CVP + adriamycin or VM 26 according to a randomized trial [1]. These different schedules of chemotherapy were given similarly in the two groups of patients. Initially, the patients received one 15-day course of chemotherapy; they were then irradiated (3500–4000 rads were given on all tumoral icebergs). Complete remission was checked immediately following radiotherapy by the same clinical and radiographic procedures as at the initial staging; patients in incomplete remission were excluded from this trial. Patients in complete remission were treated again with one course of chemotherapy as aforementioned.

These patients were then randomized to receive either BCG therapy or no further treatment. BCG was given by skin scarification according to the Villejuif method [5] (Fig. 1). The BCG used was produced by the Institut Pasteur, BCG-S, until December, 1975 and thereafter lyophilized Immuno-BCG.F, since BCG-S was no longer produced. These scarifications were done weekly over a period of 3 years and were then discontinued. In case of relapse, BCG was discontinued for the treated patients and replaced by standard anticancer therapy such as that given to control patients.

Results

Out of 28 evaluable patients, 10 relapsed: 2 out of 11 BCG treated patients and 8 out of 17 control patients. Figure 2 shows the actuarial curves of complete remission (or relapse-free survival). There is a difference of about 30% in favor of patients treated with BCG. This difference is not significant. For BCG-treated patients we have not observed any relapse after 18 months, and seven patients have exceeded this date. For control patients, relapse-free survival is close to the expected value. Only four deaths occurred, all of them attributed to malignant lymphoma: one in the BCG group and three in the control group. Until now, the difference in crude survival is thus very slight and again not significant.

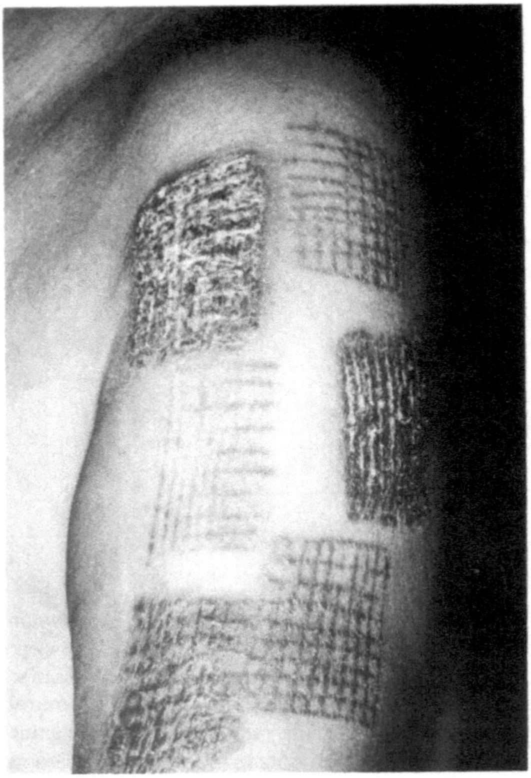

Fig. 1. Skin scarifications on a left arm

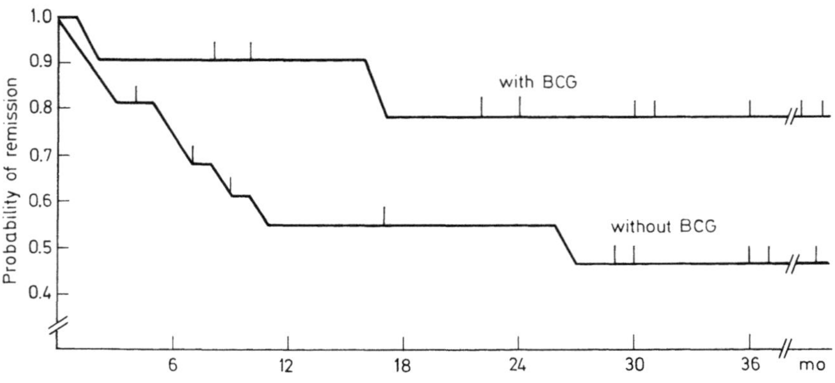

Fig. 2. Actuarial complete remission (relapse-free survival) curves of BCG-treated and control patients. Each stick represents one patient in complete remission

Comments

The present results indicate that BCG might be useful in preventing relapses in about one-third of the patients, but these results are not yet significant. This trial must be continued to obtain results on a larger number of patients. There are few data in the literature on BCG and non-Hodgkin's malignant lymphomas. The study of MATHÉ et al. [6] concerns lymphosarcoma after leukemic transformation, but it is not a randomized study. The trial of JONES et al. in this volume includes a great number of patients in whom complete remission is induced by chemotherapy without radiotherapy; these patients are in part older than 65 years and BCG is only given monthly. We think that radiotherapy is useful and perhaps necessary in order to reduce the number of malignant cells as much as possible. In any case, we shall have to wait some months or even years to have some answers to present questions about the usefulness of BCG in the management of malignant lymphomas, at least under the conditions in our trial.

Summary

Thirty-three patients exhibiting non-Hodgkin's malignant lymphoma with one or more criteria of poor prognosis and in whom complete remission had been induced by an association of chemo + radio + chemotherapy were randomized to either receive BCG or no further treatment. The present results indicate that BCG may be useful to maintain remission in about one-third of the patients, but these results are not yet significant.

References

1. CHAUVERGNE, J., DURAND, M., HŒRNI, B., HŒRNI-SIMON, G., BRUNET, R., LAGARDE, C.: Induction chemotherapy of non-Hodgkin's malignant lymphomas. Eur. J. Cancer, *13*, 399–400 (1977)
2. CHAUVERGNE, J., HŒRNI, B., DURAND, M., HŒRNI-SIMON, G., LAGARDE, C.: Chimiothérapie des réticulosarcomes. Résultats d'un essai contrôlé portant sur 60 malades. Nouv. Presse Med., *2*, 2039–2042 (1973)
3. HŒRNI, B., CHAUVERGNE, J., HŒRNI-SIMON, G., DURAND, M., LAGARDE, C.: BCG in the immunotherapy of malignant lymphomas. Current results of a controlled trial. Cancer Immunol. Immunother., *3*, 57–60 (1977)
4. LENNERT, K., STEIN, H., KAISERLING, E.: Cytological and functional criteria for the classification of malignant lymphomas. Br. J. Cancer, *31*, Suppl. II, 29–43 (1975)
5. MATHÉ, G., AMIEL, J. L., SCHWARZENBERG, L. et al.: Les diverses approches immunologiques du traitement des cancers humains, XXXVIIe Congr. Fr. Med., Paris, Masson pub. 1969
6. MATHÉ, G., BELPOMME, D., POUILLART, P., SCHWARZENBERG, L., MISSET, J. L., JASMIN, C., MUSSET, M., CATTAN, A., AMIEL, J. L., SCHNEIDER, M.: Preliminary results of an immunotherapy trial on terminal leukaemic lymphosarcoma. Biomedicine, *23*, 465–467 (1975)
7. ROSENBERG, S. A.: Report of the committee on the staging of Hodgkin's disease. Cancer Res., *26*, 1310 (1966)

Chemoimmunotherapy Versus Chemotherapy for Remission Induction in Patients With Non-Hodgkin's Lymphoma: Progress Report of a Southwest Oncology Group Study

S. E. JONES

Introduction

In October, 1974, the Southwest Oncology Group (SWOG) initiated a large-scale, controlled clinical trial of chemoimmunotherapy in advanced non-Hodgkin's lymphomas (NHL). The protocol (SWOG 7426/7427) compares three remission-induction treatment regimens: one consisting of combination chemotherapy plus Bacillus Calmette-Guérin (BCG) with two other regimens consisting of combination chemotherapy alone. Patients achieving complete remission were then rerandomized to unmaintained remission or immunotherapeutic maintenance with monthly BCG scarifications. The study was based in part on the following observations:

1. Some patients with NHL (particularly those with diffuse histologic types) manifest severe immunodeficiency [8]
2. Evidence of therapeutic effect of BCG in other neoplasms such as acute leukemia and melanoma [4, 14].
3. A suggestion of prolonged remission duration in patients with a variety of lymphomas, including Hodgkin's disease [16]

In this trial, major efforts were made to insure quality control by incorporating for the first time routine submission of pathologic material for expert histopathologic review [7] and the use of systematic restaging to more accurately define complete remission [5]. The documentation of complete remission through restaging was considered to be an essential decision point prior to discontinuation of chemotherapy and allocation to either unmaintained remission or BCG maintenance immunotherapy.

We have reported on the preliminary results of this ongoing trial at recent meetings [9, 10]. In those earlier analyses, we observed a significantly higher overall response rate (partial plus complete responses) in patients receiving chemoimmunotherapy compared with those receiving chemotherapy. We also noted that survival appeared to be superior in patients with nodular lymphoma who received chemiommunotherapy for remission induction. In this paper, we will present the most recent results of this trial based on a statistical analysis performed in April, 1977.

Patients and Methods

Only patients with biopsy-proven stage III or IV NHL without prior chemotherapy were eligible for this study. Cases were entered by investigators from 34 SWOG institutions. All lymphomas were classified according to the criteria of RAPPAPORT [15], and original biopsy material from each patient was submitted for additional review by the Lymphoma Pathology Panel and Central Repository [7]. Patients were evaluated for extent of disease prior to treatment [6] and staged according to the criteria of the Ann Arbor Conference [1]. After obtaining informed written consent, patients were then assigned at random to one of three chemoimmunotherapy or chemotherapy programs intended to induce a complete remission (randomizations were stratified by nodular or diffuse histologic pattern). The details of these three treatments are as follows:

1. COP-bleomycin (four drugs): *cyclophosphamide* (C), 125 mg/m^2 given orally daily for 14 days starting on day 1, *vincristine* (Oncovin [0]), 1.4 mg/m^2 given i.v. on days 1 and 8 (maximum of 2 mg per injection), *prednisone* (P), 100 mg/day given orally on days 1–5, and *bleomycin* (Bleo), 4 mg/m^2 given i.v. on days 1 and 8. Courses were repeated every 28 days if the peripheral blood counts were adequate. (Patients with preexisting cardiac disease or mycosis fungoides were assigned to treatment with COP- bleomycin and are listed as "other" in results).
2. CHOP-bleomycin (five drugs): *cyclophosphamide*, 750 mg/m^2 given i.v. on day 1, *doxorubicin* (hydroxyldaunorubicin, Adriamycin [H]), 50 mg/m^2 given i.v. on day 1, *vincristine*, 1.4 mg/m^2 given i.v. on day 1 (maximum of 2 mg per injection), *prednisone*, 100 mg/day given orally on days 1–5, and *bleomycin*, 4 mg/m^2 given i.v. on day 1. Courses were repeated every 21 days if the blood counts were adequate [13].
3. CHOP-BCG (five drugs): same regimen as in CHOP-bleomycin therapy except for substitution of high viability Pasteur BCG (Bacillus Calmette-Guérin) for bleomycin. BCG was given by scarification at a dose of 1 ampule ($6 \pm 4 \times 10^8$ viable units of Pasteur lyophylized BCG) on days 8 and 15 of each 21-day treatment cycle. BCG scarifications were performed on extremities with a standard 5 × 5 cm grid of ten scratches in each of two perpendicular directions. BCG sites were rotated with each dose so that all major lymphoid drainage pathways from upper and lower extremities were repetitively challenged. Doses of drugs and BCG were modified in accord with standard SWOG guidelines based on toxicity. For example, BCG was reduced to a single day 15 administration per treatment course if a moderate reaction (i.e., erythema or induration extending more than 1 cm beyond the site with or without mild systemic symptoms) occurred with the previous BCG administration. If the reduced frequency failed to reduce the intensity of reactions, specially planned reductions in dose of BCG were also recommended. BCG was to be discontinued when there were signs or symptoms of systemic BCG infection [17]. Although not addressed in this paper, patients underwent immunologic testing including a skin test battery (multiple recall antigens) and studies of circulating lymphocytes and immunoglobulins. These studies were carried out prior to treatment, at the time of restaging and 6 months thereafter.

The basic design of this study is shown in Figure 1. Remission induction therapy for responding patients consisted of eight courses of treatment given at 3–4 week intervals, followed by "systematic restaging" if all clinical signs and symptoms of lymphoma had disappeared [5]. Patients considered to be free of disease after completing restaging (this was the definition of "complete remission" used in this study) were then assigned at random to receive either no further therapy or BCG by scarification at monthly intervals for 18 months with close follow-up for signs of relapse. Patients who experienced only a "partial response" (at least a 50% regression of all measurable sites of involvement) after the first eight courses of treatment or those who were found to have persistent disease at restaging received another three courses of the same treatment. If a documented complete remission was achieved after 11 courses of induction treatment, patients were then eligible for randomization into the maintenance phase. Patients who failed to achieve at least a partial response after four courses of induction treatment were considered to be "nonresponders" and were taken off this treatment ("off-study").

A comprehensive, computerized "updated study analysis" has been performed by the SWOG Statistical Office every 4 months since the study was begun. Several tests of significance have been employed in these analyses. The χ^2 method was employed to compare differences in response rates. Survival and remission duration were calculated by the method of Kaplan and Meier [11], and comparison of survival or remission duration between various groups of

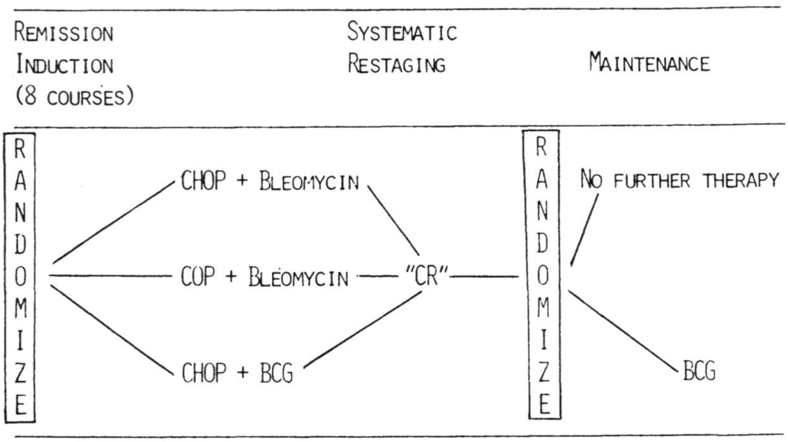

Fig. 1. Schematic representation of the treatment plan in the SWOG study 7426/7427 for patients with advanced non-Hodgkin's lymphoma (October, 1974–July, 1977)

patients was made with GEHAN's [2] modified Wilcoxon test. The data in this report are based on an analysis performed in April, 1977 on clinical records through March, 1977. Only patients with a "final evaluation" (those who have completed induction treatment) are considered for the purposes of this report.

Results

As of April, 1977, 669 patients have been entered into this study, and 420 patients have had final evaluations. The clinical and pathologic characteristics of patients in the three treatment groups are comparable. The preliminary results according to induction treatment are shown in Table 1. There is no difference in complete remission rates. Although the overall remission rate (partial plus complete responses) is higher for patients receiving CHOP + BCG (87%) compared with those receiving CHOP + bleomycin (79%) or COP + bleomycin (82%), these are not now significantly different. Among patients with final evaluations and completed hematopathology review, there is a significant difference ($p < 0.02$) in complete remission rates for those with nodular lymphoma (63%) compared with diffuse lymphoma (49%). Within each major histologic type of lymphoma, however, there is no significant difference in complete remission rates with respect to the type of induction regimen.

All three induction treatment regimens were generally well-tolerated with the major toxicity being leukopenia. The COP + bleomycin regimen was associated with significantly less

Table 1. Chemoimmunotherapy of non-Hodgkin's lymphoma: SWOG 7426/7427 (4/77). Preliminary results: remission induction

Treatment	No. of patients (final evaluation)	Percentage with		
		CR	PR	CR + PR
CHOP + BCG	112	59	28	87
CHOP + bleomycin	129	53	26	79
COP + bleomycin	143	55	27	82
COP + bleomycin (cardiac)	36	17[a]	53	70

[a] CR rate significantly less ($p < 0.05$).

toxicity ($p < 0.001$) than CHOP + bleomycin or CHOP + BCG. There was no difference in hematologic toxicity between CHOP + bleomycin or CHOP + BCG treatment. The administration of BCG was well-tolerated as shown in Table 2. Fifty-five percent of patients experienced no toxicity requiring modification of BCG frequency or dose. Less than 1% of patients were suspected of having systemic BCG infection, and no fatal BCG reactions were encountered.

As of April, 1977, 203 patients who achieved complete remission documented by restaging have been registered on the unmaintained vs. BCG immunotherapy maintenance program. Of these, 154 are currently evaluable. Forty-eight relapses to date have occurred with similar frequency in groups receiving BCG immunotherapy or in unmaintained remission status (Table 3). There is no difference in duration of complete remission according to the use of monthly BCG immunotherapy or no additional treatment.

Overall survival by initial induction treatment is not different at this time; however, survival for patients with nodular lymphoma has proven to be superior to that associated with diffuse lymphoma ($p < 0.01$). Relapses after complete remission and the number of deaths for each of the three major treatment arms are shown in Table 4. Although these figures favor the chemoimmunotherapy treatment group, there are no significant differences at this time.

Finally, we compared overall survival of all patients entered into this study with survival of the fully evaluable patients from the most recently completed SWOG study in which patients

Table 2. Chemoimmunotherapy of non-Hodgkin's lymphoma: SWOG 7426/7427 (4/77). BCG toxicity during induction

Worst degree of toxicity	Patients on CHOP + BCG (%)
None (local inflammatory response ± systemic symptoms)	55
Mild (requires BCG dosage modification)	33
Moderate (local BCG abscess formation)	8
Severe (regional lymph node involvement + abscess formation)	3
Life-threatening (systemic BCG disease)	1
Fatal	0

Table 3. Chemoimmunotherapy of non-Hodgkin's lymphoma: SWOG 7426/7427 (4/77). Preliminary results: maintenance phase

	No. patients	No. relapses[a]
No further treatment	78	25 (32%)
BCG monthly	69	22 (32%)
Refused BCG (not randomized)	7	1 (14%)

[a] No significant differences.

Table 4. Chemoimmunotherapy of non-Hodgkin's lymphoma: SWOG 7426/7427 (4/77). Relapses and deaths by induction treatment

Treatment	No. of patients (preliminary and final)	No. of	
		Relapses after CR	Deaths (overall)
CHOP + BCG	153	13/76 (17%)	20 (13%)
CHOP + bleomycin	173	21/89 (24%)	36 (21%)
COP + bleomycin	175	31/90 (34%)	35 (20%)

received induction chemotherapy with CHOP (without bleomycin or BCG) followed by maintenance chemotherapy for 18 months [13]. These two groups of patients are identical in terms of clinical and pathologic characteristics, and the rates of complete remission are also similar. Nonetheless, overall survival in this current program remains superior to that observed in the former study ($p = 0.03$).

Discussion

Nonspecific immune stimulation with BCG has received considerable attention in recent years as a form of cancer therapy. Chemoimmunotherapy with BCG has been evaluated in various types of cancers including melanoma, acute leukemia, breast cancer, and Burkitt's lymphoma [3, 4, 12, 14]. In most of these trials, survival or duration of remission has been improved by the addition of BCG to chemotherapy, but rates of complete remission have not been increased. These observations may eventually be confirmed in this study of chemoimmunotherapy for patients with NHL but the results are still too preliminary to be certain. With final evaluations of about one-half of the cases entered on this study, we have demonstrated a significant improvement in overall survival compared with our most recently completed and otherwise comparable trial [13]. However, we have not observed any significant differences in remission rates for the three types of induction treatment. There is also a suggestion (not yet significant) that survival of patients with nodular lymphoma might be improved by the addition of BCG to CHOP chemotherapy compared to the regimens without BCG. This is interesting because nodular lymphoma patients appear to be more immunocompetent at the time of presentation [8] and may have better preservation of the T-dependent areas of lymphoid organs. This could be relevant if the BCG immunotherapeutic effect is mediated through T-lymphocytes.

After induction of complete remission, we have not yet been able to demonstrate any advantage in terms of prolonging duration of complete remission by administering BCG at monthly intervals by scarification compared to no further treatment. The majority of relapses observed to date have occurred early—average time from restaging to relapse is 4 months (range 1–12 months)—and many of the relapses appear to have occurred in patients whose restaging evaluations were not sufficiently thorough to detect persistent lymphoma [5]. Our choice of administering BCG at monthly intervals after restaging, in retrospect, may have been inadequate to enhance immunoreactivity in patients who did not receive the more intensive BCG stimulation during the remission induction phase. It might have been more appropriate to begin maintenance BCG at weekly intervals until strong reactions occurred, followed by reductions in frequency of administration or dose thereafter.

It must be reinterated that the results of this study are still quite tentative as only half of the patients have been fully analyzed, and the length of follow-up, even of these patients, is still short. Much longer periods of observation and analysis of all cases in this ongoing trial will be of critical importance in eventually assessing the value of BCG in either remission duration or survival in patients with non-Hodgkin's lymphoma.

Summary

The Southwest Oncology Group is conducting a controlled clinical trial for patients with all types of advanced non-Hodgkin's lymphoma in which chemoimmunotherapy (CHOP + BCG) is being compared with chemotherapy alone (CHOP + bleomycin or COP + bleomycin) for remission induction. Patients achieving a complete remission confirmed by systematic restaging are then randomly assigned to maintenance BCG or to no further therapy. As of April, 1977, 669 patients had been registered on this trial and 420 were fully evaluable. No significant differences in response rates between the three remission induction regimens are apparent. After restaging, early relapses have occurred with equal frequency in the BCG and no-further-therapy groups. Longer follow-up and further analysis will be required to fully evaluate the potential effects of BCG on remission duration or survival in this study.

Acknowledgements

The author's work was supported in part by research grants from the National Institutes of Health: CA-13612 and CA-12014.

References

1. Carbone, P. P., Kaplan, H. S., Musshoff, K., et al.: Report of the Committee on Hodgkin's Disease Staging Classification. Cancer Res. *31*, 1860–1861 (1971)
2. Gehan, E. A.: A generalized Wilcoxon test for comparing arbitrarily singly-censored samples. Biometrika *52*, 203–223 (1965)
3. Gutterman, J. U., Mavligit, G. M., Burgess, M. A. et al.: Immunotherapy of breast cancer, malignant melanoma, and acute leukemia with BCG: Prolongation of disease free interval and survival. Cancer Immunol. Immunother. *1*, 99–107 (1976)
4. Gutterman, J. U., Mavligit, G. L., Gottlieb, J. A. et al.: Chemoimmunotherapy of disseminated malignant melanoma with dimethyltriazenoimidazole carboxamide and Bacillus Calmette-Guérin. N. Engl. J. Med. *291*, 592–597 (1974)
5. Herman, T. S., Jones, S. E.: Systematic restaging in the management of non-Hodgkin's lymphomas. Cancer Treat. Rep. *61*, 1009–1015 (1977)
6. Jones, S. E.: Non-Hodgkin lymphomas. JAMA *234*, 633–638 (1975)
7. Jones, S. E., Butler, J. J., Byrne, G. E. Jr. et al.: Histopathologic review of lymphoma cases from the Southwest Oncology Group. Cancer *39*, 1071–1076 (1977)
8. Jones, S. E., Griffith, K., Dombrowski, P. et al.: Immunodeficiency in patients with non-Hodgkin's lymphomas. Blood *49*, 335–344 (1977)
9. Jones, S. E., Salmon, S. E.: Adjuvant immunotherapy with BCG in lymphoma. In: Adjuvant Therapy of Cancer. Salmon, S. E., Jones, S. E. (eds.). Amsterdam, Holland: North Holland Press, 1977, pp. 549–556
10. Jones, S. E., Salmon, S. E., Moon, T. E. et al.: Chemoimmunotherapy of non-Hodgkin's lymphoma with BCG. A preliminary report. In: Immunotherapy of Cancer: Present Status of Trials in Man (Progress in Cancer Research and Therapy, volume 6). Terry, W. D., Windhorst, D. (eds.), New York, Raven Press, 1978, pp. 519–528
11. Kaplan, E. L., Meier, P.: Non-parametric estimations from incomplete observations. J. Am. Stat. Assoc. *53*, 457–482 (1958)
12. Magrath, I. T., Ziegler, J. L.: Failure of BCG immunostimulation to affect the clinical course of Burkitt's lymphoma. Br. Med. J. *1*, 615–618 (1976)
13. McKelvey, E. M., Gottlieb, J. A., Wilson, H. E. et al.: Hydroxyldaunomycin (adriamycin) combination chemotherapy in malignant lymphoma. Cancer *38*, 1484–1493 (1976)
14. Powles, R. L., Crowther, D., Bateman, C. J. T. et al.: Immunotherapy for acute myelogenous leukaemia. Br. J. Cancer *28*, 365–376 (1973)
15. Rappaport, H., Winter, W. J., Hicks, E. B.: Follicular lymphoma: A reevaluation of its position in the scheme of malignant lymphoma, based on a survey of 253 cases. Cancer *9*, 792–821 (1956)
16. Sokal, J. E., Aungst, C. W., Snyderman, M.: Delay in progression of malignant lymphoma after BCG vaccination. N. Engl. J. Med. *291*, 1226–1230 (1974)
17. Sparks, F. C., Silverstein, M. J., Hunt, J. S. et al.: Complications of BCG immunotherapy in patients with cancer. N. Engl. J. Med. *289*, 827–830 (1973)

Complications of Total Abdominal and Spleen Irradiation in Patients With Lymphomas

J. P. LE BOURGEOIS, M. MEIGNAN, P. LASSER, C. PARMENTIER, F. PENE, and M. TUBIANA

Exploratory laparotomy has shown that, in patients with non-Hodgkin's lymphomas, involvement of para-aortic nodes is associated with positive mesenteric nodes in 80% of well-differentiated nodular or diffuse lymphocytic lymphomas and in 50% of cases of histiocytic lymphoma [10]. Current treatment regimens stipulate that when there is supra- or infradiaphragmatic involvement, "icebergs" shall be irradiated after initial chemotherapy. Thus, in addition to the classic mantle and inverted Y treatments, we now routinely have to irradiate the whole abdomen, and this may present problems because of the large volume to be irradiated, the sensitivity of healthy organs within the field, and previous treatments which the patients have received.

Irradiation of the spleen is carried out in the normal manner, especially for the patients with Hodgkin's disease. The left kidney is partly included in the treatment volume and may, therefore, be damaged by the irradiation. We carried out a study to investigate the complications arising after total abdominal irradiation and the possible effects of radiations on the upper pole of the left kidney.

Total Abdominal Irradiation

Materials and Methods

Between January, 1973 and January, 1977, 50 patients with histologically confirmed non-Hodgkin's lymphoma have been treated by irradiation of the whole abdomen. All patients who had been irradiated in part of the abdomen only or who had been treated palliatively have been excluded from this study. Our group comprised 31 men and 20 women (age range 8–73 years) with a mean age of 43 years. Twenty-six patients had had abdominal surgery before any treatment; in 20 cases this was necessary for diagnostic purposes as the first symptom of the disease was either an abdominal mass or an obstruction; in six cases a classic exploratory laparotomy was performed.

After clinical examination, E.N.T. examination, chest x-rays, lymphangiography, laboratory studies, and liver and bone marrow biopsies, the patients are staged according to the Ann Arbor classification [2]. In our 50 cases, there were 27 stage II or IIe infradiaphragmatic (14 diagnostic and four exploratory laparotomies), 16 stage III (two diagnostic and two exploratory laparotomies), and seven stage IV cases (four diagnostic laparotomies).

Techniques of Treatment

Radiotherapy

For all patients, the aim of irradiating the whole abdomen was to sterilize known or suspected mesenteric node involvement. All were irradiated in the same way with 25 MV x-rays from a linear accelerator. Anterior and posterior opposing fields were used, the upper limit being the diaphragm and the lower pubis. The liver was only protected after 2000 rad. The kidneys were shielded posteriorly only from the start of treatment. Patients were treated four times a week with a daily dose of 185 rad with both fields treated each day. The total dose in the midline was 3000 rad, and at the end of this irradiation, a further 1000 rad were given to the para-aortic and iliac regions. The inguinal region was irradiated separately with 13 Mev electrons. Antiemetics were prescribed at the beginning of treatment as well as a low-residue, low-fat diet without gluten or milk products [3]. Only some patients in this study received this diet.

During irradiation a blood count with platelets was done each week. Patients undergoing intensive chemotherapy had more frequent blood tests because of the risk of aplasia. Digestive tolerance was estimated each week according to the following criteria: vomiting, diarrhea, degree of anorexia, and weight. Three groups of patients were thus defined:

1. Poor tolerance: continuous vomiting, profuse diarrhea, intravenous feeding required.
2. Moderate tolerance: vomiting after each treatment, diarrhea two or three times a day, anorexia++.
3. Good tolerance: no vomiting or diarrhea, anorexia ±.

Chemotherapy

Twenty-four patients were treated with chemotherapy before radiotherapy was begun. The usual schedule was eight cycles of a combination of adriamycin, VM 26, cyclophosphamide, and prednisone. At the end of irradiation, patients continued for 1 year on a maintenance therapy with oncovin, cyclophosphamide, and prednisone.

Surgery

The diagnostic laparotomies, which were usually performed as an emergency, did not allow full investigation of the abdominal lesions. On the other hand, during the exploratory laparotomies, bone biopsy of the anterior superior iliac spine, splenectomy, hepatic biopsy, and sampling of the mesenteric para-aortic and iliac nodes were possible. Metal clips were used to mark sampled nodes or inoperable masses.

Results

Digestive Tolerance During Irradiation

Table 1 shows the frequency of gastrointestinal problems during treatment; 62% of the patients suffered from vomiting and diarrhea. For 20% of these patients, these symptoms were severe enough to warrant stopping treatment or starting intravenous feeding. Weight loss was greatest when tolerance was poor. Among the 15 patients who received a low-residue diet, ten had good and five average tolerance. This diet therefore seems to us important in preventing the gastrointestinal side-effects of treatment. Diabetics should be observed especially carefully

Table 1. Digestive tolerance during irradiation (50 patients)

	Mean weight loss (kg)	No. of patients
Poor	4.5	10 (20%)
Average	3.1	21 (42%)
Good	2	19 (38%)

because the risk of decompensation is considerable. In this series, two patients on insulin were hospitalized throughout their treatment to regulate their dosage. Finally, it should be noted that early gastrointestinal effects were not correlated with previous abdominal surgery.

Hematologic Tolerance

Irradiation was interrupted if medullary hypoplasia occurred: 500 neutrophils or 50,000 platelets. In the 26 cases without chemotherapy before radiotherapy, only one (stage IIe infradiaphragmatic) developed hypoplasia at 1000 rad. This returned to normal after 5 weeks, and treatment was then completed uneventfully. Twenty-four patients had intensive chemotherapy before radiotherapy. Seven developed severe hypoplasia, and in four cases treatment had to be stopped definitively at 1000 or 2000 rad. One of these patients died several months later of aplasia. In general, in spite of the relatively advanced age of the patients, previous intensive chemotherapy did not prevent total abdominal irradiation or the continuation of maintenance chemotherapy afterward. Maintenance chemotherapy was, however, impossible after hypoplasia had developed during irradiation.

Late Effects of Irradiation

Fourteen patients out of 50 developed problems of varying severity after irradiation which could have been due to the irradiation alone or its association with other methods of treatment (Table 2).

Table 2. Late complications in 50 patients

Lower limb edema	3
Radiation nephritis	1
Gastroduodenal ulcers	2
Small bowel obstruction	6
Small bowel obstruction with rectosigmoid stenosis	1
Chylous ascites	1
Total	14

Lower Limb Edema

Three patients had lower limb edema due to lymphatic block after irradiation of the inguinal region. In all cases, a node biopsy had been performed before treatment. There is, therefore, a direct relationship between surgery, radiotherapy (4000 rad with 13 MeV electrons), and inguinal lymphatic sclerosis.

Radiation Nephritis

One patient aged 64 years with stage III disease developed radiation nephritis after receiving 2000 rad in 11 fractions and 19 days without renal protection because of the size of the tumor volume. Nine months later he developed proteinuria and 14 months later renal failure with arterial hypertension 200/100, anemia, raised BUN, microscopical hematuria, raised serum creatinine, etc. The retina showed stage II changes; IVP was normal. Histology of the renal biopsy showed chronic interstitial changes, glomerular as well as ischemic lesions, and mesangial hypertrophy compatible with radiation nephritis. In spite of symptomatic treatment, the renal failure progressed, and the patient died 22 months after his first symptom. Another patient with a gastric lymphoma received 3000 rad to the abdomen and a further 1500 rad to the left hemiabdomen without left renal protection. Thirty-six months after the end of treatment, he had no signs of renal failure. The left kidney was silent on scanning, and there was no compensatory hypertrophy of the right kidney. The first observation confirms the fact that a dose of 2000 rad in 2 weeks to both kidneys produces irreversible changes, while the second case shows that much higher doses to one kidney only do not lead to clinical signs of renal failure.

Gastroduodenal Ulcers

Two patients developed gastroduodenal ulcers after the end of radiotherapy. In the first case, an ulcer appeared on the lesser curvature of the stomach 2 months after treatment. No chemotherapy had been given. Prolonged medical treatment led to permanent healing within several weeks. In the second case, total abdominal irradiation was followed by maintenance chemotherapy with cyclophosphamide, vincristine, and prednisone. Eleven months after the end of radiotherapy, the patient had a massive hematemesis, and at operation a large crater was found on the posterior wall of the first part of the duodenum. The patient died of a catastrophic hemorrhage. Continuous steroid administration was certainly an important cause of this duodenal ulcer which became clinically symptomatic 1 month after the end of irradiation.

Intestinal Complications

Intestinal and mesenteric complications were the most serious. Seven patients developed obstruction between 1–20 months (mean 8 months) after irradiation, and one patient developed chylous ascites 6 months later. In all cases, the cause was determined by surgical intervention (Table 3). The chylous ascites was due to a mesenteric lymphatic block, and an attempted derivation into the saphenous vein was unsuccessful. Four of the seven obstructions were due to stenosis; two patients still had pathologic nodes. In all case the small intestine was normal. Three of these obstructions were radiation-induced. Once there was partial radiation damage to the small intestine in a loop which had been previously involved with tumor. Resection and end-to-end anastomosis was performed. In the two other cases, the whole small intestine showed posttreatment changes and one patient had an associated rectosigmoidal stenosis. There was no recurrence in the initial mesenteric sites of involvement. Attempted bypass was unsuccessful, and the patient died in the postoperative period. The other is alive and on a strict diet.

Table 3. Causes of small bowel obstructions

Stenosis	2
Stenosis and tumor	2
Partial intestinal radiation damage	1
Total intestinal radiation damage	1
Total intestinal radiation damage and rectosigmoidal narrowing	1
Total	7

Case Reports

Case No. 1—MS IGR 74.11120 WB—39-year-old Man

In November, 1974, he developed right inguinal lymphadenopathy and a diagnosis of nodular non-Hodgkin's lymphoma was made. An exploratory laparotomy in February, 1975, showed infiltration of the root of the mesentery by a large node mass which was marked with clips. In March, 1975, the whole abdomen was irradiated to a dose of 3000 rad and this was followed by 1000 rad to an inverted Y-field. Chemotherapy with cyclophosphamide, vincristine, and prednisone was continued for 1 year. In April, 1976, because of digestive symptoms and signs of obstruction, barium studies were performed and showed areas of narrowing of the small intestine with proximal dilatation and a tight rectosigmoid stenosis (Figs. 1 and 2).
In spite of symptomatic treatment and strict diet, his digestive problems became worse, and on November 8, 1976 surgery was performed for intestinal obstruction. The whole of the small intestine was distended with thickened pale walls with adhesions between loops and between them and the parietal peritoneum. There was no evidence of recurrence at the root of the mesentery. Because of the widespread nature of the irradiation damage, no bypass procedure was possible, and a temporary gastrostomy was performed. Postoperative recovery was uneventful, and the patient is now well, although he has to stick to a very strict diet to avoid recurrence of his abdominal pain.

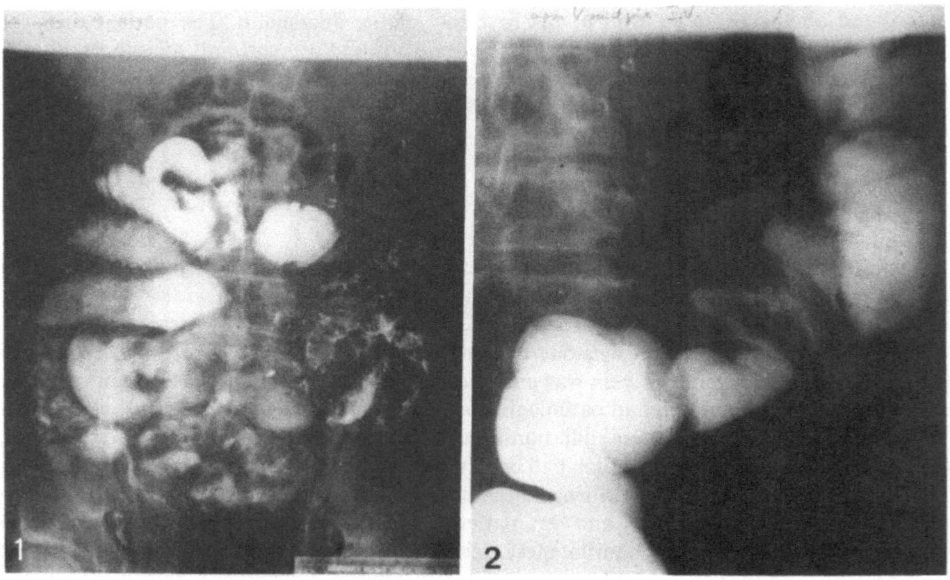

Figs. 1 and 2. Small bowel barium radiograph showing areas of narrowing of the small intestine with proximal dilatation and a tight rectosigmoid stenosis

Case No. 2—PD IGR 76.01043 DP—18-year-old Youth

This patient underwent exploratory laparotomy on February 10, 1976 because of a fluctuating fever and a suspicious lymphangiogram for which no cause had been found. This was completely negative (nodes, spleen, liver, and bone marrow normal), but later he developed abdominal pain, and a left paraumbilical mass was found. This was shown at operation to be a mass of nodes infiltrating the root of the mesentery and the majority of the free mesentery with involvement by continuity of an intestinal loop.

Biopsy showed non-Hodgkin's lymphoma; 3000 rad were given to the whole abdomen and a further 1000 rad to an inverted Y-field from August 25, 1976–September 30, 1976. Digestive tolerance of this irradiation was very poor. Subsequently, chemotherapy with adriamycin, VM 26, cyclophosphamide, and prednisone was started. One month after the end of the radiation, the patient underwent emergency surgery for small intestinal obstruction. The occlusion was found to be due to an obviously radiation-damaged intestinal loop with a whitish appearance in the middle part of the small intestine. This was resected and an anastomosis performed. In addition, there was fibrosis of the mesentery without obvious tumor. It is likely that the radiation-induced lesion corresponded with the loop previously described as being involved in continuity. Postoperative recovery was uneventful. Histologic examination of the specimen showed as a very important edema separating the mucosa from the muscle and a thickening and hyalinization of the vessel walls.

Survival

Fifty-eight percent of the patients (29/50) were alive on January 1, 1977, with a mean follow-up time of 20.5 months. Seven died of complications (Table 4). Radiotherapy was directly responsible for nephritis, radiation damage to the intestine, and lymphatic block. In the other cases, chemotherapy or previous surgery were disposing factors.

Table 4. Deaths due to complications

Total number of deaths	21/50
Died of complications	7/21
Radiation nephritis	1
Marrow failure	1
Duodenal ulcer	1
Mesenteric lymphatic block	1
Intestinal radiation damage	1
Obstruction due to stenosis	1
Obstruction due to stenosis and tumor	1

Discussion

All these patients were irradiated with the same energy, to the same doses, with the same fractionation. We must ask, therefore, what other factor could be responsible for these intestinal complications. The only predisposing factor we found was an exploratory or a diagnostic laparotomy in the weeks preceding irradiation. The 24 patients who did not undergo surgery did not have any complications (Table 5), whereas there was one radiation-damaged intestine after six laparotomies done during the initial work-up and four obstructions, two cases of radiation intestinal damage, and one lymphatic block in 20 patients operated on for

Table 5. Relationship of obstructions and radiation damage to the mesentery and previous laparotomy

No laparotomy	0/24
Exploratory laparotomy (radiation-damaged intestine)	1/6
Diagnostic laparotomy (six obstructions, one mesenteric lymphatic block)	7/20

abdominal problems which were often acute. In the latter situation, the size of the abdominal tumor and the bowel infiltration may account for the radiation damage seen. The appearance of digestive complications is not correlated with:

1. Patient's age
2. Previous surgery, such as appendicectomy
3. Immediate digestive tolerance—the three cases of radiation damage were seen in patients who had tolerated radiotherapy well
4. Dietary regimen.

On the other hand, in all the cases of obstruction due to stenosis or radiation damage, the patients had received chemotherapy with vincristine after radiotherapy. This drug, whose paralysing effect on smooth muscle is well-known, may have been a predisposing factor. Several factors must be considered in the prevention of these side-effects:

1. Avoidance of laparotomy when the lymphangiogram is pathologic, because the chances of mesenteric involvement in these cases are very high.
2. Decreasing the radiation dose. As things are at present, nobody knows definitely if doses of 2000 rad are sufficient to cure the nodular forms of non-Hodgkin's lymphomas when radiotherapy is given initially with curative intent. It is probable, however, for patients in complete remission after eight courses of chemotherapy that 2000 rad are enough to sterilize microscopic foci of disease.
3. Decreasing the dose per session. Patients are treated as present with four fractions of 185 rad per week by anterior and posterior opposing fields treated the same day. After laparotomy, this weekly dose of 750 rad could be given in five fractions.

Spleen Irradiation

Materials and Methods

Since 1972, we have undertaken a prospective study of renal function by means of clinical examination, radiology, and scanning in patients with lymphoma whose left kidneys have been partially irradiated during radiotherapy to the spleen [6]. Seventy-five patients have been studied; 63 with Hodgkin's disease and 12 with non-Hodgkin's lymphomas. There were 50 men and 25 women, and the mean age was 30 ± 14 years with a range from 4–67 years.

Radiotherapy Techniques

The spleen was irradiated by anterior and posterior fields with a linear accelerator with 25 MV x-rays. The midline dose was 4000 rad in 4 weeks. The upper and outer limits were 1–2 cm of the left lung base and the left thoracic wall. The medial margin was that of the lateral edge of the lumboaortic field, and the lower border was determined from the scan. The amount of left kidney irradiated varied from 30%–80% with a mean value of 50%.

Methods of Investigation

Renal function was studied in all patients by clinical examination, biologic and radiologic investigation, and scanning. This was done before irradiation, at 6 weeks, 6 months, and then yearly. Clinical examination consisted of taking the blood pressure after the patient had been lying down for 15 min. Biologic tests included blood urea and creatinine, creatinine and urea clearance at 3 h, 24-h urine testing for proteinuria, red and white cell counts/min in the urine, and plasma renin estimation. Radiography consisted of standard intravenous pyelogram. Early nephrotomography was performed in 14 patients. Several types of isotopic examinations were performed:

1. Scanning with ^{197}Hg neohydrin. The aim of this scan, which uses a posterior incidence, is to compare the uptake in one kidney relative to the other or in different parts of the same kidney. Subsequent computer analysis permits, in addition to classic analogue scanning, a quantitative comparison between activity in different regions of the kidneys. The program also calculates the area of the irradiated zone of the left kidney and the number of impulses in this zone as well as the ratio of impulse density/unit area in the irradiated region and the right kidney.
2. Dynamic study with the γ-camera using Hippuran^{131}I and DTPA Tc99^{m}. This measured renal plasma flow and glomerular filtration.

Results

By July 1, 1977, 75 patients had been studied. Seventy-four have been studied since 1972 and have a mean follow-up time of 36 months (range 6–66 months). One patient has been followed for 11 years, but the first renal studies were done 9 years after irradiation. The following results were obtained. The blood pressure was unchanged in all patients. We have seen three cases of proteinuria of less than 1 g/24 h and seven times a urinary leukocyte count of between 2000 and 20,000 WBC/min. In two cases, this was accompanied by microscopic hematuria of 4600 and 20,000 red cells/min. No other changes were seen in any patients, neither in proteinuria, red and white cell counts/min, creatinine, or clearance rates. In five cases where they were measured after irradiation plasma, renin levels were normal or at the upper limit of normal. Standard urography showed no abnormalities of secretion, but from the 30th month after irradiation there was a progressive although variable decrease in the size of the irradiated kidney. In 14 patients who had early nephrotomography, cortical atrophy of the upper pole with decrease in the cortical index were seen 17 months after irradiation together with rigidity and stenosis of the branches of the upper and middle calyceal system and flattening of the calyceal outlines.

Results of Analogue Scanning with ^{197}Hg Neohydrine

From the 8th months onward, there is diminished uptake of the isotope in the irradiated area sometimes associated with a decrease in size of the kidney which becomes constant 20 months after irradiation.

Results of Numerical Scanning with ^{197}Hg Neohydrine

This showed a significantly lower uptake by the irradiated kidney than by the healthy kidney from the 8th month after irradiation. This became more evident up to the 24th month when it reached 50% of the initial activity before stabilizing. In the irradiated area, the decrease in uptake was of the order of 70%. No compensatory hypertrophy of the right kidney or the nonirradiated part of the left kidney was noted.

Results of Hippuran ^{131}I Nephrograms and DTPA $Tc99^m$ Studies (11 Patients)

Analysis of the curves sometimes showed both a delay in clearance of the Hippuran in the irradiated kidney of about 2 min on average and also a decrease in amplitude of this peak relative to the normal kidney of 30%–80%. In addition, the amplitude of this peak is less at the upper pole of the irradiated kidney, while at the lower pole it is less than that at the lower pole of the nonirradiated kidney. Three months after irradiation, one patient showed low uptake in the upper pole of the irradiated kidney on DTPA scans, while the neohydrine scans were normal.

Discussion

These results confirm the conclusions of a preliminary study of 16 patients [7] but call for some comment.

Blood Pressure and Plasma Renin Levels

The absence of hypertension in these patients may be explained either by the destruction by irradiation of renin-producing sites in the juxtaglomerular apparatus or by a protective effect exerted by the controlateral nonirradiated kidney [4]. All the levels of plasma renin measured were normal, excluding any frank rise after radiotherapy.

Biologic Testing

The rare changes that we found suggested an interstitial nephropathy and are often seen after bilateral irradiation [8]. Their intermittent nature perhaps explains why they have not been found more often [9].

Radiologic Investigations and Scanning

The results show the sensitivity of isotopic methods in demonstrating postradiation changes [11]. Decreased uptake on scans with ^{197}Hg neohydrine and DTPA Tc99 occurs even when there is no radiologic lesion visible on intravenous urography or nephrotomography. In fact, there is often good opacification of the renal cavities on urography because of the increased concentration of the contrast medium which is excreted in a reduced fluid volume [1]. Changes in nephrotomograms appear at the stage of sclerosis and show atrophy of the upper pole sometimes with a high-riding kidney. Once the lesions have developed, they do not change [5]. Isotopic studies give information about renal function, proximal tubular functions by the neohydrine scan and glomerular by the DTPA. Glomerulotubular lesions 8 months after irradiation are only shown by isotopic methods.

Compensatory Hypertrophy

Our results do not show any compensatory hypertrophy of the controlateral kidney or of the nonirradiated left renal segments. These findings suggest that overall function of the two kidneys is maintained.

Conclusion

Total abdominal irradiation in patients with non-Hodgkin's lymphoma should be undertaken with great care. Whereas our present technique enables us to deliver a dose of 3000 rad without causing any digestive problems in patients who have not had surgery, this is not so when laparotomy has been performed before the radiotherapy. In these patients, the present treatment plan should be modified by decreasing the doses and prolonging the fractionation. It should be noted that all the complications seen in these patients (except for a case of radiation nephritis) were due to combination of radiotherapy with either chemotherapy or surgery or both.

Partial irradiation of the left kidney, which is inevitable when irradiating the spleen, produces no clinical or biochemical consequences within a mean follow-up time of 33 months. Only the isotopic investigations with ^{197}Hg neohydrine, hippuran ^{131}I, and DTPA Tc99 show postirradiation changes of decreased uptake at the 8th month and a fall in renal plasma flow in the irradiated area. Radiologic studies do not show changes until very late.

Summary

Fifty patients with non-Hodgkin's lymphoma were treated with total abdominal irradiation to a dose of 3000 rad by anterior and posterior fields treated the same day. Fourteen patients developed complications, four with intestinal obstruction due to stenosis and three with total or partial intestinal irradiation damage. These bowel complications were only seen in patients who had previously had a laparotomy. The ways of preventing these complications are discussed. We have studied renal function by means of clinical examination, biologic and radiologic investigations, and scanning in 75 patients who have received splenic irradiation to a dose of 4000 rad. With a mean follow-up time of 36 months, this study has shown that there was no significant change in blood pressure or in biochemical measurements. However, at the 17th month, nephrotomograms demonstrated cortical atrophy of the upper pole of the kidney; at the 8th month, low uptake in the irradiated area was seen on ^{197}Hg neohydrine scanning and a decrease in renal plasma flow in the left kidney during dynamic studies with Hippuran.

References

1. Bitker, M., Chatelain, C., Guedon, J., Kuss, R.: L'urographie dans certaines néphropathies unilatérales. J. Urol. Néphrol. *75*, 76–89 (1969)
2. Carbone, P. P., Kaplan, H. S., Musshoff, K., Smithers, D. W., Tubiana, M.: Report of the committee on Hodgkin's disease staging classification. Cancer Res. *31*, 1860–1861 (1971)
3. Donaldson, S. S., Jundt, S., Ricour, C., Sarrazin, D., Lemerle, J., Schweisguth, O.: Radiation enteritis in children. A retrospective review, clinicopathologic correlation and dietary management. Cancer *35*, 1167–1178 (1975)
4. Fischer, E. R., Hellstrom, H. R.: pathogenesis of hypertension and pathologic changes in experimental renal irradiation. Lab. Invest. *19*, 530–538 (1968)
5. Kunkler, P. B., Farr, R. F., Luxton, R. W.: The limit of renal tolerance to X-rays. An investigation into renal damage occurring following the treatment of tumours of the testis by abdominal bath. Br. J. Radiol. *25*, 190–201 (1952)
6. Le Bourgeois, J. P., Meignan, M., Parmentier, C., Tubiana, M.: Renal consequences of spleen irradiation. (Submitted paper)

7. Le Bourgeois, J. P., Godefroy, D., Di Paola, M., Parmentier, C., Tubiana, M.: A propos des néphrites post-radiothérapiques. Etude du retentissement rénal de l'irradiation de la rate dans les hématosarcomes. J. Radiol. Electrol. *56*, 826–829 (1975)
8. Luxton, R. W.: Radiation nephritis. Q.J. Med. *22*, 215–242 (1953)
9. Luxton, R. W.: Effects of irradiation on the Kidney. In: Disease of the Kidney, Strauss, M. B., Welt, L. G. (eds.) 1049–1070 2eme Edit. 1971—Boston: Little Broom Edit.
10. Morane, M., Ultmann, J. E., Ferguson, D. J., Hoffer, P. B., Ranulger, K., Rappaport, H.: Staging laparotomy in non Hodgkin's lymphoma. Br. J. Cancer, 31 Suppl. *II*, 228–236 (1975)
11. Quinn, J. L., Meschan, I., Blake, D. D., Witcovski, R. L.: The usefulness of the radioisotopic renogram in radiation therapy. Radiology *78*, 266–268 (1962)

Effects of Treatment of Malignant Lymphomas on the Granulocytic Progenitor Cells (CFU_c)

C. Parmentier, D. Maraninchi, N. Morardet, J. P. Droz, and P. Charbord

Introduction

Study of the after-effects of therapy on the healthy organs is one of the main preoccupations of oncology. Although progress in therapeutics has clearly improved the prognosis for malignant lymphomas, the after-effects of these treatments, notably the hematologic ones, are occasionally serious. The hematologic effects were approached essentially by cytologic, histologic, and isotopic methods; these only allow study of a differentiated compartment and do not always reflect the state of the true medullary reserves, i.e., the hematopoietic progenitors. In this work, the granulocytic progenitor cell (CFU_c) compartment of 14 patients with malignant lymphomas was studied after radiotherapy, associated or unassociated with chemotherapy.

Materials and Methods

In Vitro Culture of CFU_c

The CFU_c were studied by culturing them in methylcellulose in the presence of a stimulating factor from normal leukocytes (CSA) [13]. Only those colonies of at least 50 cells were counted after 10 days of culture. All the results were obtained with the same batch of CSA, which enables one to assure a constant plating efficiency in all of the cultures [6].

Modes of Expressing the Results

In addition to the number of colonies per 10^5 medullary cells plated, two other modes of expression were used.

1. The number of CFU_c per 10^5 metamyelocytes plated enabled us to correct the dilution of the medullary samples, which is not reproducible [8, 12]. Moreover, this mode of expression limits, in our experience (unpublished data), the disparity in the medullary distribution of CFU_c observed by others [11]. Although data are still scarce in this field and further investigation is needed, several studies enable one to accept that there is a slight variability in the mean transit time of metamyelocytes in the bone marrow [2, 7, 10]. This variability does not explain the variations in the numbers of CFU_c per 10^5 metamyelocytes encountered clinically [18]. Therefore, it can be assumed that the number of CFU_c per 10^5 metamyelocytes gives information on the number of mitoses inserted between the stem cell and the differentiated cell. Reduction in the number of CFU_c per 10^5 metamyelocytes suggests an increased efficiency of granulopoiesis by an increase in the number of mitoses in the line. Increase in the number of CFU_c suggests either a reduction in the number of mitoses or ineffective granulopoiesis.

2. Many studies [4, 5, 14, 19] enable one to accept the existence in normal subjects of a constant of proportionality (K) between the total number of medullary metamyelocytes (M) and the number of circulating granulocytes (G) (measurable by a blood count and calculation of the blood mass) which leads to the relationship

$$M = K \times G$$

where from the average of the results in the literature, K is virtually equal to 10. It is possible by the above equation to calculate the total number of medullary CFU_c (N) by the equation

$$N = \text{number of } CFU_c \text{ per } 10^5 \text{ metamyelocytes} \times 10^{-5} \times 10 \times G$$

and to normalize this value by kg body weight so as to be able to compare it with the results found in a normal reference population [17, 18].

This calculation only gives an order of magnitude of the total number of CFU_c as their plating efficiency is not known and is probably subject to a certain variability. In addition, the total number of metamyelocytes not being measurable, it is necessary to accept the existence of the same constant K in normal and pathologic subjects. This hypothesis can only be accepted under certain conditions. The possible variability in the mean transit time of metamyelocytes in the bone marrow has already been discussed. The problems posed by the peripheral kinetics must not be underestimated [1, 8]. Shortening of the life span of granulocytes is exceptional except in hypersplenism [8] and the major granulopathies. The balance between the marginal and circulating granulocytic pools can be affected by transitory causes such as anxiety and is subject to a certain physiologic variability. It is, nevertheless, possible to reduce these artifacts by standardizing the hours of sampling and by controlling the constancy of the number of circulating granulocytes by several counts. The calculation of the total number of CFU_c thus appears rather rough, but it is clinically useful and able to provide better information than that provided by the number of colonies per 10^5 medullary nucleated cells [18]. In irradiated patients, the granulocytic production of the irradiated and nonirradiated zones was calculated, taking into account the medullary volume irradiated, according to the data of MECHANIK [21] and a formulation described in detail elsewhere [9].

Ferrokinetic Measurements

Seven patients had a ferrokinetic study with ^{59}Fe at the same time as the culture. The external counting from irradiated and nonirradiated zones served as a control of the erythropoietic activity of these zones [17]. The erythropoietic activity was judged null (o), weak (+), normal (+ +), or raised (+ + +) (Table 1) as a function of the radioactivity effectively fixed by the bone marrow 24 h after the injection of ^{59}Fe.

Patients Studied

Fourteen patients who had received no treatment for some time were studied 1–6.5 years after the end of radiotherapy (Table 1). Five had had mantle irradiation, three mantle and lomboaortic irradiation, and six total lymphoid irradiation. Seven of these patients had had complementary chemotherapy for 2 years with vinblastine (6 mg/m^2/week) according to an EORTC clinical trial.

Results

The concentration of circulating granulocytes, the results of CFU_c cultures, and the external ^{59}Fe counting are given in Table 1. All the patients had a concentration of circulating

Table 1. Hematologic effects in malignant lymphomas after radiotherapy alone or associated with chemotherapy

Case	Treatment	Diagnosis	Time lapse between end of radiotherapy and culture (years)	Peripheral blood			Irradiated areas			Nonirradiated areas			Total No. of CFU_c/kg × 10^5
				Hemoglobin (g/100 ml)	Granulocytes/mm^3 × 10^3	Platelets/mm^3 × 10^3	$CFU_c/10^5$ nucleated cells	$CFU_c/10^5$ metamyelocytes	^{59}Fe (external counting)	$CFU_c/10^5$ nucleated cells	$CFU_c/10^5$ metamyelocytes	^{59}Fe External counting)	
1	Radiotherapy (mantle fields)	HD	6.5	10.5	4.8	260	0	0		43	253		80
2		HD	1	15	8.3	210	2	125		11	85		46
3		HD	6	13	3.7	190	1	200	+	21	184	+++	45
4	Radiotherapy (mantle fields + 2 years vinblastine	HD	4	12	4.2	270	0	0		6	86		24
5		HD	5	11.5	4.3	180	1	50		10	53		15
6	Radiotherapy (mantle fields + inverted Y)	HS	2	14	2.7	100	13	310	++	25	132	++	28
7		HD	1.5	12.5	2.3	150	4	83	+	6	65	+++	11
8		HD	6	14	8	250	11	550	++	32	571	++	301
9		LS	5.5	14	3.8	880	8	35		15	100		10
10	Radiotherapy mantle fields + lomboaortic + 2 years vinblastine	HD	2.75	12.5	5	290	0	0		5	50		10
11		HD	2.8	13	3.6	200	0	0	0	8	138	+++	33
12		HD	3.3	15	2.1	150	0	0		0.6	7		1
13	Radiotherapy mantle fields + Inverted Y + 2 years vinblastine	HD	2.25	14	4	410	0	0	0	19	240	++	64
14		HD	2.5	14	5	210	0	0	0	23	120	++	40

HD = Hodgkin's disease.
LS = Lymphocytic sarcoma well differentiated.
HS = Histiocytic sarcoma poorly differentiated.

granulocytes above 2000/mm^3, which is within the normal limits. Three patients (1, 2, and 3) treated by moderate radiotherapy had, in the nonirradiated zone, normal numbers of colonies for 10^5 medullary cells and for 10^5 metamyelocytes; calculation of the total number of CFU_c gave a normal value. In contrast, two patients (4 and 5) treated by moderate radiotherapy followed by continuous chemotherapy had reduced cloning values in the nonirradiated zones and a reduced total number or CFU_c, contrasting with the normal concentration of circulating granulocytes. In the four patients treated by total lymphoid irradiation alone, three (6, 7, and 9) had, despite a variable cloning ability in the nonirradiated zone, a reduced total number of CFU_c which could be explained by the large medullary volume irradiated. One patient (8), the only one in our sample in relapse at the time of culture, had the cloning ability and the total number of CFU_c raised. Three patients (10, 11, and 12), in whom extensive irradiation (mantle and lomboaortic fields) was associated with continuous chemotherapy, had reduced cloning ability as well as a reduction in their total number of CFU_c. Finally, patients 13 and 14, who had received a very aggressive treatment, had normal cloning ability and total number of CFU_c.

The hematopoietic activity in the nonirradiated and irradiated zones could be studied in every patient by culture of CFU_c and in seven patients (3, 6, 7, 8, 11, 13, and 14) by ^{59}Fe external counting. Medullary regeneration, granulocytic as well as erythropoietic, appeared weak when the patient was treated only by irradiation of a limited medullary target volume. On the other hand, when the treatment consisted of extensive pure irradiation, the regeneration of the two cell lines was clearly evident. In our sample, in all the patients treated by chemotherapy associated with radiotherapy, whatever its extent, *we observed an absence of medullary regeneration* in both the granulocytic and red cell lines.

Discussion

The CFU_c compartment can be markedly reduced subsequent to radiotherapy or associated radio- and chemotherapy. With radiotherapy alone, possible after-effects appear to be directly correlated with the volume irradiated. We have not seen a significant deficit with limited radiotherapy ($\leq 25\%$ of the hematopoietic bone marrow), whereas total lymphoid irradiation ($\geq 60\%$ of the medullary volume) can bring about a big reduction in the number of granulocytic progenitor cells. In many cases, we have found a reduction in the number of CFU_c when long-term chemotherapy is associated with radiotherapy, even inextensive radiotherapy. These findings must, however, be qualified by three considerations:

1. Certain patients having undergone an aggressive treatment protocol had nevertheless, 3 years later, a normal CFU_c count, which leads one to assume that individual responses are very variable (patients 13 and 14).
2. The study of the number of CFU_c per 10^5 metamyelocytes suggests a powerful correction mechanism by mitotic amplification. Certain bone marrows have, therefore, probably lost their ability for adaptation but remain capable of producing a sufficient number of granulocytes.
3. The results of the cultures after treatment must be interpreted cautiously. In fact, the cloning ability is often low in hematosarcomas before treatment [3, 9].

   In a series of 23 hematosarcomas, we found significant reductions in cloning values and total numbers of CFU_c (Table 2). Nevertheless, the post-therapeutic reduction does not seem to us to be in doubt for two reasons: 1) the distribution of the cloning ability and the number of CFU_c were reported after the first phase of treatment when the evolutive phase of the disease was attenuated [3, 9] and 2) in our sample, we were able to culture samples from patients 12 and 13 before any treatment and during the evolution of their disease (Table 3).

Table 2. Comparison of the CFU_c of 26 normal subjects and 23 patients with malignant lymphomas before treatment

	Blood granulocytes/ mm^3	$CFU_c/10^5$ nucleated cells	$CFU_c/10^5$ metamyelocytes	$CFU_c/kg \times 10^5$
26 normal subjects	4448 ± 1440	18 ± 8	287 ± 100	84 ± 40
23 untreated malignant lymphomas	3850 ± 700	6 ± 2	83 ± 47	25 ± 14

Means ± 2 SD.

The secondary reduction in CFU_c in these patients not receiving any treatment, in complete remission, and who had had normal numbers of CFU_c during the evolution of their disease seems to well reflect the true effects of treatments received.

Patient 8 probably had ineffective leukopoiesis. Let us remember that it concerns the only patient in this group in evolutive phase of disease at the time of culture. This patient died 1 month after culture with disseminated Hodgkin's disease. This suggests that a similar hematologic profile would be indicative of a poor prognosis.

Among the possible compensatory mechanisms for a post-therapeutic attack of hematopoiesis, we were able to study, besides the granulocytic mitotic amplification, medullary regeneration. In both the erythrocytic and granulocytic lines, the regeneration appeared to be a function of the volume irradiated in the case of radiotherapy alone. Weak or inexistent with limited irradiation, regeneration clearly became a compensatory mechanism in the case of total lymphoid irradiation [9, 15, 16, 20].

When continuous chemotherapy is associated with irradiation, we have established, in our sample, the absence of medullary regeneration irrespective of the irradiated volume or the hematopoietic count. This finding needs confirmation by the study of other patients, as much for its reproducibility as for its significance: abolition of regeneratation by the toxicity of chemotherapy for the residual stem cells or simply retardation of regeneration?

Table 3. Evolution of the total number of CFU_c after radiotherapy and chemotherapy in two patients with Hodgkin's lymphoma

Case	Time lapse between diagnosis and culture	Culture time in the therapeutic scheme	Granulocytes/ mm^3	$CFU_c/kg \times 10^5$
12	0	Before treatment	4600	141
	1 month	After mantle fields RT	3600	10
	3 months	After lomboaortic RT	3000	20
	5 months	2 months after completion of RT	4500	70
	48 months	43 months after completion of RT and 15 months after the end of a complementary 2 years VLB course	2100	1
13	0	Before treatment	6700	9
	1 month	After mantle fields RT	5800	10
	3 months	2 months after mantle fields RT	6000	120
	5 months	4 months after mantle fields RT	5000	150
	36 months	35 months after mantle fields, 27 months after inverted Y and 3 months after the end of a complementary 2 years VLB course	4500	64

RT: radiotherapy; VLB: vinblastine.

Summary

The goal of this work was to appraise the after-effects of radiotherapy and associated radio- and chemotherapy on hematosarcomas by studying the granulocytic progenitor cells (CFU_c). The bone marrow of 14 subjects was cultured in methylcellulose 1–6.5 years after completion of radiotherapy. The results were recorded as the number of CFU_c per 10^5 nucleated medullary cells plated and per 10^5 metamyelocytes plated, and the total number of medullary CFU_c was calculated. These different modes of expression are discussed.

The post-radiotherapeutic effects appeared to be closely correlated with the volume irradiated. Chemotherapy seemed in several cases to accentuate the effects. Nevertheless, the organism can operate a powerful compensatory mechanism by means of increased mitosis, and in addition, certain subjects are able to maintain a normal number of CFU_c after an aggressive treatment. It was possible in certain cases to study the medullary regeneration of the irradiated zone by culture of the CFU_c and by the ^{59}Fe external counting. Its extent after radiotherapy seemed for both the granulocytic and the red cell line to be correlated with the volume irradiated. Subject to the study of new cases, regeneration appears to be very reduced when chemotherapy is associated with radiotherapy.

References

1. Athens, J. W., Haab, O. D., Raab, S. O., Mauer, A. M., Ashenbrucker, H., Cartwight, G. E., Wintrobe, M. M.: Leucokinetic studies IV the total blood circulating and marginal granulocyte pools and the turn over rate in normal subjects. J. Clin. Invest. *40*, 989–985 (1961)
2. Bishop, C. R., Rothstein, G., Ashenbrucker, A. E., Athens, J. N.: Leucokinetic studies XIV. Blood neutrophil kinetics in chronic steady state neutropenia. J. Clin. Invest. *50*, 1678–1689 (1971)
3. Bull, J. M., De Vita, V. T., Carbone, P. P.: In vivo granulocyte production in patients with Hodgkin's disease and lymphocytic, histiocytic and mixed lymphomas. Blood *45*, 833–842 (1975)
4. Dancey, J. T., Deubelbeiss, K. A., Harker, L. A., Finch, C. A.: Neutrophil kinetics in man. J. Clin. Invest. *85*, 705–715 (1976)
5. Donohue, D. M., Gabrio, B. W., Finch, C. A.: Quantitative measurement of hematopoietic cells of the marrow and blood. J. Clin. Invest. *37*, 1564–1570 (1958)
6. Douglas, I. D. C., Pickering, B. M. J.: The effect of various sources of colony stimulating activity on normal human bone marrow in agar culture. Exp. Cell Res. *104*, 95–99 (1977)
7. Dresh, C., Faille, A., Bauchet, J., Najean, Y.: Studies of granulocyte kinetics in normal and granulopoietic subjects. Biomedicine *22*, 145–157 (1975)
8. Dresh, C., Najean, Y.: Cinétique des polynucléaires neutrophiles chez l'homme. Rev. Eur. Etudes Clin. Biol. *15*, 729–739 (1970)
9. Droz, J. P., Parmentier, C., Morardet, N., Maraninchi, D., Gardet, P., Tubiana, M.: Effects of radiotherapy on the bone marrow granulocytic progenitor cells CFU_c) of patients with malignant lymphomas. Part I—Short term effects. Int. J. Radiat. Oncology Biol. Phys, 1978, in press
10. Fieschi, A., Sachetti, C.: Clinical assessment of granulopoiesis. Acta Haematol. *31*, 150–155 (1964)
11. Gordon, M. Y., Douglas, I. D. C., Clink, H. M., Pickering, B. M. J.: Distribution of granulopoietic activity in the human skeleton, studied by colony growth in agar diffusion chambers. Br. J. Haematol. *32*, 537–542 (1976)
12. Gruppo, R. A., Lampkin, B. C., Granger, S.: Bone marrow cellularity determination: comparison of the biopsy, aspirate and buffy coat. Blood *49*, 29–31 (1976)
13. Iscove, N. N., Senn, J. S., Till, J. E., McCulloch, E. A.: Colony formation by normal and leukemic human marrow cells in culture: effect of conditioned medium from human leucocytes. Blood *37*, 1–5 (1971)
14. Killman, S. A., Cronkite, E. P., Fliedner, T. M., Bond, V. P.: Mitotic indices of human bone marrow cells. I. Number and cytologic distribution of mitoses. Blood *19*, 743–750 (1962)
15. Knospe, W. H., Rayndu, V. M. S., Cardello, M., Friedman, A. M., Fordham, E. W.: Bone marrow scanning with 52 Iron (^{52}Fe). Cancer *37*, 1432–1442 (1976)

16. MORARDET, N., PARMENTIER, C., FLAMANT, R.: Etude par le Fer 59 des effets de la radiotherapie étendue des hématosarcomes sur l'érythropoïèse. Biomedicine *18*, 228–234 (1974)
17. PARMENTIER, C., DROZ, J. P., SUBTIL, E., MOREL-BROSSEL, S., GARDET, P., MORARDET, N., CHARBORD, P., TUBIANA, M.: In vitro culture of normal human bone marrow granulocytic stem cells (CFU_c), how to express the results? Exp. Hematol. *4*, suppl., 131 (1976)
18. PARMENTIER, C., DROZ, J. P., TUBIANA, M.: Ways of expressing results of human bone marrow progenitor cell culture. B. J. Haematol. *40*, (1978) in press
19. PATT, H. M.: A consideration of myeloid-erythroid balance in man. Blood *12*, 777–787 (1957)
20. RUBIN, P., LANDMAN, S., MAYER, E., HELLER, B., CICCIO, S.: Bone marrow regeneration and extension after extended field irradiation in Hodgkin's Disease. Cancer *32*, 699–711 (1973)
21. WOODWARD, H. Q., HOLODNY, E.: A summary of the data of Mechanik on the distribution of human bone marrow. Phys. Med. Biol. *5*, 57–59 (1960)

Preliminary Results of Chemoradiotherapy Followed (or Not) by Active Immunotherapy of Stage III and IV Lymphosarcoma and Reticulosarcoma: Correlation of the Results With WHO Categorization

J. L. Misset, G. Mathé, M. Tubiana, B. Caillou, F. de Vassal, P. Pouillart, M. Gil, C. Tentas, M. Hayat, L. Schwarzenberg, C. Jasmin, M. Delgado, D. Machover, P. Ribaud, and M. Musset

Introduction

Stages III and IV lymphosarcoma (LS) and reticulosarcoma (RS) are disseminated diseases that are typical indications for chemotherapy. Utilizing the drugs vincristine, cyclophosphamide, prednisone (12), adriamycin (6), bleomycin (4), nitrosoureas (5), VM 26 (20), and/or a few others (see [7] and [18]) and combinations of these drugs (8, 9, 10, 21, 22, 23, 24), chemotherapy has been shown to be able to induce a high rate of remission and to significantly but variably prolong survival due to several factors, the major factor being histologic classifications. One group [1] applied Lennert's classification [11]. Most others used the classic Rappaport classification [25], including in the so-called "histiocytic" type several different types, some of which may have good prognosis, e.g., diffuse large cell prolymphocytic (centrofollicular) LS, some of which may have very severe prognosis, e.g., immunoblastic LS [15], and a few of which may have intermediate prognosis, e.g., RS, as discussed in this paper. The present work assesses the value of the WHO categorization [19] in which 1) tumors of the lymphocytic series are called LS and those of the fixed, so-called mononuclear phagocytes [32] (e.g., reticular cells, dendritic cells), which are not in fact macrophages [see 29, 30, 31], are called RS and 2) types of LS are distinguished according to the cell differentiation stages. Among the common varieties, the prolymphocytic (centrofollicular) nodular or diffuse type, the lymphoblastic type, and the immunoblastic type are recognized.

This paper also appraises a strategic regimen comprising an initial chemotherapy, a complementary radiotherapy, a supplementary chemotherapy, and an active systemic immunotherapy, the last being applied to one randomized group of patients out of two. The preliminary results were published [21]; they were encouraging and are confirmed by the present evaluation.

Methods and Patients

This therapeutic study concerns 101 patients who received the predetermined regimen mentioned above and described in Fig. 1. The treatment started with a combination of four drugs shown to be active when given singly: adriamycin (6), VM 26 (20), cyclophosphamide (12), and prednisone (12). Thus, as chemotherapy obeys first-order kinetics [26, 27, 28] and as relapses after chemotherapy mainly occur in the sites of larger masses, after 8 months of the preceding chemotherapy, we applied radiotherapy localized on the "icebergs," i.e., on the detectable tumors; then we applied a complementary chemotherapy less intensive than the first, combining vincristine, cyclophosphamide, and prednisone [22] for 12 months. The patients were then randomized to either receive active immunotherapy comprising the application of BCG and the injection of irradiated leukemic LS cells [13] or to stop treatment.

PROTOCOL OF TREATMENT FOR LYMPHOSARCOMA AND RETICULOSARCOMA
STAGE III AND IV - (PILOT STUDY)

INDUCTION CHEMOTHERAPY									RADIOTHERAPY	COMPLEMENTARY CHEMOTHERAPY					IMMUNOTHERAPY
A	A	A	A	A	A	A	A	A	on "Icebergs" 3000 to 4000 rads	V	V	V	V	to be followed for one year	BCG + leukemic cells (beginning after about 20 months of chemotherapy)
VM	VM	VM	VM	VM	VM	VM	VM	VM		C	C	C	C		
C	C	C	C	C	C	C	C	C		P	P	P	P		
P	P	P	P	P	P	P	P	P							
0	1	2	3	4	5	6	7	8		0	1	2	3		

(time in months)

A	Adriamycin	50 mg/m2	D 1
VM	VM 26	60 mg/m2	D 2
C	Cyclophosphamide	300 mg/m2	D 3-4
P	Prednisone	40 mg/m2	D 3-7

V	Vincristine	1,5 mg/m2	D 1
C	Cyclophosphamide	300 mg/m2	D 2-5
P	Prednisone	40 mg/m2	D 2-6

Fig. 1. Scheme of the protocol

This group of patients is different from the one studied by us for immune markers [2, 3, 14, 16, 17], although some patients were included in both investigations. Some of the patients in the present group were not submitted to cell surface marker determination because the biopsy had already been carried out when they were referred to our service. However, the sections of all patients included in this study were reviewed at the WHO Reference Center for the Classification of Neoplasias of Hematopoietic and Lymphoid tissues [19].
The distribution of the group according to age, sex, stage, perceptible phase of the disease (first presentation or relapse), and the WHO classification are given in Table 1. The correlation between the WHO classification, sex, and stage is given in Table 2. The present results are still preliminary since the action of immunotherapy has not been evaluated. However, the data

Table 1. Patient data

Patients	101
Age	5–70 years
Sex	
Female	39
Male	62
Stage III	44
Stage IV	57
Perceptible phase	
First presentation	69
Relapse	32
Typing according to the WHO categorization	
Lymphosarcomas	
Prolymphocytic (centrofollicular)	36
Nodular	19
Diffuse	14
Non-diffuse	3
Lymphoblastic	15
Immunoblastic	18
Unclassified	21
Reticulosarcoma	11

[a] Median age: 43 years; ten patients were younger than 15 years.

collected already do allow one to correlate the results with the categorization of the WHO Reference Center for the Classification of Neoplasias of Hematopoietic and Lymphoid Tissues [19].

Table 2. Stratification of the patients: correlation between sex, stage, and WHO typing

	Age (extremes)	Median age	Male	Female	Stage III	Stage IV
Lymphosarcomas						
Prolymphocytic (centrofollicular)	19–67	48				
Nodular			13	6	13	6
Diffuse			10	7	5	12
Lymphoblastic	3–62	22	10	5	4	11
Immunoblastic	4–69	45	10	8	9	9
Reticulosarcoma	15–63	44	6	5	4	7

Results

Tolerance

Tolerance was generally good. No death occurred which could be related to the treatment. Alopecia was the most frequent side-effect. Leukopenia at the end of at least one interval which was severe enough to slightly delay the next cycle was observed in 41% of the patients. It was complicated by regressive infections in six patients (Table 3).

Table 3. Tolerance

Alopecia	85%
Leukopenia < 1500 WBC	41%
Thrombocytopenia < 50,000 Platelets	12%
Regressive infection	6 patients
Moderate nausea	6 patients
Heart failure	1 patient
Asthenia	0
Severe diabetes	1 patient
Hemorrhagic cystitis	1 patient
Acute intolerance to VM 26	3 patients
Renal failure	1 patient
Death due to the treatment	0

Overall Remission Induction: LS vs RS

The incidence of complete remission was 79% (71/90) and that of partial remission 9% for LS (Table 4). It was not different for RS (8/11 = 73%).

Overall Rate of Remission Duration and Survival: LS vs RS

The cumulative curves of remission established according to the direct method are shown for stage III and IV LS and RS in Fig. 2. One sees that the median is about 2 years for the three

Table 4. Therapeutic responses

	No. of patients	Complete remission	Partial remission	Failure
Lymphosarcomas				
Prolymphocytic				
(centrofollicular)	36	31	2	3
Nodular	19	19	0	0
Diffuse	14	9	2	3
Lymphoblastic	15	15	0	0
Immunoblastic	18	12	2	4
Unclassified	21	13	4	4
Reticulosarcoma	11	8	1	2
Total	101	79 (78%)	9 (9%)	13 (13%)

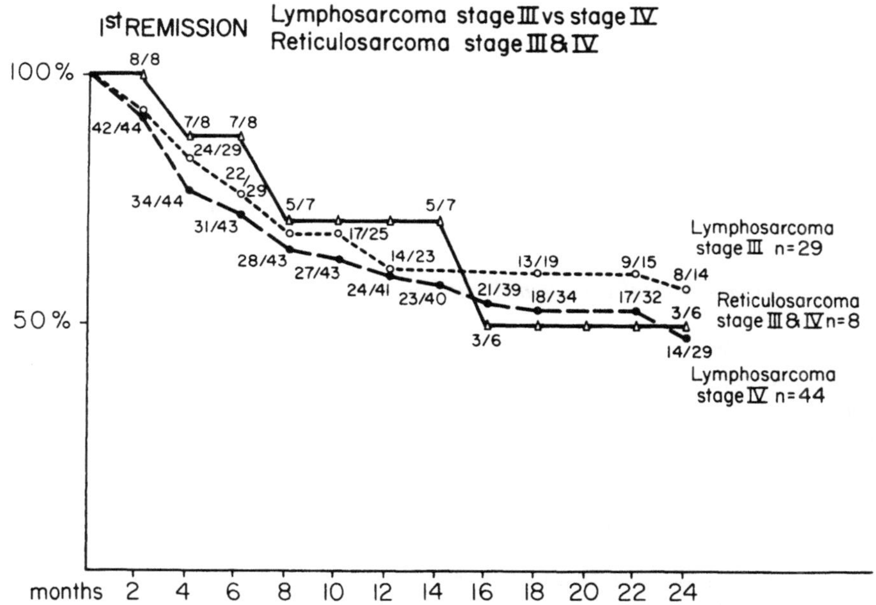

Fig. 2. Direct curves of cumulative duration of first remission of overall LS and RS patients

categories of patients. There is no significant difference between the three curves, which tend to flatten out after ca. 16 months, nor is there significant difference between the cumulative survival curves of stage III and stage IV LS patients and RS patients (Fig. 3). However, the median of survival of LS patients is not attained at 2 years, while that of RS patients is reached at 16 months.

Remission Induction According to WHO Histocytologic Types of LS

A complete remission was obtained in 31 patients out of 35 prolymphocytic (centrofollicular) cases (19 out of 19 nodular and 9 out of 14 diffuse), in 15 out of 15 lymphoblastic cases, and in 12 out of 18 immunoblastic cases.

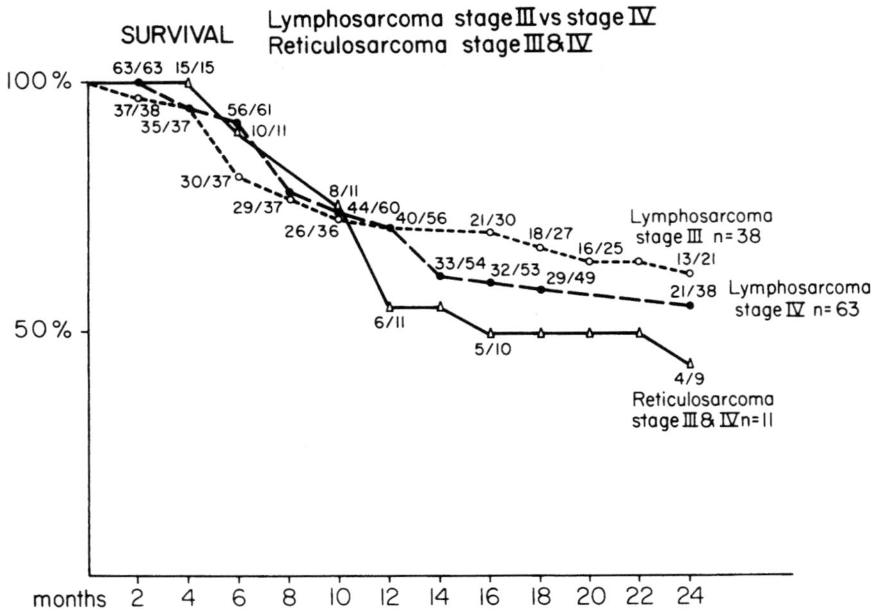

Fig. 3. Direct curves of cumulative duration of survival of overall LS and RS patients

Remission and Survival Duration According to WHO Histocytologic Types of LS

One first remarks that the remission duration curve is significantly higher for the nodular prolymphocytic (centrofollicular) form (88% at 18 months) (median not reached) than for the diffuse prolymphocytic (centrofollicular) form (median 14 months) ($p < 0.05$) (Fig. 4). The survival curves of these two forms also differ, but the difference is not significant (Fig. 5).

The second observation concerns the differences between the three WHO types of LS: the prolymphocytic (centrofollicular), the lymphoblastic, and the immunoblastic types. The remission curve is much more favorable for the prolymphocytic (centrofollicular) type than for the lymphoblastic type (the difference is significant, $p = 0.025$), the curve for which appears a little more favorable than that for the immunoblastic type, although the difference between these two last types is not significant (Fig. 6).

The same phenomenon appears for the survival curves: the curve for the prolymphocytic type is more favorable than that for the lymphoblastic type (the difference is highly significant, $p < 0.025$), which seems more favorable than that for the immunoblastic type, but the difference is not significant (Fig. 7).

One should stress that the results obtained in the cases of RS are intermediate between the best and the poorest prognostic types of LS, i.e., similar to those of the lymphoblastic type, a fact which illustrates the practical importance of distinguishing immunoblastic LS from RS as does the WHO Reference Center [15].

Summary

One hundred and one patients with advanced (stage III and IV) LS and RS at the first presentation of the disease or on relapse were treated with a regimen combining initial

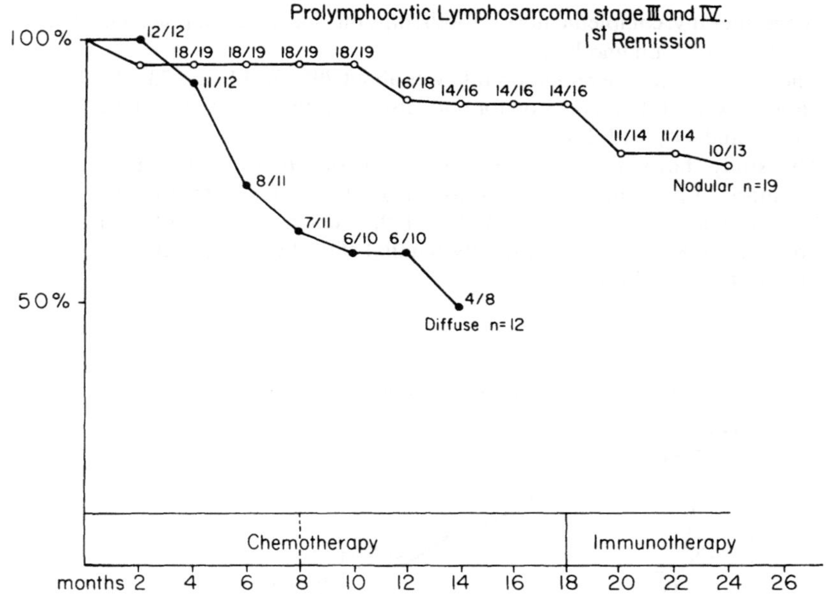

Fig. 4. Comparative duration of first remission of nodular and diffuse prolymphocytic (centrofollicular) LS patients

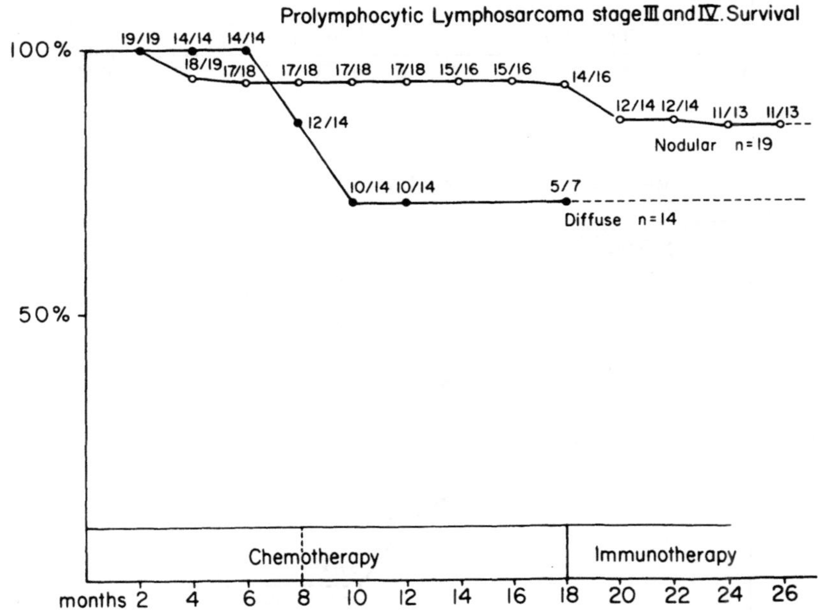

Fig. 5. Comparative duration of survival of nodular and diffuse prolymphocytic (centrofollicular) LS patients

chemotherapy, complementary radiotherapy on "icebergs," supplementary chemotherapy, and finally, active immunotherapy.

The overall complete remission rate was about 79% for LS and 73% for RS. About 50% of the patients were still in remission for both diseases after 2 years; 60% with LS were still alive after 2 years and 44% with Rs.

This study shows the useful prognostic value of the WHO classification for LS and RS: the prognosis of prolymphocytic (centrofollicular) LS is far better than that of the lymphoblastic type, which is itself better than that of the very poor prognostic immunoblastic type. The prognosis of RS is intermediate between that of the best prognostic type and that of the poorest prognostic type of LS.

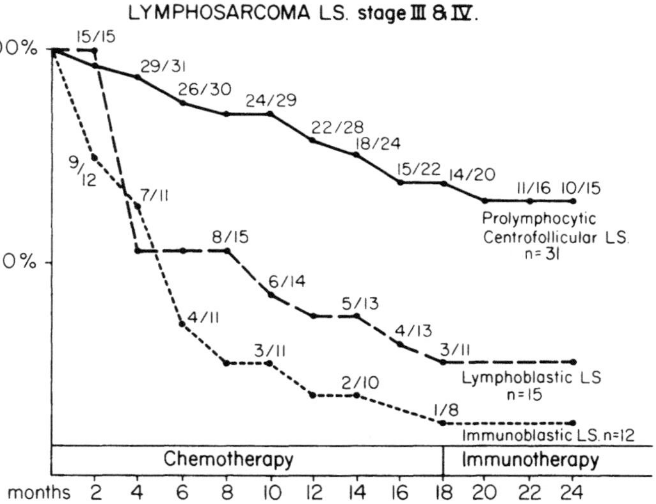

Fig. 6. Cumulative duration of first remission of LS patients according to the WHO histocytologic typing

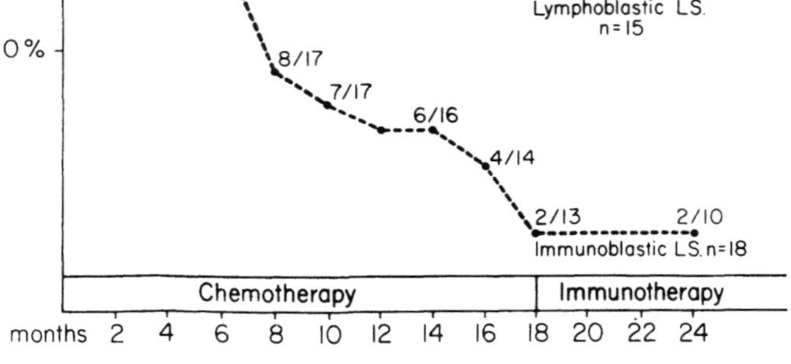

Fig. 7. Cumulative duration of survival of LS patients according to the WHO histocytologic typing

References

1. BARTELLS, H., BRENER, K., BRITTINGER, G., BURGER, A., DRUHMKE, E., GUNZER, U., KONIG, E., STACHER, A., THEML, H., WALDNER, R.: Clinical significance of the Kiehl classification of the Non-Hodgkin's lymphomas. Abstract S-19-5, p. 60. In: Abstracts of the 16th International Congress of Haematol., Kyoto, 1976
2. BELPOMME, D., LELARGE, N., MATHÉ, G., DAVIES, A. J. S.: Etiological clinical and prognostic significance of the T-B immunological classification of primary acute lymphoid leukemias and non-Hodgkin's lymphomas. pp. 33–45. In: "Immunological Diagnosis of Leukemias and Lymphomas" (THIERFELDER, S., RODT, H., THIEL, E. eds.) Heidelberg, New York: Springer, 1977
3. BELPOMME, D., CAILLOU, B., LELARGE, N., BOTTO, I., GERARD-MARCHANT, A., RAPPAPORT, H., DAVIES, A. J. S., MATHÉ, G.: Prognostic value and clinical significance of the T-B-"null" immunological classification of non-Hodgkin's lymphomas: its correlation with other classifications. In: "Lymphoid Neoplasias II" (RRCR) (MATHÉ, G., SELIGMANN, M., TUBIANA, M. eds.), pp. 28–40. Berlin-Heidelberg-New York: Springer, 1978
4. BLUM, R. H., CARTER, S. K., AGRE, K.: A clinical review of bleomycin, an antineoplastic agent. Cancer, *31*, 309 (1973)
5. CARTER, S. K.: An overview of the status of the nitrosoureas in other tumours. Cancer Chemother. Rep., Part 3, 4, 35 (1973)
6. CARTER, S. K., DI MARCO, A., GHIONE, M., KRAKOFF, I. H., MATHÉ, G. (eds.): Adriamycin. Berlin-Heidelberg-New York: Springer, 1972
7. CLARYSSE, A., KENIS, Y., MATHÉ, G.: Cancer chemotherapy (its role in the treatment strategy of hematologic malignancies and solid tumors). In: RRCR, Berlin-Heidelberg-New York: Springer, 1976, Vol. 53
8. DE VITA, V. T., CANELLOS, G. P., CHABNER, B. A., SCHEIN, P., HUBBARD, S. P., YOUNG, R. C.: Advanced histiocytic lymphoma, a potentially curable disease: Results with combination chemotherapy. Lancet, *1*, 248–250 (1975)
9. GARRET, T. J., GEE, T. S., DOWLING, M. D., LEE, B. J., MIDDLEMAN, M. P., CLARKSON, B. D., YOUNG, C. W.: Cyclophosphamide L2 Protocol: A combination chemotherapeutic regimen for advanced non-Hodgkin's lymphomas, Cancer Treat. Rep., *61*, 7–16 (1977)
10. GORIN, N. C., DAVID, R., STACHOWIAK, J., NAJMAN, A., DUHAMEL, G.: Combination of cyclophosphamide, vincristine and prednisone, followed by maintenance chemotherapy, with and without radiotherapy, in the management of patients with Non-Hodgkin's lymphomas. Med. Pediatr. Oncol., *3*, 41–51 (1977)
11. LENNERT, K., MOHRI, N., STEIN, H., KAISERLING, E.: The histopathology of malignant lymphoma. Brit. J. Haematol., *31*, Suppl. 193 (1975)
12. LIVINGSTON, R. B., CARTER, S. K.: Single Agents in Cancer Chemotherapy. New York: Plenum Press 1970
13. MATHÉ, G.: Cancer active immunotherapy, immunoprophylaxis and immunorestoration. An introduction. In: RRCR, Berlin-Heidelberg-New York: Springer, 1976, Vol. 55
14. MATHÉ, G., BELPOMME, D., DANTCHEV, D.: Les hématosarcomes non-hodgkiniens (classification du Centre de Référence de l'O.M.S.) Ann. Anat. Pathol., *21*, 285–300 (1976)
15. MATHÉ, G., BELPOMME, D., DANTCHEV, D., KHALIL, A., AFIFI, A. M., TALEB, N., POUILLART, P., SCHWARZENBERG, HAYAT, M., DE VASSAL, F., JASMIN, C., MISSETT, J. L., MUSSET, M.: Immunoblastic lymphosarcoma, a cytological and clinical entity? Biomedicine, *22*, 473–488 (1975)
16. MATHÉ, G., BELPOMME, D., DANTCHEV, D., POUILLART, P.: Progress in the classification of lymphoid and/or monocytoid leukemias and or lympho- and reticulosarcomas. Biomedicine, *22*, 177–185 (1975)
17. MATHÉ, G., BELPOMME, D., MISSET, J. L.: Integration of modern data in W.H.O. categorisation of lymphosarcomas. Its value for prognosis prediction and therapeutic adaptation to prognosis. Biomedicine, 1977. (In press)
18. MATHÉ, G. and KENIS, Y.: La Chimiothérapie des Cancers (Leucémies, Hématosarcomes et Tumeurs Solides). 3ème ed., Paris. Expansion Scientifique Française, 1975, 1 vol.
19. MATHÉ, G., RAPPAPORT, H., O'CONOR, G. T., TORLONI, H.: Histological and cytological typing of neoplastic diseases of haematopoietic and lymphoid tissues. Geneva: W.H.O., 1976
20. MATHÉ, G., SCHWARZENBERG, L., POUILLART, P., OLDHAM, R., WEINER, R., JASMIN, C., ROSENFELD, C., HAYAT, M., MISSET, J. L., MUSSET, M., SCHNEIDER, M., AMIEL, J. L., DE VASSAL, F.: Two epipodophyllotoxin derivatives VM26 and VP 16213, in the treatment of leukemias, hematosarcomas and lymphomas. Cancer, *34*, 985–992 (1974)
21. MISSET, J. L., POUILLART, P., AMIEL, J. L., SCHWARZENBERG, L., HAYAT, M., DE VASSAL, F., MISSET, M., BELPOMME, D., JASMIN, C., ALBAHARY, C., DEPIERRE, R., MATHÉ, G.: Combinaison d'adrimaycine, de VM26, de cyclophosphamide et de prednisone (AVmCP) pour la chimiothérapie des lymphoréti-

culosarcomes disséminés (Stades ou formes topographiques III et IV). Nouv. Presse. Méd., *4*, 3117–3120 (1975)

22. Monfardini, S., Tancini, G., De Lena, M., Villa, E., Valagussa, P., Bonadonna, G.: Cyclophosphamide, vincristine, and prednisone (CVP) versus adriamycin, bleomycine, and prednisone (ABP) in stage IV non-Hodgkin's lymphomas. Med. Pediatr. Oncol., *3*, 67–74 (1977)
23. O'Connell, M. J., Silverstein, M. N., Kiely, J. M., White, W. L.: Pilot study of two adriamycin-based regimens in patients with advanced malignant lymphomas. Cancer Treat. Rep., *61*, 65–68 (1977)
24. Portlock, C. S., Rosenberg, S. A.: Combination chemotherapy with cyclophosphamide, vincristine and prednisone in advanced non-Hodgkin's lymphomas. Cancer, *37*, 1275–1282 (1976)
25. Rappaport, H.: Tumours of the hematopoietic system. Washington D. C., Armed Forces Institutes of Pathology, 1966, pp. 91–206
26. Skipper, H. E., Schabel, F. M., Wilcox, W. S.: Experimental evaluation of potential anticancer agents. XIII. On the criteria and kinetics associated with "curability" of experimental leukemia. Cancer Chemother. Rep., *35*, 1–111 (1964)
27. Skipper, H. E., Schabel, F. M., Wilcox, W. S.: Experimental evaluation of potential anticancer agents. XIV. Further study of certain basic concepts underlying chemotherapy of leukemia. Cancer Chemother. Rep. *45*, 5–28 (1965)
28. Skipper, H. E., Schabel, F. M., Wilcox, W. S.: Experimental evaluation of potential anticancer agents. XXI. Scheduling of arabinosylcytosine to take advantage of its S-phase specificity against leukaemic cells. Cancer Chemother. Rep., *51*, 125–165 (1967)
29. Steinman, R. M., Adams, J. C., Cohn, Z. A.: Identification of novel cell type in peripheral lymphoid organs of mice. III. Identification and distribution in mouse spleen. J. Exp. Med., 141, 808, 1975
30. Steinman, R. M., Cohn, Z. A.: Identification of a novel cell type in peripheral lymphoid organs of mice. I. Morphology, quantification, tissue distribution. J. Exp. Med., *137*, 1142 (1973)
31. Steinman. R. M., Lustig, D. S., Cohn, Z. A.: Identification of a novel cell type in peripheral lymphoid organs of mice. II. Functional properties in vivo. J. Exp. Med., *139*, 1431 (1974)
32. van Furth, R., Cohn, Z. A., Hirsch, J. G., Humphrey, J. H., Spector, W. G., Langevoort, H. L.: The mononuclear phagocyte system: a new classification of macrophages, monocytes and their precursor cells. Bull. W.H.O., *48*, 845–852 (1972)

Outline of a Prospective Multicentric Study on the Clinical Significance of the Kiel Classification of Non-Hodgkin's Lymphomas[1]

G. Brittinger (for the Kiel Lymphoma Study Group)[2]

After the Kiel classification of non-Hodgkin's lymphomas had been proposed [12, 20] a multicentric cooperative group of clinicians in Germany and Austria, the Kiel Lymphoma Group, has analyzed retrospectively the clinical features of 405 patients who had been diagnosed according to this histopathologic scheme [5, 6, 7, 31]. In these patients, staging evaluation had not been performed regularly, and treatment protocols were different in the various centers. As shown in Fig. 1, differences in the survival probabilities could be evidenced among the lymphomas of low-grade malignancy. In contrast, patients with the high-grade malignant immunoblastic and lymphoblastic lymphomas showed an almost identically poor prognosis. The data obtained from this analysis suggested the clinical relevance of the Kiel classification. Therefore, on October 1, 1975 the Kiel Lymphoma Group initiated a prospective study which follows a single diagnostic and therapeutic protocol and has as its aim the further

---

1 Supported by the Deutsche Krebshilfe e.V., Bonn.

2 Members of the Kiel Lymphoma Group: Berlin: II. Innere Abteilung des Städt. Krankenhauses Moabit: Dr. H. H. Fülle, Dr. S. Mende, Prof. Dr. W. Pribilla, Dr. I. Weißenfels; Abteilung für Strahlentherapie und Nuklearmedizin des Städt. Krankenhauses Moabit: Dr. U. Rühl; II. Innere Abteilung des Städt. Krankenhauses Neukölln: Prof. Dr. I. Boll, Dr. K.-M. Koeppen; Hämatologische Abteilung, Klinikum Steglitz der Freien Universität: Prof. Dr. H. Brücher, Dr. M. Pfoch; Strahlenabteilung, Klinikum Steglitz der Freien Universität: Prof. Dr. H. Ernst, Dr. B. Wenzel-Hora; Hämatologisch-Onkologische Abteilung, Klinikum Westend der Freien Universität: Dr. B. Bombik, Prof. Dr. H. Gerhartz, Dr. J. Oertel.—Bremen: Medizinische Klinik der Evangelischen Diakonissenanstalt: Prof. Dr. M. Schmidt.—Essen: Hämatologische Abteilung der Medizinischen Klinik und Poliklinik, Universität Essen (Gesamthochschule): Dr. W. Augener, Dr. K. Bremer, Prof. Dr. G. Brittinger, Dr. S. Dabag, Dr. R. Donhuijsen-Ant, Priv.-Doz. Dr. E. König, Dr. P. Meusers, Dr. U. Schmalhorst; Strahlenklinik und Poliklinik, Radiologisches Zentrum, Universität Essen (Gesamthochschule): Dr. H. Holfeld, Prof. Dr. E. Scherer, Dr. U. Schulz.—Flensburg: Innere Abteilung des St. Franziskus-Hospitals: Prof. Dr. L. Nowicki.—Freiburg i. Br.: Zentrum für Innere Medizin der Universität: Dr. H. Common, Prof. Dr. G. W. Löhr; Abteilung für Strahlentherapie, Zentrum für Radiologie der Universität: Dr. H. Leopold, Prof. Dr. K. Musshoff, Prof. Dr. M. Wannenmacher.—Gießen: Zentrum für Innere Medizin der Universität: Dr. M. Graubner, Prof. Dr. H. Löffler, Priv.-Doz. Dr. H. Pralle.—Homburg/Saar: Innere Medizin I der Medizinischen Universitätsklinik: Prof. Dr. A. Pappas, Dr. H. W. Pees, Prof. Dr. G. Scheurlen.—Kiel: Pathologisches Institut der Universität: Dr. D. Helbron, Dr.med.habil. E. Kaiserling, Prof. Dr. K. Lennert, Dr. E. W. Schwarze, Dr.med.habil. H. Stein, Prof. Dr. H.-J. Stutte, Dr. G. Tolksdorf; Radiologische Universitätsklinik: Dr. E. Dühmke, Prof. Dr. H. Gremmel.—Linz: Medizinische Klinik des Öffentlichen Krankenhauses der Barmherzigen Schwestern: Prof. Dr. H. Huber.—Lübeck: I. Medizinische Klinik der Medizinischen Hochschule: Dr. H. Bartels, Dr. H. Rengshausen.—Marburg/Lahn: Medizinische Universitätsklinik: Dr. M. Begemann, Dr. G. Glaas, Prof. Dr. K. Havemann.—München: Medizinische Klinik Innenstadt der Universität: Dr. F. Brunswicker, Prof. Dr. E. Buchborn; III. Medizinische Klinik der Universität, Klinikum Großhadern: Priv.-Doz. Dr. D. Huhn, Prof. Dr. W. Wilmanns; I. Medizinische Abteilung des Städt. Krankenhauses Schwabing: Prof. Dr. H. Begemann, Dr. A. Burger, Dr. W. Kaboth, Dr.med.habil. H. Theml.—Ulm: Hämatologische Abteilung, Zentrum für Innere Medizin und Kinderheilkunde der Universität: Prof. Dr. H. Heimpel, Prof. Dr. B. Kubanek, Dr. A. Schoengen.—Wien: III. Medizinische Abteilung des Hanusch-Krankenhauses und Ludwig-Boltzmann-Institut für Leukämieforschung und Hämatologie: Dr. R. Heinz, Prof. Dr. A. Stacher, Dr. R. Waldner.—Würzburg: Medizinische Universitätsklinik: Dr. U. Gunzer, Dr. R. Nürnberger; Pathologisches Institut der Universität: Prof. Dr. H.-W. Altmann, Doz. Dr. W.-D. Heine.

clarification of the clinical and prognostic features of the lymphoma entities diagnosed according to the Kiel classification.

The histopathologic evaluation is performed by Professor Dr. K. LENNERT at the Institute of Pathology, University of Kiel. In addition, Professor Dr. H. RAPPAPORT, Duarte, Calif., has consented to analyze the material according to his classification criteria so that a comparison between the Kiel and the Rappaport classification [28, 29] can also be made from a clinical point of view.

All consecutive, untreated patients admitted to the various centers are included in the study and are staged according to a modification by MUSSHOFF [25] of the Ann Arbor classification [9]. As obligatory diagnostic measures, the initial staging evaluation comprises a complete history and physical examination, the hemogram and the usual clinical chemistries including quantitative and immunoelectrophoretic analysis of serum immunoglobulins, a radiograph of the chest (including a hilar tomogram), a bilateral pedal lymphangioadenogram, a spleen scan if this organ is not palpable, a bone marrow aspiration, a rhinolaryngologic examination, and a lumbar puncture if a lymphoblastic lymphoma is present. If bone marrow aspiration cytology is negative a bilateral iliac crest bone marrow biopsy is performed using the Jamshidi technique [15]. If bone marrow biopsy is also negative a percutaneous liver biopsy and, if still negative, a laparoscopy with multiple liver biopsies are made. If all these examinations do not reveal a stage IV of the disease staging laparotomy including complete abdominal exploration, wedge liver biopsies from both lobes, splenectomy, splenic, portal, mesenteric and retroperitoneal lymph node biopsies, and oophoropexy if indicated has to be considered. Staging laparotomy is recommended in all patients with clinical stages I–III having no contraindications against

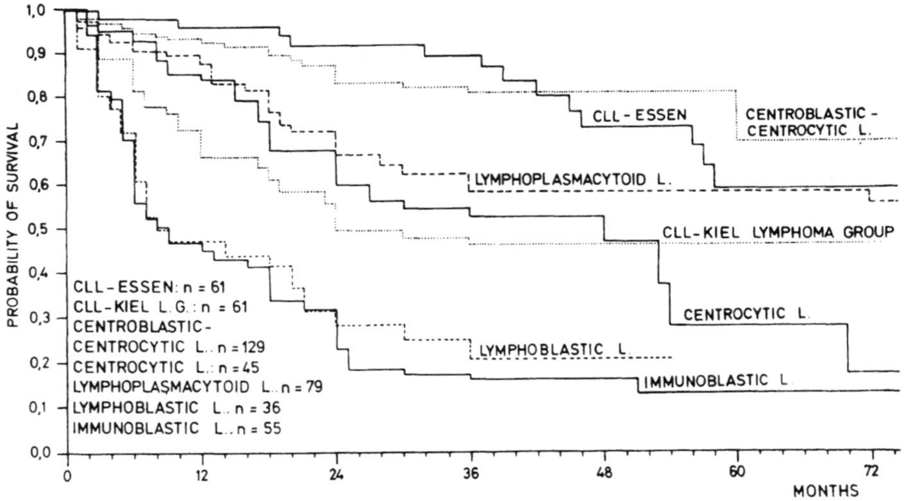

Fig. 1. Probability of survival of 405 patients with non-Hodgkin's lymphomas diagnosed according to the Kiel classification (retrospective study of the Kiel Lymphoma Group). CLL-Essen: patients with chronic lymphocytic leukemia observed at the Department of Medicine, University of Essen. In these patients diagnosis was made by cytologic, immunologic and biochemical criteria and only in part by lymph node biopsy. CLL-Kiel Lymphoma Group: patients with chronic lymphocytic leukemia diagnosed histologically by lymph node biopsy. Statistical analysis of differences in probability of survival between patients with various lymphoma entities: centroblastic-centrocytic (CB-CC) vs. CLL-Essen (CLL-E): not significant (NS); CB-CC vs. lymphoplasmacytoid (LP): NS; CB-CC vs. CLL-Kiel Lymphoma Group (CLL-L): $p < 0.01$; CB-CC vs. centrocytic (CC): $p < 0.001$; CB-CC vs. lymphoblastic (LB): $p < 0.001$; CB-CC vs. immunoblastic (IB): $p < 0.001$; CLL-E vs. LP: NS; CLL-E vs. CLL-L: $p < 0.05$; CLL-E vs. CC: $p < 0.05$; CLL-E vs. LB: $p < 0.001$; CLL-E vs. IB: $p < 0.001$; LP vs. CLL-L: NS; LP vs. CC: NS; LP vs. LB: $p < 0.01$; LP vs. IB: $p < 0.001$; CLL-L vs. CC: NS; CLL-L vs. LB: NS; CLL-L vs. IB: $p < 0.05$; CC vs. LB: $p < 0.05$; CC vs. IB: $p < 0.05$; LB vs. IB: NS

this surgical intervention but it is considered mandatory in clinical stages I–III of centroblastic-centrocytic lymphoma and in stages I and II of other non-Hodgkin's lymphomas (excluding lymphoblastic lymphoma in patients below 30 years of age) since, according to the treatment protocol assigned for the study, in these cases therapeutic consequences may arise from the result of explorative laparotomy. In patients beyond 60 years of age, however, staging laparotomy is generally considered a facultative diagnostic measure.

As this prospective study does not represent a comparative therapeutic trial, no randomizations are made with regard to treatment. The therapeutic protocol is considered as a contribution to evaluate the validity of the hypothesis that like Hodgkin's disease non-Hodgkin's lymphomas, at least in part, arise as localized nodal (intralymphatic) or extranodal (extralymphatic) tumors and that spread originates at the initial site of involvement, frequently contiguously via lymph channels [11, 16, 24, 25, 26]. It is further assumed that in extranodal disease first evidence of extension occurs in the regional lymph nodes [4, 24, 27]. Thus, in stages I and II of all histopathologic types—excluding lymphoblastic lymphoma arising in children and young adults which apparently tends to disseminate early [18, 23]—long-term control or even cure should be possible by radiotherapy alone [2, 8, 21, 25, 26]. This might also be true for stage III [13] of the highly radiosensitive centroblastic-centrocytic type [10, 26] which is believed to correspond to the majority of nodular lymphomas according to Rappaport [11, 20, 28, 29]. On the other hand, stages I–III of lymphoblastic lymphoma [18, 23], as well as stage III of all other histopathologic types, must be considered as potentially generalized [13] and are treated like all stage IV types by chemotherapy followed by irradiation of at least the remnant lymphomas and/or extranodal tumors; in chronic lymphocytic leukemia (CLL), however, additional radiotherapy is facultative.

In stages I and II of low-grade malignant lymphomas such as lymphoplasmacytoid and centrocytic lymphomas extended field irradiation using 3600–4400 rad [4, 26] is performed including additional chemotherapy if mesenteric lymph nodes are involved. In stages III and IV including CLL chemotherapy is given if indications are present which are defined as follows: progression of disease within 12 weeks (increase of lymph node and/or spleen size and/or blood lymphocyte count); presence of significant anemia (hemoglobin <10 g/dl in females, <11 g/dl in males) and/or thrombocytopenia ($<100{,}000/\mu l$) and/or other complications such as autoimmune hemolytic anemia; total serum protein $>9{,}0$ g/dl if monoclonal gammopathy is present, e.g., in lymphoplasmacytoid lymphoma. In such cases, intermittent chlorambucil + prednisone [14, 17] is considered as the treatment of first choice, followed by administration of cyclophosphamide + vincristine + prednisone (CVP) [1] if the former regimen fails. After adequate chemotherapy in stages III and IV, at least the remnant lymphomas and/or extranodal tumors are irradiated with 3600–3800 rad; however, radiotherapy of all sites initially involved is desirable.

In stages I and II of centroblastic-centrocytic lymphoma extended field irradiation with 2500 rad and in stage III total lymphoid irradiation (including abdominal bath) with 2500 rad is administered [26]. Stage IV patients are treated as patients with other lymphomas of low-grade malignancy. Additional radiotherapy is performed again with 2500 rad.

In stages I and II of the high-grade malignant centroblastic and immunoblastic lymphomas extended field irradiation with at least 4500 rad [26] is carried out and additional chemotherapy is given if mesenteric lymph nodes are affected. In stages III and IV, however, chemotherapy and additional radiotherapy are considered necessary. If the initial treatment with CVP fails after two cycles, CVP + methotrexate (0.5 mg/kg on day 1) are started. If still not effective enough after two more cycles, adriamycin + bleomycin + prednisone (ABP) [3] are given and, if failure occurs again after two cycles, other combinations such as CHOP [22], BACOP [30] etc., are used. Additional radiotherapy follows the principles outlined above for the low-grade malignant lymphomas except for a higher radiation dose of 3600–4500 rad.

In children and young adults (up to 30 years of age), therapy of stages I–IV of lymphoblastic lymphoma is performed in analogy to the treatment of childhood acute lymphoblastic leukemia and consists of three phases [modification of a schema proposed by LANDBECK, 19]. During phase 1 (days 1–28), for remission induction, vincristine (2 mg/week i.v. × 5), prednisone (2 mg/kg/day p.o.) and, if no sufficient regression of disease is reached until day 14, adriamycin (0.4 mg/kg/day i.v. on days 15 and 16) are used. On days 28–56 (phase 2a) 6-thioguanine (2 mg/kg/day p.o.) and prednisone (2 mg/kg on alternate days p.o.) are administered. In addition, cytosine arabinoside (3 mg/kg/day i.v. on days 29–31) is given if bone marrow aspirate performed on day 28 reveals no hypoplasia. Cranial irradiation with 2000 rad is considered obligatory if the initial blood leukocyte count exceeds 100,000/µl and/or cerebrospinal fluid suggests the presence of meningeal infiltration on day 28. It is performed from days 35 to 56. In all patients 5 intrathecal injections of methotrexate (maximum dose 7.5 mg/m^2 per injection) are given. During phase 2b (days 56–84) 6-thioguanine (2 mg/kg/day p.o.) and involved field irradiation with 3500–4000 rad (1000 rad/week) are administered. Maintenance therapy during phase 3 (days 84–814) is performed with 6-thioguanine (2 mg/kg/day p.o.) and methotrexate (0.5 mg/kg/week p.o.). In addition, every 3 months a pulse with vincristine (2 mg/week × 3 i.v.) + prednisone (1.5mg/kg/day p.o. on days 1–15) or CVP is given alternately. When pulses are administered, 6-thioguanine and methotrexate are discontinued. During phases 2a and 2b and until the end of the 1st month of phase 3 antimicrobial prophylaxis with cotrimoxazole has to be considered.

In adult patients over 30 years of age with lymphoblastic lymphoma the chemotherapeutic regimen is identical with that used in other lymphomas of high-grade malignancy. Restaging evaluation (including repetition of all obligatory examinations performed before therapy, control of all examinations which had initially yielded pathologic results, and biopsy of remnant lymphomas—no exploratory relaparotomy) is performed after 12 cycles of chlorambucil + prednisone or 10 cycles of CVP or 2 cycles of CVP + 8 cycles of CVP + methotrexate or 2 cycles of CVP, 2 cycles of CVP + methotrexate and 6 cycles of ABP. If complete remission has been achieved, intermittent chlorambucil + prednisone will be continued for a further 6 months whereas maintenance therapy with CVP or CVP + methotrexate is performed at 3 monthly intervals.

At present, no detailed data are available from the study, but it is expected that this will be the case in about 1 year from now.

Note added in proof:

Recent experience of the Kiel Lymphoma Group suggests more aggressive chemotherapy in high-grade malignant lymphomas. Therefore, CVP has been replaced by C-MOPP (DeVita, V.T. et al.: Ann.Intern.Med. *73*, 881–895, 1970) as treatment of first choice in stages III and IV.

In order to increase the rate of complete remissions in lymphoblastic lymphoma of children and younger adults administration of adriamycin is now considered obligatory on days 15 and 16 or earlier. In addition, obligatory cranial irradiation in phase 2a is discussed.

Summary

Retrospective analysis of 405 patients suggested the clinical relevance of the Kiel classification of non-Hodgkin's lymphomas. In order to further clarify the clinical and prognostic features of the lymphoma entities diagnosed according to this histopathologic scheme, a prospective multicentric study was initiated by the Kiel Lymphoma Group. Initial staging evaluation is performed according to the Ann Arbor classification. On the basis of the hypothesis that like Hodgkin's disease non-Hodgkin's lymphomas originate, at least in part, as localized nodal or extranodal tumors, extended field irradiation is performed in localized disease (stages I and II) (with the exception of lymphoblastic lymphoma in children and young adults) whereas in more widespread disease (stages III and IV) (with the exception of stage III of centroblastic-centrocytic lymphoma) chemotherapy with additional radiotherapy is applied.

References

1. Bagley, C. M., De Vita, V. T., Berard, C. W., Canellos, G. P.: Advanced lymphosarcoma: Intensive cyclical combination chemotherapy with cyclophosphamide, vincristine, and prednisone. Ann. Intern. Med. *76*, 227–234 (1972)
2. Bitran, J. D., Kinzie, J., Sweet, D. L., Variakojis, D., Griem, M. L., Golomb, H. M., Miller, J. B., Oetzel, N., Ultmann, J. E.: Survival of patients with localized histiocytic lymphoma. Cancer *39*, 342–346 (1977)
3. Bonadonna, G., De Lena, M., Lattuada, A., Milani, F., Monfardini, S., Beretta, G.: Combination chemotherapy and radiotherapy in non-Hodgkin's lymphomata. Br. J. Cancer *31*, Suppl. II, 481–488 (1975)
4. Bonadonna, G., Lattuada, A., Banfi, A.: Recent trends in the treatment of non-Hodgkin's lymphomas. Europ. J. Cancer *12*, 661–673 (1976)
5. Bremer, K., Bartels, H., Brittinger, G., Burger, A., Dühmke, E., Gunzer, U., König, E., Stacher, A., Theml, H., Waldner, R. (Kiel Lymphoma Group): Clinical significance of the Kiel classification of the non-Hodgkin's lymphomas (NHL). In: Topics in Hematology. Seno, S., Takaku, F., Irino, S. (eds.), International Congress Series, Amsterdam: Excerpta Medica 1977, Nr. 415, p. 352–355
6. Brittinger, G., Bartels, H., Bremer, K., Dühmke, E., Gunzer, U., König, E., Stein, H. (Kieler Lymphomgruppe): Klinik der malignen Non-Hodgkin-Lymphome entsprechend der Kiel-Klassifikation: Centrocytisches Lymphom, centroblastisch-centrocytisches Lymphom, lymphoblastisches Lymphom, immunoblastisches Lymphom. In: Maligne Lymphome und monoklonale Gammopathien. Löffler, H. (ed.), Hämatologie und Bluttransfusion, München: Lehmann 1976, Vol. 18, p. 211–223
7. Brittinger, G., Bartels, H., Bremer, K., Burger, A., Dühmke, E., Gunzer, U., König, E., Stacher, A., Stein, H., Theml, H., Waldner, R. (Kieler Lymphomgruppe): Retrospektive Untersuchungen zur klinischen Bedeutung der Kiel-Klassifikation der malignen Non-Hodgkin-Lymphome. Strahlentherapie *153*, 222–228 (1977)
8. Bush, R. S., Gospodarowicz, M., Sturgeon, J., Alison, R.: Radiation therapy of localized non-Hodgkin's lymphoma. Cancer Treat. Rep. *61*, 1129–1136 (1977)
9. Carbone, P. P., Kaplan, H. S., Musshoff, K., Smithers, D. W., Tubiana, M.: Report of the committee on Hodgkin's disease staging classification. Cancer Res. *31*, 1860–1861 (1971)
10. Cox, J. D., Koehl, R. H., Turner, W. M., King, F. M.: Irradiation in the local control of malignant lymphoreticular tumors (non-Hodgkin's malignant lymphoma). Radiology *112*, 179–185 (1974)
11. Fuks, Z., Glatstein, E., Kaplan, H. S.: Patterns of presentation and relapse in the non-Hodgkin's lymphomata. Br. J. Cancer *31*, Suppl. II, 286–297 (1975)
12. Gérard-Marchant, R., Hamlin, I., Lennert, K., Rilke, F., Stansfeld, A. G., Van Unnik, J. A. M.: Classification of non-Hodgkin's lymphomas. Lancet *II*, 406–408 (1974)
13. Glatstein, E., Fuks, Z., Goffinet, D. R., Kaplan, H. S.: Non-Hodgkin's lymphomas of stage III extent. Is total lymphoid irradiation appropriate treatment? Cancer *37*, 2806–2812 (1976)
14. Han, T., Ezdinli, E. Z., Shimaoka, K., Desai, D. V.: Chlorambucil vs. combined chlorambucil-corticosteroid therapy in chronic lymphocytic leukemia. Cancer *31*, 502–508 (1973)
15. Jamshidi, K., Swaim, W. R.: Bone marrow biopsy with unaltered architecture: A new biopsy device. J. Lab. clin. Med. *77*, 335–342 (1971)
16. Jones, S. E.: Clinical features and course of the non-Hodgkin's lymphomas. Clin. Haematol. *3*, 131–160 (1974)
17. Knospe, W. H., Loeb, V. Jr., Huguley, C. M. Jr.: Bi-weekly chlorambucil treatment of chronic lymphocytic leukemia. Cancer *33*, 555–562 (1974)
18. Landbeck, G., Gaedicke, G., Winkler, K., Stein, H.: Besonderheiten der malignen Lymphome im Kindesalter. In: Maligne Lymphome und monoklonale Gammopathien. Löffler, H. (ed.), Hämatologie und Bluttransfusion, München: Lehmann 1976, Vol. 18, p. 225–235
19. Landbeck, G.: Personal communication
20. Lennert, K., Mohri, N., Stein, H., Kaiserling, E.: The histopathology of malignant lymphoma. Br. J. Haematol. *31*, Suppl., 193–203 (1975)
21. Levitt, S. H., Bloomfield, C. B., Lee, C. K. K., Nesbit, M. E., McKenna, R. W.: Extended field radiotherapy in non-Hodgkin's lymphomas. Radiology *118*, 457–459 (1976)
22. McKelvey, E. M., Gottlieb, J. A., Wilson, H. E., Haut, A., Talley, R. W., Stephens, R., Lane, M., Gamble, J. F., Jones, S. E., Grozea, P. N., Gutterman, J., Coltman, C. Jr., Moon, T. E.: Hydroxyldaunomycin (adriamycin) combination chemotherapy in malignant lymphoma. Cancer *38*, 1484–1493 (1976)
23. Murphy, S. B.: The management of childhood non-Hodgkin's lymphoma. Cancer Treat. Rep. *61*, 1161–1173 (1977)

24. Musshoff, K., Schmidt-Vollmer, H.: Prognostic significance of primary site after radiotherapy in non-Hodgkin's lymphomata. Br. J. Cancer *31*, Suppl. II, 425–434 (1975)
25. Musshoff, K.: Die Strahlenbehandlung der Non-Hodgkin-Lymphome. In: Maligne Lymphome und monoklonale Gammopathien. Löffler, H. (ed.), Hämatologie und Bluttransfusion, München: Lehmann 1976, Vol. 18, p. 315–328
26. Musshoff, K., Slanina, J.: Maligne Systemerkrankungen. In: Strahlentherapie. Radiologische Onkologie. Scherer E. (ed.), Berlin-Heidelberg-New York: Springer 1976, p. 705–788
27. Peters, M. V., Bush, R. S., Brown, T. C., Reid, J.: The place of radiotherapy in the control of non-Hodgkin's lymphomata. Br. J. Cancer *31*, Suppl. II, 386–401 (1975)
28. Rappaport, H.: Tumors of the hematopoietic system. In: Atlas of Tumor Pathology, sect. III, fasc. 8, Washington, D.C.: Armed Forces Institute of Pathology, 1966, p. 91–156
29. Rappaport, H.: Roundtable discussion of histopathologic classification. Cancer Treat. Rep. *61*, 1037–1048 (1977)
30. Skarin, A. T., Frei, E. III, Moloney, W. C., Gutterman, J. U.: New agents and combination chemotherapy of non-Hodgkin's lymphoma. Br. J. Cancer *31*, Suppl. II, 497–504 (1975)
31. Stacher, A., Waldner, R., Theml, H. (Kieler Lymphomgruppe): Klinik der malignen Non-Hodgkin-Lymphome entsprechend der Kieler Klassifikation: Lymphoplasmozytoides Lymphom (LPL) und chronisch lymphatische Leukämie (CLL). In: Maligne Lymphome und monoklonale Gammopathien. Löffler, H. (ed.), Hämatologie und Bluttransfusion, München: Lehmann 1976, Vol. 18, p. 199–209

On the Question of the Tumoricidal Dose in Non-Hodgkin's Lymphomas

K. MUSSHOFF and H. LEOPOLD

We would like to address an open question on the radiotherapy of non-Hodgkin's lymphomas, the question regarding the tumoricidal dose level that yields permanent eradication of the tumor in a high percentage of cases. VAN DER WERF-MESSING [9] found that in patients with reticulum cell sarcoma and lymphosarcoma, 2000–4000 rad can be sufficient for a local focal dose. We, ourselves, together with SCHMIDT-VOLLMER and MERTEN [6], found that in patients with reticulum cell sarcoma and lymphoreticular sarcoma, who were treated with 4500 rad and more, only one relapse occurred, and that following a dose of 6000 rad. But there were also many involved regions in our patient group that were controlled with a dose of less than 4500 rad.

COX and co-workers [2] discovered in a series of patients with lymphosarcoma, reticulum cell sarcoma, and giant follicle lymphomas that there was a correlation between radiation sensitivity and the histologic pattern, either nodular or diffuse of the RAPPAPORT classification [7]. The eradication dose consisted of 2200 rad for the nodular and 4400 rad for the diffuse tumors (Fig. 1). But here, too, there were a considerable number of nodular tumors that were held under control with a dose of less than 2200 rad, as well as diffuse tumors with a dose of less than 4400 rad.

If one subdivides the lymphomas of the diffuse pattern according to their cytologic structure into a lymphocytic and undifferentiated cell group on the one hand and into a histiocytic on the other, as COX et al. have done, it becomes apparent that the diffuse lymphocytic and the undifferentiated cell groups show a sensitivity similar to that of the nodular forms and that only the histocytic lymphomas require a dose of 4400 rad for their eradication (Fig. 2).

All the results appear to indicate that the eradication dose for the different malignant lymphomas varies according to the histiopathologic pattern as well as the cell type of the tissue. If we remember the results of Dr. KAPLAN's first lecture (in this volume) that histopathologic entities may contain different kinds of cells (with possible different degrees of radiosensitivity), then it is not astonishing that there is a variation in the eradication doses.

Patients, Methods, and Results

In pursuing this question further, we have conducted experiments in the last couple of years in which patients with non-Hodgkin's lymphomas of low-grade malignancy of the centroblastic-centrocytic type in the Kiel classification, [4], corresponding to the nodular form of the RAPPAPORT classification, were irradiated with doses of 2500–3000 rad. Extended field to total nodal irradiation was performed with a pilot trial of five patients in stages PS II–III of the Ann Arbor classification [1].

In the subsequent observation period of about 2 years, which, however, is rather short for nodular or follicular tumors, we have not observed any true relapses. In the following, We shall present the findings obtained from one of these patients. The patient concerned is a 36-year-old

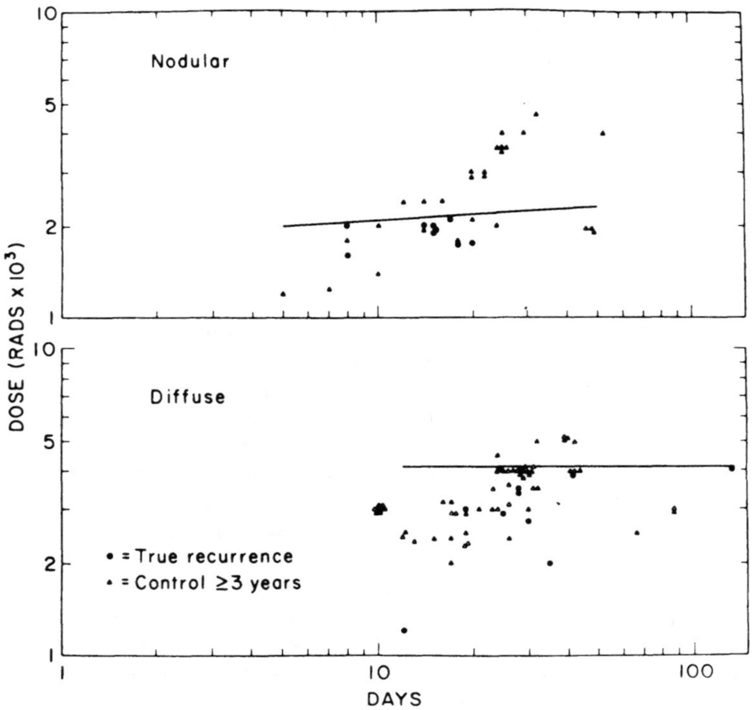

Fig. 1. Malignant non-Hodgkin's lymphomas. Time-dose scattergrams of true recurrences and minimum 3-year controls. Nodular and diffuse tumors: dose in rad vs. time. (By courtesy of J. D. Cox)

male with centroblastic-centrocytic lymphomas in stage PS III $A_{N+S-H-M}$ with predominantly abdominal involvement, in whom the abdominal lymph node tumors had caused hydronephrosis on the right side with anuria (Fig. 3A). In this case, the treatment consisted of total nodal irradiation plus an abdominal bath with a focal dose of 2500 rad with photons from a 4 Mev. linear accelerator. In the last 2 years since therapy, the patient has been in complete remission, whereby there has been a normalization of all findings and complete restoration of physical and mental capacities. The pyelogram gives no indication of pathologic findings (Fig. 3b).

Discussion

In the radiologic treatment of the non-Hodgkin's lymphomas, it must be taken into consideration that the extent of lymphatic irradiation extends considerably beyond that necessary for treating Hodgkin's disease, the side-effects of which, as joint investigations with SLANINA et al. [8] have shown, are considerable. In addition to supradiaphragmatic mantle and infradiaphragmatic inverted Y-field irradiation, the treatment includes the abdominal bath and, often, irradiation of the auricular lymph nodes, Waldeyer's lymphatic ring, and the epitrochlear and popliteal lymph nodes. Every rad that can be eliminated in this extensive irradiation treatment reduces the rate of side-effects. We should, therefore, devote more attention to the clarification of this question.

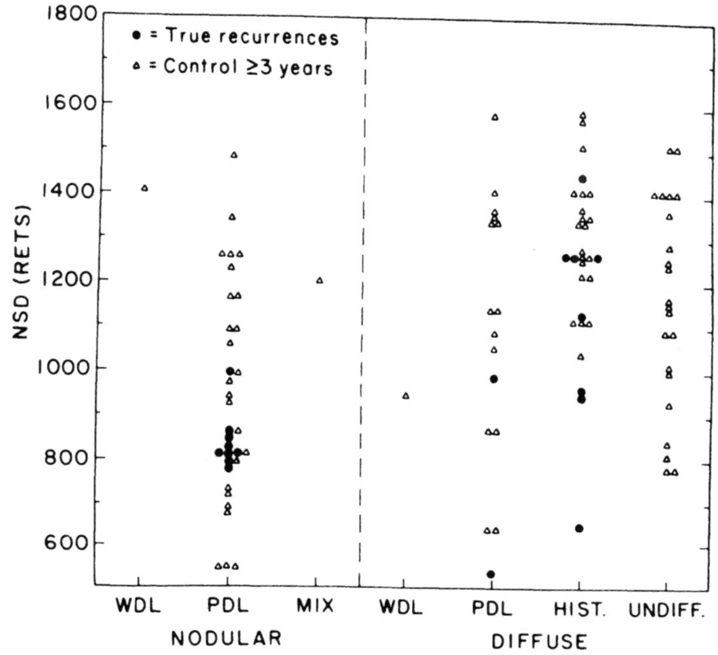

Fig. 2. Malignant non-Hodgkin's lymphomas. True recurrences and minimum 3-year controls by cytologic subtype. NSD: nominal standard dose by Ellis; RET: rad-equivalent therapy; WDL: well-differentiated lymphocytic; PDL: poorly differentiated lymphocytic; MIX: mixed; UNDIFF: undifferentiated lymphomas of the Rappaport classification. (By courtesy of J. D. Cox)

In undertaking this task, it would be advisable, on the basis of the results to date, to subdivide the total group of patients into the following three groups, in which differences in radiation sensitivity can possibly be expected:

1. The nodular forms of the Rappaport classification (lymphocytic, histiocytic, and mixed lymphocytic-histiocytic) and the follicular forms of the Kiel classification (centroblastic-centrocytic). It is not yet quite clear whether the two groups of the Rappaport and the Kiel classifications are identical in all cases, as was shown in the comparative tables of Dorfman, or whether there are nodular forms of the Rappaport classification which do not correspond to the centroblastic-centrocytic group of the Kiel classification, as was shown in a new pilot investigation [5].
2. The diffuse nonhistiocytic forms of the Rappaport classification, which, according to the findings of Cox et al., are more sensitive to irradiation than the diffuse histiocytic lymphomas.
3. The diffuse histiocytic lymphomas of the Rappaport classification, which correspond in almost all cases to the immunoblastomas of the Kiel classification and which are the least sensitive to irradiation. The dose necessary for their eradication possibly corresponds to the dose which is currently considered to be the eradication dose for the entire disease group.

Acknowledgements

This study was supported, in part, by "Kampf dem Krebs" of the German Cancer Society.

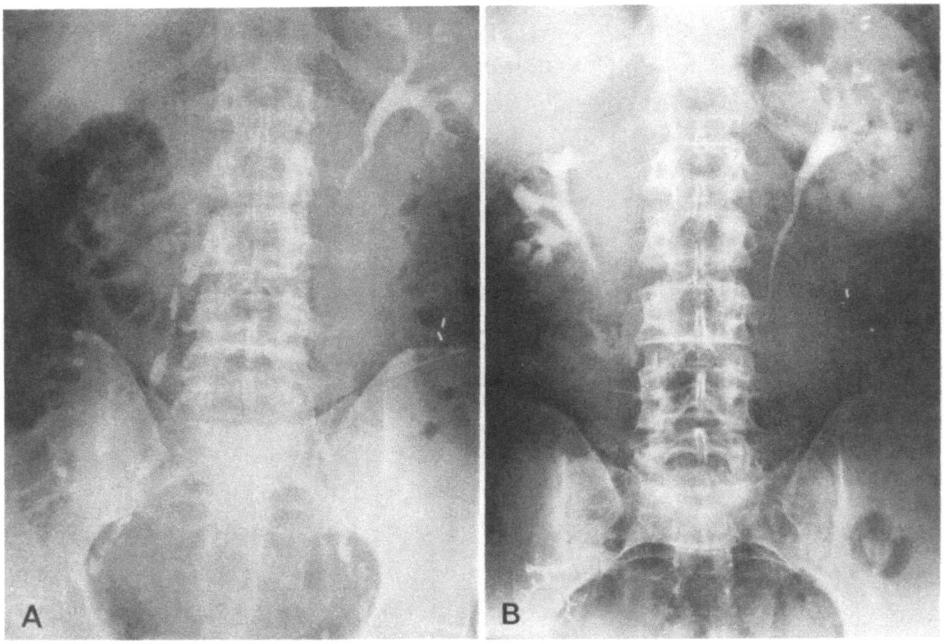

Fig. 3. G.W., born 24.1.1939, 36-year-old male with low-grade malignant lymphoma of the centroblastic-centrocytic type in the Kiel classification and stage PS III $A_{N+S-H-M-}$ in the Ann Arbor classification.
(A) Lymphangiogram and urogram before irradiation.
(B) Two years after irradiation

References

1. Carbone, P. P., Kaplan, H. S., Musshoff, K., Smithers, I. W., Tubiana, M.: Report of the Hodgkin's disease staging classification committee. Conference on staging in Hodgkin's disease. Ann Arbor, April 26–28, 1971. Cancer Res. *31*, 1860–1861 (1971)
2. Cox, J. D., Koehl, R. H., Turner, W. M., Kind, F. M.: Irradiation in the local control of malignant lymphoreticular tumors (non-Hodgkin's malignant lymphoma). Radiology *112*, 179–185 (1974)
3. Dorfman, R. F.: Invitational workshop for the planning of retrospective and prospective studies to delineate optimal classifications of the non-Hodgkin's lymphomas. September 4–5, 1975, Warrenton, Virginia, U.S.A., Airlie House
4. Gerard-Marchant, R., Hamlin, I., Lennert, K., Rilke, F., Stansfeld, A. G., van Unnik, J. A. M.: Classification of non-Hodgkin's lymphomas. Lancet 1974 *II*, 405–408 (1974)
5. Musshoff, K.: Vergleich der Kiel- und Rappaport Klassifikation. In Lymphknoten tümore. Stacher and Höcker (eds.). 1 Forumdiskussion. München: Urban und Schwarzenberg (In Press)
6. Musshoff, K., Schmidt-Vollmer, H., Merten, D.: Reticulum cell sarcoma: An oncological model for a system of classifying the malignant lymphoma. Eur. J. Cancer *7*, 451–457 (1971)
7. Rappaport, H.: Tumors of the hematopoetic system. Sect. 3, fasc. 8, Washington D.C.; Armed Forces Institute of Pathology, 1966, pp. 91–156
8. Slanina, J., Musshoff, K., Rahner, T., Stiasny, R.: Long-term side effects in irradiated patients with Hodgkin's disease. Int. J. Radiation Oncology Biol. Phys., *2*, 1–19, (1977)
9. van der Werf-Messing, B.: Reticulum cell sarcoma and lymphosarcoma. A retrospective study of potential survival in luco-regional disease. Eur. J. Cancer *4*, 549–557 (1968)

Combined Modality Therapy of Childhood Non-Hodgkin's Lymphoma

S. B. MURPHY

Introduction

The survival of children with non-Hodgkin's lymphoma (NHL) has improved in the recent past through the systematic application of intensive therapy employing involved field radiation plus combinations of drugs. A comprehensive review of combined modality therapy of NHL in childhood has been published recently [9]. Table 1, which outlines the 2-year survival by stage of disease at diagnosis from selected representative series [1, 2, 5, 7, 10, 13], shows that as many as 80%–90% of children with stage I disease are curable with such an approach. Also shown is a remarkably uniform overall success rate of roughly 30% and a depressingly high rate of treatment failures in patients with generalized disease (stages III–IV).

Table 1. The 2-year survival, according to the Ann Arbor classification [3] of stage of disease at diagnosis, from five recent series of children with NHL. Survival is stage dependent

<table>
<tr><th rowspan="2">No. of patients</th><th colspan="6">Percent surviving</th></tr>
<tr><th>Stage I</th><th>Stage II</th><th>Stage III</th><th>Stage IV</th><th>Overall</th><th>Reference</th></tr>
<tr><td>31</td><td colspan="2">50%</td><td colspan="2">7.7%</td><td>32%</td><td>10</td></tr>
<tr><td>32</td><td>55%</td><td>38%</td><td>33%</td><td>0%</td><td>31%</td><td>5</td></tr>
<tr><td>172</td><td>58%</td><td>24%</td><td colspan="2">8%</td><td>27%</td><td>7</td></tr>
<tr><td>64</td><td>92%</td><td>20%</td><td>11%</td><td>0%</td><td>30%</td><td>13</td></tr>
<tr><td>25</td><td>80%</td><td>26%</td><td>—</td><td>—</td><td>30%</td><td>1,2</td></tr>
</table>

The challenge of management of these children today lies primarily in improvement in results in poor prognosis patients. The prognostic features associated with an unfavorable outcome of therapy in children with NHL have been reviewed [8] and include extensive or generalized disease, particularly involvement of the central nervous system (CNS), diffuse histology, and location of primary tumor within the mediastinum or abdomen. In these poor prognosis patients, in particular, optimal combined modality therapy remains ill-defined. The relative contributions of multiple-agent chemotherapy for induction and maintenance of remission, radiotherapy for known areas of bulky tumor involvement and for prophylaxis of CNS disease and surgery, particularly for primary abdominal disease, require critical testing in the setting of controlled clinical trials.

Therapy for children with localized disease with a good prognosis, such as a completely resected ileocecal tumor, or a localized primary in the head and neck region, is more likely to be crowned with success in achieving long-term survival but no less subject to a requirement for analysis of critical variables contributing to such success. The current tendency in some centers is toward overtreatment of such patients, which courts the hazard of unacceptable acute and late effects of therapy, such as infectious complications, leukoencephalopathy, growth retardation, sterility, second malignancies, etc. For example, NELSON and co-workers [11] determined that, of 40 children with localized resectable gastrointestinal tract tumors treated by a combination of modalities, there was not a single instance of CNS disease as the initial site of treatment failure. In a smaller series, HUTTER et al. [6] made the same observation. The logical conclusion of such analyses is that children with localized completely resectable gastrointestinal tract tumors should not receive CNS prophylaxis.

That example merely serves to illustrate the obvious point that childhood NHL is a heterogenous disorder, not only in terms of relapse patterns, but also in light of clinicopathologic correlations of location of primary tumor, histopathology, blast cell surface markers, etc. Recognition of such heterogeneity would suggest that the therapy for children with NHL should somehow reflect and accommodate the variable features of disease exhibited.

Despite this, most regimens in current use [9] treat every child with NHL uniformly. The LSA_2-L_2 protocol developed by WOLLNER et al. is an example, as all children are treated with a complex ten-drug regimen plus intrathecal methotrexate and radiation to single or multiple sites [16, 17]. Although the results reported are superior to historical and literature controls, the series is difficult to compare with others reported [9], and the actual contribution of each of the many agents employed difficult to assess because concurrent controls, treated adequately but less intensively, are lacking. Current studies in progress [9] may help to clarify some of the issues outlined above.

This paper will describe the approach to management of children with NHL at St. Jude Children's Research Hospital (SJCRH) which bases therapy on a staging system that recognizes the location of primary tumor and extent of disease. Preliminary results are presented of a randomized trial in progress designed to evaluate 1) the adjuvant effect of involved field radiation in poor prognosis patients during induction, in addition to combination drugs and 2) the influence of cranial irradiation plus intrathecal methotrexate during early remission on the frequency of CNS disease and the duration of complete remission.

Methods

All untreated patients, aged 18 years or younger, with biopsy-proven NHL of any histologic type or anatomic presentation are eligible, provided they are not in a leukemic phase of NHL at diagnosis. For purposes of this study, "leukemia" was arbitrarily defined as presence of circulating blast cells or more than 25% replacement of marrow with blasts.

Patients are clinically staged on the basis of the usual procedures, including hemogram, bone marrow aspirate, and percutaneous biopsy, roentgenograms of the chest, skeleton and skull, IVP, lumbar puncture with cytocentrifuge examination of cerebrospinal fluid, and scans of liver-spleen, bone, and whole body (^{67}Ga). Patients with head-neck primaries have additional roentgenograms of the facial bones, mandible, and soft-tissue views of the nasopharynx. Upper and lower gastrointestinal tract series are performed in patients with abdominal disease. Bilateral lower extremity lymphangiography is performed in patients whose clinically apparent disease is supradiaphragmatic but not in patients with mediastinal primaries or obviously disseminated disease. Staging laparotomy and splenectomy are not performed. On the basis of this pretreatment evaluation, a stage is assigned (Table 2). Treatment is based on stage of disease and is outlined in Table 3.

Definitions of complete reponse, remission, and survival durations are conventional. Calculations of actuarial estimates of remission and survival are performed by standard statistical techniques and comparisons of the differences in remission and survival according to the nonparametric log rank test [12].

Table 2. The staging classification for children with NHL in use at St. Jude Children's Research Hospital

Stage I
A single tumor (extranodal) or single anatomic area (nodal), with the exclusion of mediastinum or abdomen
Stage II
A single tumor (extranodal) with regional node involvement
Two or more nodal areas on the same side of the diaphragm
Two single (extranodal) tumors with or without regional node involvement on the same side of the diaphragm
A primary gastrointestinal tract tumor, usually in the ileocecal area, with or without involvement of associated mesenteric nodes only.
Stage III
Two single tumors (extranodal) on opposite sides of the diaphragm
Two or more nodal areas above and below the diaphragm
All the primary intrathoracic tumors (mediastinal, pleural, thymic)
All extensive primary intra-abdominal disease
Stage IV
Any of the above with initial CNS and/or bone marrow involvement

Table 3. The schema for treatment of childhood NHL according to a randomized clinical trial currently in progress at St. Jude Children's Research Hospital

Phase I induction (6–9 weeks)

Stages I–II	Stages III–IV
Vincristine 1.5 mg/m² i.v. weekly × 6	Same as stages I–II plus
Cyclophosphamide 1200 mg/m² i.v. every 3 weeks × 3	Adriamycin 45 mg/m² i.v. every 3 weeks × 3
Prednisone 40 mg/m² daily orally × 28 days	Randomize ± for involved field radiotherapy (3500–4000 rad)
Involved field radiotherapy (3500–4000 rad)	

Phase II CNS prophylaxis (2–3 weeks)

Stage I—No prophylaxis
Stages II[a]–III–IV—Randomize ± for
cranial irradiation (2400 rad) + intrathecal methotrexate 12 mg/m² × 5

Phase III maintenance (18 months)

Stages I–IV
6-mercaptopurine 75 mg/m² orally daily
Methotrexate 30 mg/m² orally weekly

[a]Stage II, completely resected, localized gastrointestinal tumor patients receive no CNS prophylaxis.

Results

Forty children have been entered on this study from March, 1975–May, 1977, and the study remains open and in progress. The stages and locations of the primary tumors are shown in Table 4. It can be seen that the majority of these children have advanced stage disease and/or unfavorable abdominal or mediastinal presentations. Thirty-nine of the 40 children had diffuse histologic sybtypes of NHL, mainly undifferentiated or lymphoblastic. One four-year-old girl had a nodular and diffuse poorly differentiated lymphocytic intestinal lymphoma. The median

Table 4. The primary anatomic location of tumor and stage of disease for 40 children with NHL enrolled in the current clinical trial in progress at St. Jude Children's Research Hospital

Location	Stage				
	I	II	III	IV	Totals
Abdominal		3	9	2	14
Mediastinal			8	3	11
Head-neck	2	2	1	5	10
Peripheral nodes	3		1		4
Bone				1	1
Totals	5	5	19	11	40

duration of time spent on study is 230 days with a range of 9+ days–701+ days. Two children have completed 2 years of treatment and are off therapy.

The results of this trial are preliminary, so firm conclusions are premature. Many subgroups of patients are represented by only small numbers, and 14 of the 40 children were diagnosed less than 1 year ago and consequently are still at significant risk of relapse.

The overall success of complete remission induction is 89%, 33 of 37 evaluable patients. The four patients failing to achieve complete remission were all boys with widespread (stage III–IV) unresectable abdominal disease. The actuarial calculation of overall survival and of survival according to stage of disease (stage I–II vs. stage III–IV) is shown in Fig. 1. Twenty-five of 40 children are currently alive. Two are still in induction, and three are alive following relapse. The remaining 20 are in remission, with no evidence of disease. A total of 15 patients have died, and 13 of the 15 who died had stage III–IV disease.

As outlined in Table 3, the induction therapy for all patients with stage III–IV disease consisted of four drugs, and patients were randomized to receive or not receive involved field

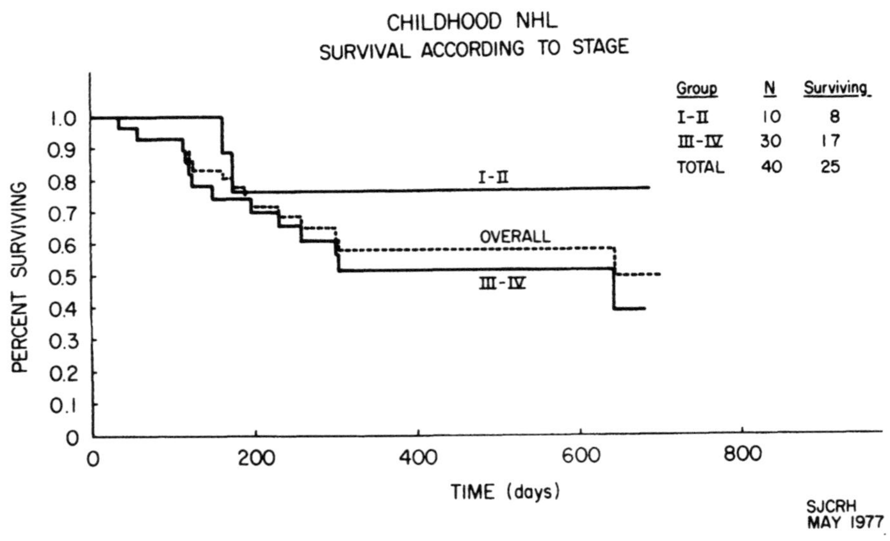

Fig. 1. The actuarial estimate of overall survival (----) and survival according to stage of disease at diagnosis (————) for children with NHL treated according to the schema outlined in Table 3. Children with localized disease have a better survival. However, the difference is not significant according to the nonparametric log rank test (P=0.2)

radiation therapy in addition. Figure 2 shows that the addition of radiation therapy to an intensive multiple drug regimen has failed to appreciably influence survival in this group of poor prognosis patients. The actuarial estimates of survival duration for the two groups are not significantly different ($P=0.6$).

Twenty-three of 35 patients with stage II, III, or IV disease have so far been eligible for randomization early in remission to receive or not to receive prophylactic treatment of the CNS with cranial irradiation (2400 rad) plus intrathecal methotrexate. The remaining 12 patients either failed to achieve remission (four cases), had initial or early lymphomatous involvement of their CNS (three cases), are still in induction (two cases), or bypassed the randomization because of parents' wishes (one case), nodular histology (one case), or preexisting anoxic encephalopathy (one case). Thus far, CNS involvement has occurred more commonly in the group not receiving prophylaxis (4 of 11 cases) than in the group receiving prophylaxis (two of 12 cases), although two of the six instances of CNS spread occurred simultaneously, with systematic relapse as well. Due to the small numbers, no firm conclusions regarding the efficacy of CNS prophylaxis in childhood NHL are yet possible, although it is evident that the complication is not completely preventable.

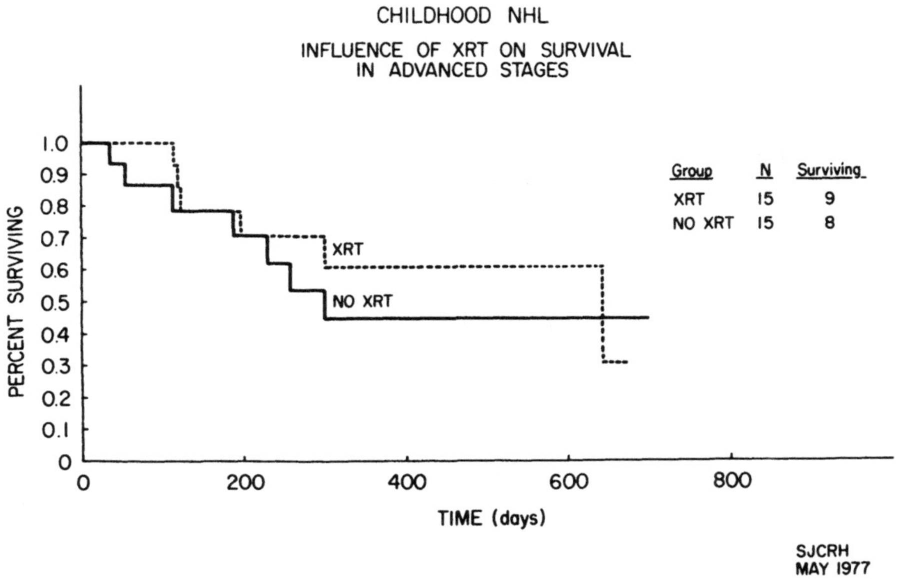

Fig. 2. The actuarial estimate of survival duration in patients with stages III and IV disease according to whether they received (----) or did not receive (————) involved field radiation therapy (3500–4000 rad) during induction. All patients were treated with the same drug regimen. The addition of radiotherapy has not influenced survival, as the curves are not significantly different ($p=0.6$)

Discussion

Currently, there seems little doubt that the results of therapy for children with NHL have improved, and that many children are potentially curable. This trend is a reflection of the abandonment of a palliative approach to treatment which historically employed radiation alone or single-agent chemotherapy. Instead, virtually all regimens now in use by major centers or cooperative groups treating substantial numbers of children with NHL employ multiple agents and use high-dose cyclophosphamide, moderate to high-dose methotrexate, adriamycin, vincristine, prednisone, and other agents combined with radiation therapy and intrathecal drugs (for a review of these regimens, see Ref. 9). Early reports of the success of such regimens, such as the 76% overall actuarial estimate of 2-year survival reported by WOLLNER with use of the LSA_2-L_2 protocol [16,17], have led to considerable enthusiasm for such approaches. Inevitably, the experience of others in the use of the LSA_2-L_2 regimen has been less uniformly successful [4, 15]. The suitability of such intensive regimens for all children with NHL, even those with a good prognosis, has been rather uncritically accepted with little attention directed to the possibility that some elements of the therapy are either unnecessary or ineffective, contributing little to the overall success and only adding to the toxicity of the regimen.

For example, the actual contribution of radiation therapy delivered to sites of bulky tumor involvement, when used in combination with a multiple drug regimen, requires some reexamination in view of the preliminary results of the St. Jude randomized trial reported above. In patients with generalized or extensive intracavitary disease (stages III–IV), those treated with multiple drugs plus radiation therapy during induction fared no better than those receiving drugs alone, administered as outlined in Table 3. The contribution of radiation therapy in mediastinal NHL, in particular, is further questioned by the results reported by WOLLNER et al. in nine children with primary mediastinal NHL treated according to the LSA_2-L_2 regimen [16, 17]. Actuarial survival was reported to be 88% 3–4 years after diagnosis, and only one patient out of nine received radiotherapy in addition to drugs during induction. However, it is not the author's intent to question the utility of radiation therapy as a modality with established curative potential in the management of lymphomas or to suggest that its use in patients with localized disease be withdrawn or reduced, possibly jeopardizing their potential for cure. It does appear though that further controlled trials which critically examine the contribution of radiation therapy to an intensive multiple drug regimen in childhood NHL are necessary.

Prophylactic treatment of the CNS in childhood NHL is rational and appears warranted, at least in certain subgroups of patients, but evidence is so far lacking that current approaches will prove uniformly efficacious in patients at high risk of this complication. For example, in the only randomized controlled trial reported to date, ZIEGLER and BLUMING treated a total of ten patients with Burkitt's lymphoma prophylactically with a combination of intrathecal methotrexate and cytosine arabinoside and compared these patients with a control group. Five out of 10 in the treatment group and 4 out of 10 in the controls subsequently developed malignant pleocytosis [18]. In the St. Jude Children's Research Hospital experience with mediastinal tumors, leukemic at diagnosis, five of 23 patients achieving remission developed CNS disease as their initial relapse on therapy, despite prophylaxis with cranial irradiation and intrathecal methotrexate [1]. SULLIVAN reports a similar experience with a small number of non-Burkitt's, convoluted cell-type cases. Active CNS disease developed in three out of seven children given prophylaxis and in three out of four not given CNS prophylaxis [14]. WOLLNER and colleagues reported spread to CNS occurring in 7 out of 43 (17.5%) patients treated with intermittent intrathecal methotrexate and the LSA_2-L_2 regimen [16, 17].

In conclusion, it is apparent that therapy for childhood NHL needs refinement. Results of controlled trials of the elements of combined modality therapy, such as the St. Jude NHL trial reported here, may assist in the rational design of future regimens.

Acknowledgements

The author acknowledges the collaboration of Drs. Omar Hustu and Warren Johnson in the design and conduct of NHL-75 and Dr. Stephen George in performance of the statistical analysis. This study was supported, in part, by Cancer Research Center Grant CA08480, by Training Grants CA05176 and CA08151 from the National Cancer Institute and by ALSAC.

References

1. AUR, R. J. A., personal communication
2. AUR, R. J. A., HUSTU, H. O., SIMONE, J. V., PRATT, C. B., PINKEL, D.: Therapy of localized and regional lymphosarcoma of childhood. Cancer *27*, 1328–1351 (1971)
3. CARBONE, P., KAPLAN, H. S., MUSSHOF, K., SMITHER, D. W., TUBIANA, M.: Report of the committee on Hodgkin's disease staging classification. Cancer Res. *31*, 1860–1861 (1971)
4. FRIAS, A., SULLIVAN, M. P.: Convoluted cell lymphoma and "T" cell leukemia: Survival, patterns of relapse, and rescue with LSA_2-L_2 therapy. (Abst. C-155) Proc. AACR and ASCO *18*, 305 (1977)
5. GLATSTEIN, E., KIM, H., DONALDSON, S., DORFMAN, R. F., GRIBBLE, T. J., WILBUR, J. R., ROSENBERG, S. A., KAPLAN, H. S.: Non-Hodgkin's lymphomas. VI. Results of treatment in childhood. Cancer *34*, 204–211 (1974)
6. HUTTER, J. J., FAVARA, B. E., NELSON, M., HOLTON, C. P.: Non-Hodgkin's lymphoma in children. Correlation of CNS disease with initial presentation. Cancer *36*, 2132–2137 (1975)
7. LEMERLE, M., GERARD-MARCHANT, R., SARRAZIN, D.: Lymphosarcoma and reticulum cell sarcoma in children. Retrospective study of 172 cases. Cancer *32*, 1499–1507 (1973)
8. MURPHY, S. B.: Prognostic Features and Obstacles to Cure of Childhood Non-Hodgkin's Lymphoma, Seminars in Oncology, *4*, 265–271 (1977)
9. MURPHY, S. B.: The management of childhood non-Hodgkin's lymphoma, Cancer Treat. Rep. *61*, 1161–1173 (1977)
10. MURPHY, S. B., FRIZZERA, G., EVANS, A. E.: A study of childhood non-Hodgkin's lymphoma. Cancer *36*, 2121–2131 (1975)
11. NELSON, D. R., CASSADY, J. R., TRAGGIS, D., BAEZ, A., VAWTER, G. F., JAFFE, N., FILLER, R. M.: The role of radiation therapy in localized resectable intestinal non-Hodgkin's lymphoma in children. Cancer *39*, 89–97 (1977)
12. PETO, R., PIKE, M. C., ARMITAGE, P., BRESLOW, N. E., COX, D. R., HOWARD, S. V., MANTEL, N., MCPHERSON, K., PETO, J., SMITH, P. G.: Design and analysis of randomized clinical trials requiring prolonged observation of each patient. Br. J. Cancer *35*, 1–39 (1977)
13. PINKEL, D., JOHNSON, W., AUR, R. J. A.: Non-Hodgkin's lymphoma in children. Br. J. Cancer *31*, Suppl., 298–323 (1975)
14. SULLIVAN, M. P.: Treatment of lymphoma. Cancer *35*, 991–995 (1975)
15. SULLIVAN, M. P., personal communication
16. WOLLNER, N., BURCHENAL, J. H., LIEBERMAN, P. H., EXELBY, P., D'ANGIO, G., MURPHY, M. L.: Non-Hodgkin's lymphoma in children. Med. Pediatr. Oncol. *1*, 235–263 (1975)
17. WOLLNER, N., BURCHENAL, J. H., LIEBERMAN, P. H., EXELBY, P., D'ANGIO, G., MURPHY, M. L.: Non-Hodgkin's lymphoma in children. A comparative study of two modalities of therapy. Cancer *37*, 123–134 (1976)
18. ZIEGLER, J. L., BLUMING, A. Z.: Intrathecal chemotherapy in Burkitt's lymphoma. Br. Med. J. *3*, 508–512 (1971)

Concluding Remarks on Malignant Lymphomas

S. K. CARTER

The malignant lymphomas are the subject of many meetings. Why do we have so many meetings on this subject and so comparatively few on cancer of the pancreas or bladder? The reason is because great success has been achieved in the treatment of the lymphomas, and it is postulated that the lessons learned in the successful control of these tumors willl be ultimately applicable to the major solid tumors which cause the greatest number of cancer deaths. In endeavoring to give concluding remarks to this excellent 3-day meeting, an attempt will be made to draw attention to certain principles which were illustrated at the therapy sessions.

The meeting contained many reports of clinical trial results. Unfortunately, while all were presented in the same verbal language (English), they were not all presented in the same scientific language. Differing terminologies were used as were differing definitions of response, calculation of duration and survival, and general data reporting techniques. In addition, the baseline information items given were not consistent. We need an international approach to standardized reporting of cancer treatment results. The WHO has recently has a meeting on this subject, and it is hoped that all of the international organizations such as UICC, WHO, EORTC, and the national organizations will ultimately get together on such an approach. It is time that standardized reporting of results was added to standardized pathology and staging definitions which have occupied past deliberations.

In attempting to analyze lymphoma trials, there are at least ten major variables that need to be considered (table 1). Pathology is one of the most critical. At this meeting, there was much debate about the optimal pathology classification for the non-Hodgkin's lymphomas in the United States. The RAPPAPORT classification has now achieved wide acceptance, and for the first time, some consistency can be seen in this aspect of clinical trial reporting. It is fervently hoped that the current NCI-sponsored study at Stanford University reviewing case material and correlating classifications with clinical results will lead to an internationally consistent classification.

Another important aspect of pathology in analyzing trials is adequate pathology review. In the United States, lymphoma review panels exist which go over the slides of study cases to confirm

Table 1. Ten critical factors in analyzing lymphoma trials

1. Adequacy of pathology review
2. Adequacy of staging procedure
3. Intensity of therapy
4. Complete remission rate
5. Definition of CR
6. Duration of remission
7. Survival
8. Acute toxicity
9. Chronic toxicity
10. Incidence of second tumors

the pathology reported. It has been consistently shown that these panels change a significant number of histologic subtype classifications.

Staging is another critical factor. The Ann Arbor classification is utilized for both Hodgkin's disease and non-Hodgkin's lymphoma. As was pointed out by ROSENBERG at the meeting, while adequate for Hodgkin's disease, the Ann Arbor staging is suboptimal for the other lymphomas since the stages do not give clean prognostic groupings. At some point in the future, thought will have to be given to a better staging system for the non-Hodgkin's lymphomas.

The staging work-up was also discussed at the meeting. It appears from the data of the Istituto Tumori de Milano and the NCI in Bethesda that laparascopy is an important staging tool and if properly utilized may obviate the need for staging laparatomies in most instances. It was emphasized again that the staging laparatomy is only indicated where a change in stages would alter the therapy to be given.

With the success of cancer chemotherapy, the importance of the complete remission has been highlighted. The complete remission has a significant implication for long-term disease-free survival, while the partial regression is of minimal impact when survival is examined. Definitions of complete response are becoming more stringent. JONES reported at this meeting data on the "restaging" of patients who were in apparent complete remission clinically. When restaged residual tumor was found in more than 20%, the complete remission rate was lowered accordingly. In comparing clinical trial data, it will be essential to delineate the criteria of complete remission including the restaging procedures which might have been done. Until restaging for delineation of complete remission is widely accepted, this will be a complicating factor in analyzing clinical trial results from various centers.

In evaluation the impact of a therapeutic regimen, the complete response rate is only the beginning of the analysis. It is absolutely essential to have data on disease-free remission and survivial before a definitive analysis can be made. One of the major complicating factors in this area is the fact that excellent salvage therapy exists after chemotherapy failure, radiation therapy failure, or combined modality treatment failure. Recently, the NCI has reported that a significant number of MOPP failures can be reinduced into complete remission with MOPP again and that some have long disease-free remissions. At Stanford, the salvage rate after failure with radiation therapy alone or radiation + MOPP is 45%. It is higher in those treated with radiation alone as compared with radiation + MOPP where only nodal relapse could be salvaged. The implication of this is that a regimen might seem superior to another in terms of relapse-free survival but show no difference in overall survival because of the ability to salvage patients in relapse. An example of this can be seen in the Stanford University study in which total nodal radiation (TNR) alone was compared to TNR + MOPP for stage I–III disease. The results with long follow-up showed that the relapse-free survival overall was 81% for TNR + MOPP and 61% for TNR alone but that the survival rate was 88% for TNR + MOPP vs. 78% for TNR alone which is not significant. Therefore, while the study could be called positive for adjuvant MOPP in terms of relapse-free survival, it was negative in terms of overall survival. This is particularly true when it is considered that 61% of the TNR alone group was exposed to MOPP, which was not necessary since TNR alone was curative. With the increasing data indicating that combined TNR and drugs leads to a significant incidence of secondary acute myeloid leukemia, this aspect of chronic toxicity will bear watching in the final analysis.

One of the important emerging concepts coming from combined modality adjuvant trials in general is that there are two phases of risk vs. benefit analysis. The first is relapse vs. acute toxicity while the second is survival vs. chronic toxicity. Too great a reliance on the first, especially early in the trial history, can lead to interpretations which will not stand the test of long-term follow-up. It will be necessary to sharpen our thinking about long-term analysis, giving thought to how to follow up on chronic organ damage and the development of second malignancies.

Chemotherapy for advanced stage lymphoma is currently at a plateau in Hodgkin's disease. No regimen has been shown to be clearly superior to the MOPP originally developed at the NCI. The Southwest Oncology Group has added bleomycin and is now evaluating a six-drug approach of MOPP + bleomycin and adriamycin. While the complete remission rate with MOPP + bleomycin appears higher than with MOPP alone, the long-term analysis data are not as yet available. The same is true for substitution approaches such as CCNU, vinblastine, procarbazine, prednisone of the cancer and leukemia group B, and the BCVPP (BCNU, cytoxan, vinblastine, procarbazine, prednisone) of the Eastern and Southeastern groups in the United States. The newest approach is the integration of noncross-resistant combinations with MOPP as exemplified by the ABVD regimen of BONADONNA (Table 2).

Table 2. Attempts to improve on initial induction potential of MOPP

MOPP

Additive

MOPP + bleomycin
MOPP + bleomycin + adriamycin

Substitution

CCNU, VLB, PP
BCNU, VLB, cytoxan, PP (BCVPP)

Noncross-resistant combinations

ABVD
ABVS (streptozotocin)

The problem of maintenance therapy still remains unresolved. There is no clear evidence that any maintenance therapy evaluated to date is superior to six courses of MOPP with no maintenance and salvage therapy upon relapse. Immunotherapy in the maintenance phase is being evaluated by several groups.

The chemotherapy of the non-Hodgkin's lymphomas is a complicated picture since one has to separate these diseases minimally into a good and poor risk category. The seminal combination regimen for NHL is cytoxan, vincristine, and prednisone, which is called either CVP or COP depending upon how the alkylating agent is given (Table 3). For the diffuse histiocytic group of lesions, the addition of adriamycin alone or with bleomycin to COP in regimens such as CHOP and BACOP has led to a significant number of long-term disease-free complete remissions which appear to be cures. It is worth noting, however, that C-MOPP (cytoxan substituted for nitrogen mustard) at the NCI has given results as good as any reported with adriamycin-containing combinations. Little data are currently available on long-term complications due to adriamycin cardiac damage or bleomycin pulmonary damage in this group of patients.

For the good risk categories, the Stanford group has shown that conservative approaches utilizing single-agent chemotherapy and occasionally even no initial therapy can give results equivalent to more intensive combinations. The NCI, however, has recently reported what appear to be high cure rates for the nodular lymphoma with combination chemotherapy, and it will be of interest to see if this can be confirmed.

As in Hodgkin's disease, there is no clear-cut evidence that combined radiation and

Table 3. Attempt to improve on initial induction potential of COP (CVP)

COP (CVP)

Substitution	Noncross resistant combination	Addition
HOP	ABV	COP + bleomycin
Streptonigrin OP		CHOP
BCNU OP		BACOP

chemotherapy gives superior results to either modality used alone as appropriate to stage. There is one positive study at the NCI in Milan but other studies are negative and the issue remains to be resolved. One of the current enigmas in cancer treatment is why the combination of drugs and radiation has not been more successful in the lymphomas since they are both so effective when used alone.

The lymphomas continue to be an area of exciting developments and lively debate, and we can all look forward to many valuable meetings in the future. It was exciting at this EORTC plenary session to see the interaction of European and American investigators, which is now becoming more and more commonplace. This international communication bodes well for progress in the future.

Recent Results in Cancer Research

Sponsored by the Swiss League against Cancer. Editor in Chief: P. Rentchnick, Genève

For information about Vols. 1—9, please contact your bookseller or Springer-Verlag.

10 Nelson, R. S.: Radioactive Phosphorus in the Diagnosis of Gastrointestinal Cancer.

11 Freeman, R. G. and J. M. Knox: Treatment of Skin Cancer.

12 Lynch, H. T.: Hereditary Factors in Carcinoma.

13 Tumours in Children, 2nd Edition. Edited by H. B. Marsden and J. K. Steward.

14 Odartchenko, N.: Production Cellulaire Erythropoïétique.

15 Sokoloff, B.: Carcinoid and Serotonin.

16 Jacobs, M. L.: Malignant Lymphomas and Their Management.

17 Normal and Malignant Cell Growth. Edited by R. J. M. Fry, M. L. Griem, and W. H. Kirsten (Symposium).

18 Anglesio, E.: The Treatment of Hodgkin's Disease.

19 Bannasch, P.: The Cytoplasm of Hepatocytes during Carcinogenesis. Electron- and Lightmicroscopical Investigations of the Nitrosomorpholine-intoxicated Rat Liver.

20 Rubidomycin. A new Agent against Cancer. Edited by J. Bernard, R. Paul, M. Boiron, C. Jacquillat, and R. Maral.

21 Scientific Basis of Cancer Chemotherapy. Edited by G. Mathé (Symposium).

22 Koldovský, P.: Tumor Specific Transplantation Antigen.

23 Fuchs, W. A., J. W. Davidson, and H. W. Fischer: Lymphography in Cancer. With contributions by G. Jantet and H. Rösler.

24 Hayward, J.: Hormones und Human Breast Cancer. An Account of 15 Years Study.

25 Roy-Burman, P.: Analogues of Nucleic Acid Components. Mechanisms of Action.

26 Tumors of the Liver. Edited by G. T. Pack and A. H. Islami.

27 Szymendera, J.: Bone Mineral Metabolism in Cancer.

28 Meek, E. S.: Antitumour and Antiviral Substances of Natural Origin.

29 Aseptic Environments and Cancer Treatment. Edited by G. Mathé (Symposium).

30 Advances in the Treatment of Acute (Blastic) Leukemias. Edited by G. Mathé (Symposium).

31 Denoix, P.: Treatment of Malignant Breast Tumors. Indications and Results.

32 Nelson, R. S.: Endoscopy in Gastric Cancer.

33 Experimental and Clinical Effects of L-Asparaginase. Edited by E. Grundmann and H. F. Oettgen (Symposium).

34 Chemistry and Biological Actions of 4-Nitroquinolin 1-Oxide. Edited by H. Endo, T. Ono, and T. Sugimura.

35 Penn, I.: Malignant Tumors in Organ Transplant Recipients.

36 Current Concepts in the Management of Lymphoma and Leukemia. Edited by J. E. Ultmann, M. L. Griem, W. H. Kirsten, and R. W. Wissler (Symposium).

37 Chiappa, S., R. Musumeci, and C. Uslenghi: Endolymphatic Radiotherapy in Malignant Lymphomas. With contributions by G. Bonadonna, B. Damascelli, G. Fava, F. Pizzetti, U. Veronesi.

38 Koller, P. C.: The Role of Chromosomes in Cancer Biology.

39 Current Problems in the Epidemiology of Cancer and Lymphomas. Edited by E. Grundmann and H. Tulinius (Symposium).

40 Langley, F. A. and A. C. Crompton: Epithelial Abnormalities of the Cervix Uteri.

41 Tumours in a Tropical Country. A Survey of Uganda (1964—1968). Edited by A. C. Templeton.

42 Breast Cancer: A Challenging Problem. Edited by M. L. Griem, E. V. Jensen, J. E. Ultmann, and R. W. Wissler (Symposium).

43 Nomenclature, Methodology and Results of Clinical Trials in Acute Leukemias. Edited by G. Mathé, P. Pouillart, L. Schwarzenberg (Symposium).

44 Special Topics in Carcinogenesis. Edited by E. GRUNDMANN (Symposium).

45 KOLDOVSKÝ, P.: Carcinoembryonic Antigens.

46 Diagnosis and Therapy of Malignant Lymphoma. Edited by K. MUSSHOFF (Symposium).

47 Investigation and Stimulation of Immunity in Cancer Patients. Edited by G. MATHÉ and R. WEINER (Symposium).

48 Platinum Coordination Complexes in Cancer Chemotherapy. Edited by T. A. CONNORS and J. J. ROBERTS (Symposium).

49 Complications of Cancer Chemotherapy. Edited by G. MATHÉ and R. K. OLDHAM (Symposium).

50 Cancer Registry. Edited by E. GRUNDMANN and E. PEDERSEN (Symposium).

51 Gliomas. Current Concepts in Biology, Diagnosis and Therapy. Edited by J. HEKMATPANAH (Symposium).

52 The Ambivalence of Cytostatic Therapy. Edited by E. GRUNDMANN and R. GROSS (Symposium).

53 A. CLARYSSE, Y. KENIS, and G. MATHÉ: Cancer Chemotherapy.

54 Malignant Bone Tumors. Edited by E. GRUNDMANN.

55 MATHÉ, G.: Cancer Active Immunotherapy, Immunoprophylaxis, and Immunorestoration.

56 Lymphocytes, Macrophages, and Cancer. Edited by G. MATHÉ, I. FLORENTIN, and M.-C. SIMMLER (Symposium).

57 Breast Cancer: A Multidisciplinary Approach. Edited by G. ST. ARNEAULT, P. BAND, and L. ISRAËL (Symposium).

58 B. S. SCHOENBERG: Multiple Primary Malignant Neoplasms.

59 Selective Heat Sensitivity of Cancer Cells. Edited by A. ROSSI-FANELLI, R. CAVALIERE, B. MONDOVI, and G. MORICCA.

60 Tumors of the Male Genital System. Edited by E. GRUNDMANN and W. VAHLENSIECK (Symposium).

61 D. METCALF: Hemopoietic Colonies.

62 Tactics and Strategy in Cancer Treatment. Edited by G. MATHÉ (Symposium).

63 Antitumor Antibiotics. Edited by S. K. CARTER, H. UMEZAWA, J. DOUROS, and Y. SAKURAI (Symposium).

64 Lymphoid Neoplasias I: Classification, Categorization, Natural History.

65 Lymphoid Neoplasias II: Clinical and Therapeutic Aspects.
Lymphoid Neoplasias I & II. Proceedings of the 1977 CNRS-EORTC International Colloquium. Editors: G. MATHÉ, M. SELIGMANN, M. TUBIANA. Devided into two volumes.

MIX
Papier aus verantwortungsvollen Quellen
Paper from responsible sources
FSC® C105338

If you have any concerns about our products,
you can contact us on
ProductSafety@springernature.com

In case Publisher is established outside the EU,
the EU authorized representative is:
Springer Nature Customer Service Center GmbH
Europaplatz 3, 69115 Heidelberg, Germany

Printed by Libri Plureos GmbH
in Hamburg, Germany